Spatial Variations

ADVANCED LABANOTATION SERIES

EDITOR
Ann Hutchinson Guest
Director, Language of Dance® Centre, London, UK

Vol. 1, 1:
Canon Forms
by Ann Hutchinson Guest
and Rob van Haarst

Vol. 1, 2:
Shape, Design, Trace Patterns
by Ann Hutchinson Guest
and Rob van Haarst

Vol. 1, 3:
Kneeling, Sitting, Lying
by Ann Hutchinson Guest
and Rob van Haarst

Issue 4:
Sequential Movements
by Ann Hutchinson Guest
and Joukje Kolff

Issue 5:
Hands, Fingers
by Ann Hutchinson Guest
and Joukje Kolff

Issue 6:
Floorwork, Basic Acrobatics
by Ann Hutchinson Guest
and Joukje Kolff

Issue 7:
Center of Weight
by Ann Hutchinson Guest
and Joukje Kolff

Issue 8:
Handling of Objects, Props
by Ann Hutchinson Guest
and Joukje Kolff

Issue 9:
Spatial Variations
by Ann Hutchinson Guest
and Joukje Kolff

Spatial Variations

BY

ANN HUTCHINSON GUEST

AND

JOUKJE KOLFF

©2002 Ann Hutchinson Guest. All rights reserved

Dance Books Ltd,
4 Lenten Street, Alton, Hampshire GU34 1HG

Printed in the United Kingdom by H. Charlesworth & Co.,
Huddersfield

ISBN: 1 85273 091 9

This book was written and produced at the Language of Dance® Centre:
  The Language of Dance® Centre
  17 Holland Park
  London W11 3TD
  United Kingdom
  T: +44 (0)20 7229 3780
  F: +44 (0)20 7792 1794
  web: http://www.lodc.org
  e-mail: info@lodc.org

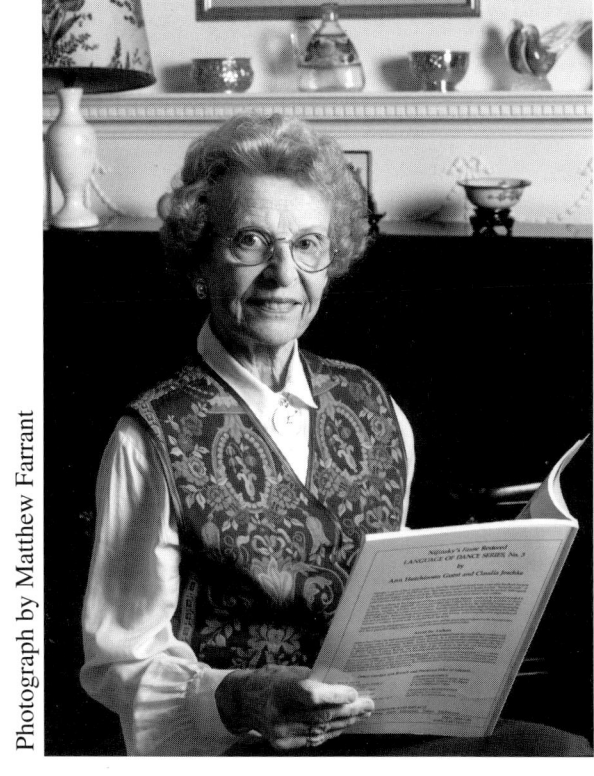

Ann Hutchinson Guest

Joukje Kolff

Contents

Introduction to the Series		xv
Preface		xvii
Acknowledgements		xix
I	MODIFICATION OF DIRECTIONS	2
1	Indication of Halfway Point; Third-way Point	2
	Intermediate Directions	2
	Between Two Cardinal Directions	2
	Moving to an Intermediate Point	2
	Between Three Cardinal Directions	2
	Directional Definition of Pins	4
	Third-way Points	4
2	Minor Modifications of a Main Direction	6
	Proximal Analysis	6
II	PATHS FOR GESTURES - STANDARD ANALYSIS	8
3	Peripheral and Central Paths	8
	Peripheral Path	8
	Central Path	8
	Standard Path	8
	Aimed Destination	8
4	Indication of Aimed Destination, Straight or Peripheral Path for Gestures	10
	Aimed Destination	10
	Passing Flexion	10
	Inward Path Indication	10
	Straight Path	12
	Peripheral Path	12
5	Timing for Third Degree Pathway	14
	Empty Direction Symbol for Pathway	14

Spatial Variations

6	General Indication of Spatially Central or Peripheral Paths	16
	Spatially Central or Peripheral Paths	16
	Degree of Curve	16
7	Sharp or Rounded Corners for Gestures	18
8	Retrace Path	20
III	DEVIATIONS FROM THE PATH OF A GESTURE	22
9	Analysis of Deviations	22
	Single Deviations	22
	Single Symmetrical Deviations	24
	Compound Symmetrical Deviations	24
10	Other Kinds of Deviations	26
	Asymmetrical Deviations	26
	Non-Centered Deviations	26
	Regressive (Jagged) Deviations	28
	Loops	28
	Reference to Standard Directions	30
	System of Reference Based on the Path	30
11	Size of Deviation from Path of Gesture	32
IV	MODIFICATION OF PATH ACROSS THE FLOOR	34
12	Veering off Normal Path	34
	Distance in Modification of Path	36
	Modification of Circular Path	36
13	Detóur to Avoid a Person or Object	38
	Timing of Detour	38
14	Displacement for Step Patterns in Place - Choice of Description	40
	Toward, Away From an Area	40
	Reaching a Destination	40
15	Displacement Paths Combined with Turning or Circling	42
	Displacement Paths Combined with Turning	42

	Displacement Paths Combined with Circling	42
V	MINOR MOVEMENTS	46
16	Displacements from a Point	46
	The Distal Center	46
	Distal Analysis	46
	Distal Displacements	46
	The Proximal Center	48
	Proximal Analysis	48
	Distal Center Key	48
	Comparison between Distal and Proximal Analyses	48
	Distal Analysis	50
	Use of Specific Directional Keys	50
	Cancellation of Minor Displacements	50
	Direction of Relationship	52
	Size of Distal and Proximal Displacements	52
	Types of Movement	52
17	Vibrating Actions	54
	Cancellation of Vibrations	54
18	Minor Circling Movements	56
	Intermediate Placements of Limb	56
	Size of Transitional Arm Deviations	58
19	Minor Shifting Actions	60
20	Deviations for Successions	62
	Overlapping Successions	62
	Retained Displacement	62
21	Timing	64
	Indication of Duration	64
	Indication of Speed	64
	Momentary Displacement	64
	Emphasis on Destination	64
22	Size of Displacement	66
	Clarification	68

Spatial Variations

23	Polar Pins	70
	The Disadvantage of Proximal and Distal Pins	70
	The Idea of Polar Pins	70
	The Signs for Polar Pins	72
	Displacement from the Poles	72
	Analysis of Spoke-like Displacements	74
	To and Fro Polar Displacements	76
	Circular Displacements	76
VI	**MOTION VERSUS DESTINATION**	78
24	Steps Versus Gestures, Direction of Progression, Shifting and Path Signs	78
	Direction in a Support Column	78
	Direction in a Gesture Column	78
	Direction of Progression	78
	Level	80
	Minor Movements	80
	Cancellation of Result of Previous Motion	80
	Shifting	82
	Motion Indicated by Path Sign	82
	Straight or Curved Direction of Progression	84
	Flexion/Extension or Distance	84
25	Toward, Away versus Destination	86
	Toward and Away	86
	Toward, Away from a Directional Point	88
	Toward, Away from the Body	88
	Away as Cancellation	88
	Destinational Statement	90
	Contraction and Extension - Destination	90
	Motion Toward a Defined State of Flexion or Extension	90
	Motion Away from a Defined State of Flexion or Extension	92
	Contracting and Extending - Motion Toward	92
VII	**PATH SIGNS FOR GESTURES**	94
26	Straight Path	94
27	Analysis of Circular Paths for Gestures	96

Advanced Labanotation

	Planal Circles	96
	Conical Circles	96
28	Indication of Circular Path for Gestures	98
	Horizontal Circular Paths	98
	Somersault Paths	98
	Cartwheel Paths	98
29	Elongated Circular Paths for Gestures	100
30	Diagonal Circles, Tilted Circles for Gestures	102
	Diagonal Circles	102
	Tilted Circles	102
31	Location and Size of Circle for Gestures	104
32	Circles Achieved Through Flexion of the Limb; Spirals	106
	Circles Achieved Through Flexion of the Limb	106
	Spiral Paths	108
	Helical Paths	108
	Three-dimensional Spiral	108
33	Indication of 'Surface' for a Gestural Circle	110
34	Circular Paths for Head, Torso and Pelvis	112
35	Circular Paths for Hands, Knees	114
36	Performance Details for Paths for Limbs	116
	Spatial Placement of a Conical Circle	116
	Spatial Retention for Direction of Gestural Path	116
	Timing of Gestural Circles	120
VIII	DISTANCE	122
37	Length of Steps	122
	Natural Step-length	122
	Standard Step-length	122
	Modifying Step-length - General Scale	124
	Modifying Step-length - Specific Scale	124

Spatial Variations

	Length of Steps - Modifying Distance	126
	Increase or Decrease of Distance	126
38	Distance, Aim of Path	128
	Distance in Terms of Units	128
	Relative Location for Aim of Path	128
39	Distance for Leg Gestures	130
	Distance for Touching Leg Gestures	130
	Distance for Leg Gestures Off the Floor	132
	Distance of Leg Gestures from the Center Line	134
40	Sign for Distance	136
IX	ORIENTATION	138
41	Focal Point	138
	Orientation in Relation to Focal Point	138
	Focal Destination for a Turn	138
	Focal Point System of Reference	140
42	Line of Dance	142
43	Front in Relation to the Path; to the Periphery	144
	Front in Relation to the Path	144
	Movements related to the Direction of the Path	144
	Front Oriented to the Periphery	146
44	Area Signs	148
	Basic Signs	148
	Application of the Stage Area Signs	148
	Intermediate Areas	152
	Use of Narrow and Wide Signs	152
	Placement of Performers	152
	Offstage Actions	154
	Further Subdivisions Using Strokes	156
	Unspecified Area	158
	Areas Above or Below Stage Level	158
	Indications for Floor, Water	158
	Miscellaneous Area Indications	160

45	Wings, Lines on Stage	162
	Indication of Wings on Stage	162
	Lines on Stage	164
	Specific Stage Diagonals	166
46	Fixed Points in a Defined Space	168
	Fixed Points in the Audience	169
X	MISCELLANEOUS	170
47	Carets, Spot Holds, Same Spot Caret	170
	Use of Ordinary Caret	170
	In Place	170
	Closed to Open	171
	Open to Closed on Two Feet	172
	From Open Position to Weight on One Foot	174
	Rise Without Adjusting the Feet	174
	Motion or Destination Description	174
	Zed Caret	176
	Retention of a Spot (Spot Hold)	176
	Same-Spot Caret	178
	Same-Spot Zed Caret	178
	Foward Reference Caret	180
	Forward Reference Caret: 'Lead Into' Zed Caret	182
48	Reading Examples	184
	Lark Ascending	184
	Roses	194
	Sorcerer's Sofa	196
	Snow Pas	200
	Parade	204
	Rooms	208
	Spanish Dance	210
	Hungarian Dance	212
	Water Study	214
	APPENDICES	216
A	The Direction System of Labanotation	216
	Definition of Direction in Labanotation	216

Spatial Variations

	Intermediate Palm Facing Directions	220
	The Standard 45° Intermediate Directions	220
	The Proposed Intermediate Direction System	222
	Chart of Directions	224
B	Categories of Pins	226
	Relationship Pins	226
	Relationship Indications	228
	Minor Displacements	228
	Minor Movements	228
	Deviations from a Path	228
	Intermediate Directions	230
	Specific Parts of the Body	230
	Degree of Turn, Circling	230
	Axis of Rotation	230
	Orientation, Front Signs	232
	Track Pins for the Legs	232
	Black Pins, Positions of the Arms	234
	Track Pins, Positions of the Arms	236
	Identifying Performers	238
	Surfaces for Design Drawing	238
	Modifying Parts of the Room/Stage	238
	Fixed Points in the Room/on Stage	238
	Pins with Dynamic Signs	238
	Polar Pins	240
C	Historical Background on Labanotation Textbooks	242
Notes		245
Bibliography		271
Index		273
Useful Contact Information		289

Introduction to the Series

The <u>Advanced Labanotation</u> series provides a detailed exposition of the many topics introduced in the chapters of the 1970 textbook *Labanotation - The System of Analyzing and Recording Movement*. To make the material immediately accessible to the reader, each book in this series begins at a basic level, thus avoiding the need for immediate reference to other texts.

Within the series each topic is published independently as soon as it is completed in order to make the information immediately available. Topics for which there is at present a lack of informaiton available, and those for which there is an immediate need, are being presented first.

Detailed theoretical exposition is supported by appropriate notated examples, and, where needed, figure illustrations of the movements and positions. A selection of reading materials from choreographic scores illustrates the different points, with the examples taken from various sources and styles of movement. Finally, a detailed index facilitates rapid access to required information and, for the researcher, meticulous endnotes and a bibliography indicate background sources.

Preface

There is a need to explore the less frequently met usages in dealing with subtle variations in spatial aspects of movement. Finding a practical and logical sequence in which to present this material is not easy. For our purposes here Intermediate Directions are dealt with first, exploring the different needs and the solutions established.

General forms of paths for a gesture are covered, together with the various types of curves along which the extremity (usually of the arm) moves. The defining of peripheral paths, central paths and what is meant by an 'aimed destination' in comparison with a straight path are also explored. While in Labanotation specific performance is usually required, usages allowing more freedom, valuable specifically in Motif Notation are introduced.

The range of deviations from the defined path of a gesture are investigated. Minor detours or undulating gestural paths are explored. Modifications of paths across the floor also need to be considered, modifications which include veering away from the standard path, a detour to avoid a person or object; gradual progression modifying a repeated step in place toward a stage area; such progressions combined with turning and also with circling.

Minor movements which are indicated with pins are explored, movements such as fluttering, vibrating, and how the directions for these are determined; minor circular movements; the range of deviations for successions and so on.

Other spatial variations include motion versus destination, orientation to less frequently used systems of reference and variations in location in the room or on stage.

During these investigations the questions of distance, size, timing and validity are also included. It must be recognized that precision in spatial placement cannot always be physically achieved. The performer intends repeatedly to produce an identical movement but the body is often not capable of such exactness. In this book definitive statements have needed to be made, degrees of distance and spatial placement for which the performer aims. In the heat of performance such perfection is rarely achieved.

Spatial Variations

The reader should be aware that, for general use, there will not be the need to include all the detailed uses given in this book. In the course of using Labanotation for many different types of movement during the decades since publication of the first Labanotation textbook in 1954, the need has been expressed to provide descriptions other than the standard, long established method. Several of these have not been generally known but exist and hence need to be included in a comprehensive book on the subject of Spatial Variations. Certain choices occur only when there is the need to indicate how to approach the movement, the intent, the inner movement idea, to achieve a particular quality. For purposes of mime, the eloquent gestures of hands, head and body, these subtleties are extremely important. In contrast, other movement descriptions are required for general movement exploration with its need for more flexible boundaries.

The expected degree of accuracy in performance needs to be considered. Why include fine differentiations if the human body, even that trained to a high degree, cannot be relied upon to achieve that particular result each time? There will always be some leeway in the actual performance of a subtle spatial difference, but the attitude of the performer, what s/he is aiming to perform, is important. If choreographers explain and ask for such subtle differences, then we must have a way of indicating these on paper.

When usages not in the mainstream are required, it is wise to give explanations of these in a glossary at the start of the score.

Acknowledgements

Details on the Spatial Variations presented in this book have come from many sources. Colleagues involved with many different aspects of movement have challenged the system to be able to describe movement in particular terms. The particular needs met in the development of the Language of Dance approach to movement analysis and exploration, for example, as set forth in the book *Your Move - A New Approach to the Study of Movement and Dance*, have required consideration and solution.

Movement analysis and descriptions used in other movement notation systems have been considered over the years and have influenced the thinking and development in finding solutions to recording different concepts and approaches to movement. Particular acknowledgement must be given to the Eshkol/Wachmann system.

The detailed recording of training methods such as ballet and contemporary dance, in particular the Graham technique, have demanded a movement analysis and precision in the notated description not usually met.

Work on this book, initially undertaken with Joukje Kolff, has been concluded through the contribution made by Rosemarie Gerhard; her joining the team has been much welcomed.

For checking the drafts of this material and for actively taking part in discussions concerning issues and problems we gratefully acknowledge the help given by our consultants, Jacqueline Challet-Haas, Ilene Fox, János Fügedi, David Henshaw, Sheila Marion and Lucy Venable. Their detailed and judicious comments contributed much to the correction and clarification of working drafts. When all appeared concluded, Jane Dulieu undertook the final review and proofreading, finding with her eagle eye further details to be corrected or improved.

The team at the Language of Dance Centre must also be given heartfelt thanks - Roma Dispirito and Cheryl Hutton for their excellent work producing the Labanotation examples on *Calaban*, and Helen Elkin for co-ordinating the compilation of the book and keeping an eye open for consistency in usage.

We also wish to express appreciation for the contribution made by Veronica Dittman in finding appropriate reading examples from choreographic scores to illustrate the movement material covered.

Spatial Variations

The research for this issue of <u>Advanced Labanotation</u> and its production have been made possible through funding from the National Endowment for the Humanities, a Fellowship awarded to Ann Hutchinson Guest by the John Simon Guggenheim Memorial Foundation and also a grant from the Arts and Humanities Research Board. We are grateful for their generous support.

To conclude, we must also express appreciation to Andy Adamson who developed the *Calaban* software used to produce the Labanotation graphics.

Spatial Variations

I MODIFICATION OF DIRECTIONS[1]

1 Indication of Halfway Point; Third-way Point

1.1. **Intermediate Directions.** Although a general cardinal directions statement may suffice, in many techniques and dance styles a slight or greater modification in directional placement is needed, thus a specific statement must be made. Intermediate directions, i.e. those between cardinal directions, are shown as: i) halfway points between two main directions, ii) third-way points from one main direction toward another, and iii) a slight displacement from a cardinal direction (discussed in Section 2). Ex. **1a** is a schematic drawing, illustrating the halfway and third-way points between the directions side low, **1b**, side middle, **1c**, and side high, **1d**. The halfway points will be dealt with first.

1.2. **Between Two Cardinal Directions.** A halfway point is indicated by a dot placed between the two main direction symbols. Ex. **1e** shows the midpoint between side low and side middle. The two directions are tied with a small vertical bow to indicate one movement to that point and one unit in timing.

1.3. If the body part is already in one of the directions, as in **1f**, then that direction need not be repeated, only the dot and the second direction need to be stated. In **1g** the arm is side middle, therefore it is enough to indicate the dot and the side low symbol. The diagram of **1h** shows these halfway points.

1.4. **Moving to an Intermediate Point.** When moving from another direction as in **1i**, the first direction symbol stated is logically that nearer the starting point, therefore **1i** is more appropriate then **1j**.

1.5. In **1k**, because the head is understood to be erect at the start, the statement of **1k** can be simplified to **1l**, only the dot and the side high symbol being written. In moving from halfway to right side high to the same point on the other side, i.e. passing through place high, the fuller statement of **1m** is reduced to **1n**, a convenient shorthand usage, illustrated in **1o**.[2]

1.6. **Between Three Cardinal Directions.** A point between three cardinal directions can be shown as in **1p**, the three points being tied together with one bow. Without the bow the arm would go up, then halfway to right side high and from there halfway to right diagonal high.[3]

Such use of halfway points is applicable to all the main directions.

Advanced Labanotation

Intermediate Directions

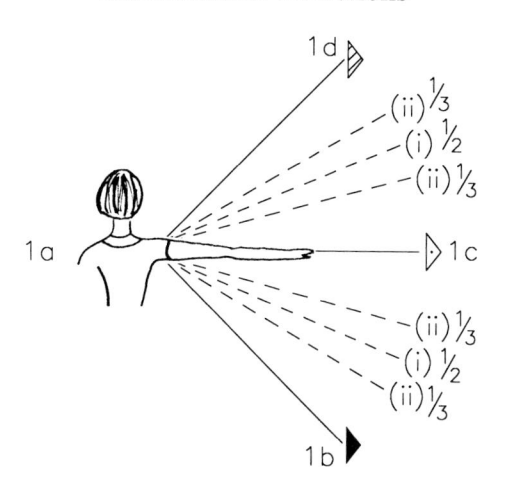

Between Two Cardinal Directions

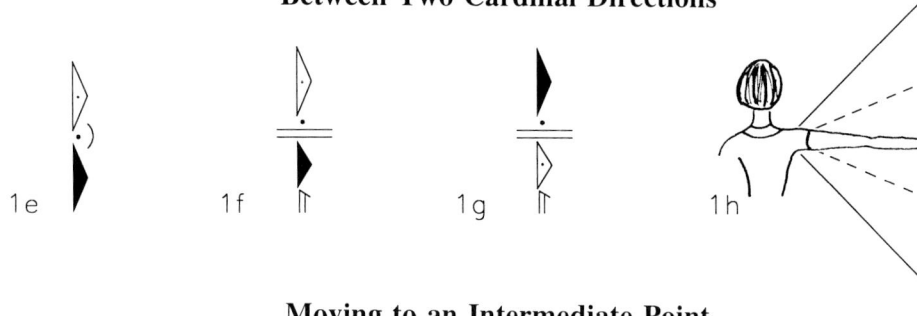

Moving to an Intermediate Point

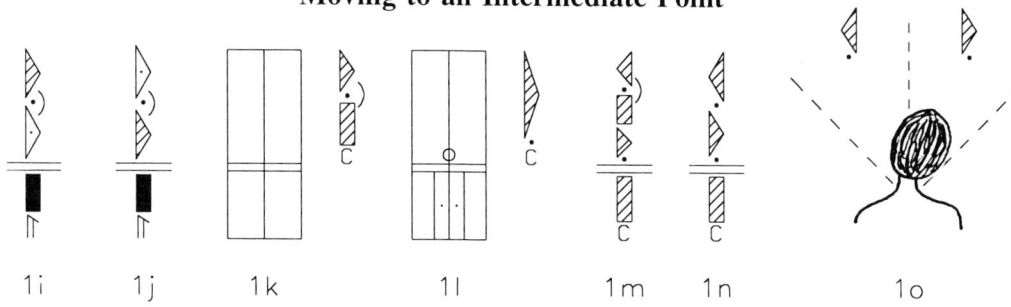

Between Three Cardinal Directions

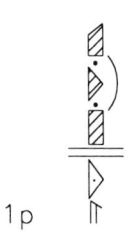

1.7. **Directional Definition of Pins.** Pins are used in specific ways to indicate modifications of major direction symbols and also minor movements. The pin itself is like a miniature direction symbol, the point of the pin indicates the direction, the head of the pin gives the level. White pins represent high level, black pins represent low level and 'tacks' (straight backed pins) represent middle level (horizontal) points. In **1q-1aa** the appropriate pin is placed next to the indication of the major direction to which it relates.

1.8. **Third-way Points.** A third-way point, that is, a 15° point located between one main direction and an adjacent (neighboring) direction, is shown by use of a pin within the main direction symbol. The advantage of this usage is that the main direction can be recorded and the modification added without the timing being affected.

1.9. It is important to remember that a *pin placed within a main direction sign refers to an adjacent main direction.* The diagram of **1ab** shows the third-way points between place high, side high, side middle, side low and place low. Note that for middle level third-way points the middle level dot is usually understood and not stated. For high and low symbols a gap in the middle of the sign is left open for placement of the pin.

1.10. The third-way point may be an adjacent direction on the same level, as in **1ac**, (middle level), **1ad** (high level) or **1ae** (low level) or it may be an adjacent direction at a different level, **1af**. The description is not in terms of a relative direction, that is the relative motion as in "lower than side high" or "higher than side low", the directions referred to are destinational points.[4]

1.11. It is also possible (but more rarely encountered) to have two pins within one direction symbol, as in **1ag**. Here the point described is between one third-way to side high and one-third to diagonal high, as illustrated in **1ah**, viewed from above, x marking the point being described. This point is closer to place high than that of **1p**.

1.12. Two pins are used in **1ai** to show a point which is a third-way toward forward low and also a third-way toward right diagonal low.

Advanced Labanotation 5

Directional Definition of Pins

1q ¢ or -o- = ▨   1r ♦ or -•- = ▮

1s ↓ = ▮   1t ⊥ = ▯   1u ↓ = ▨   1v ✓ = ▮   1w ✓ = ▯   1x ✓ = ▨

1y .— = ▶   1z ⊢ = ▷   1aa -o- = ▷

Third-way Points

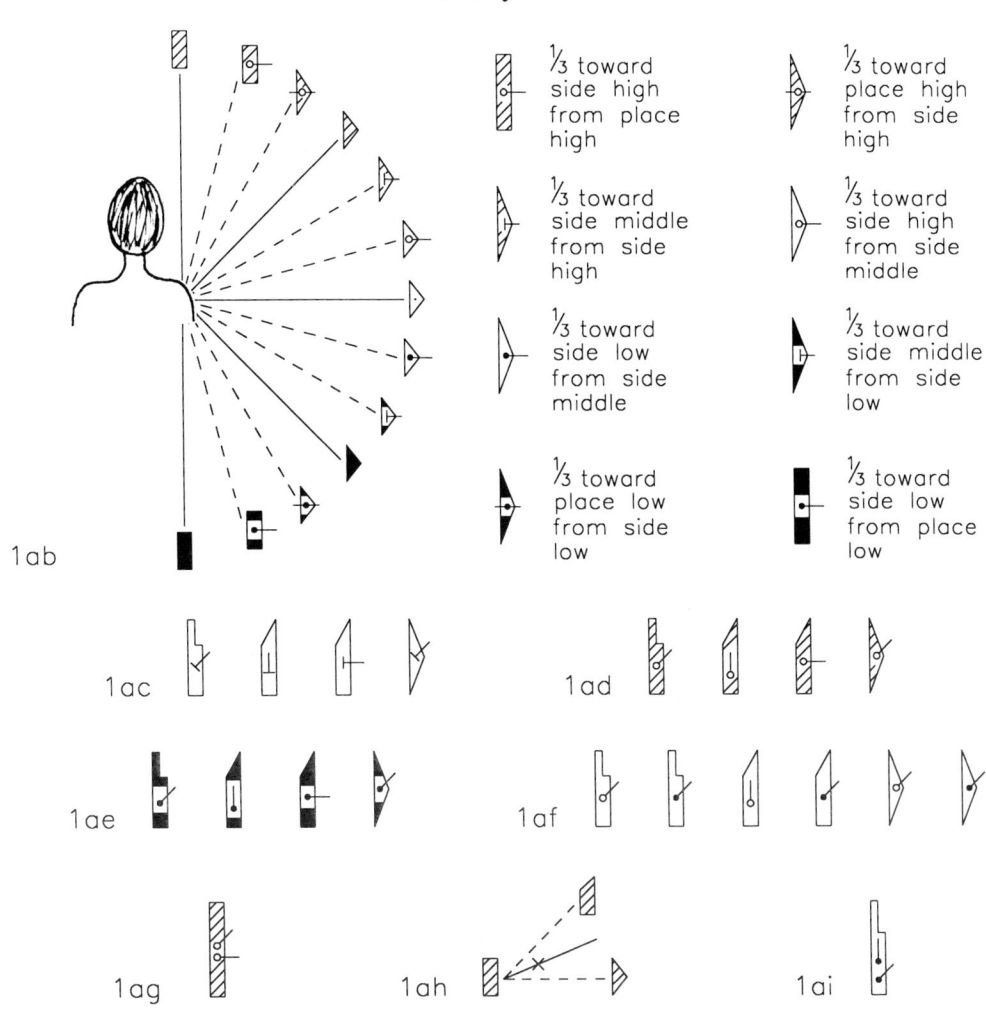

1ab

⅓ toward side high from place high

⅓ toward side middle from side high

⅓ toward side low from side middle

⅓ toward place low from side low

⅓ toward place high from side high

⅓ toward side high from side middle

⅓ toward side middle from side low

⅓ toward side low from place low

1ac

1ad

1ae

1af

1ag

1ah

1ai

2 Minor Modifications of a Main Direction

2.1. **Proximal Analysis.** A pin, placed next to a direction sign and tied to it by a small horizontal bow, indicates a minor modification of that direction, a point closer than the third-way points. The pin next to the direction symbol is understood to be part of that symbol in respect to timing. These pins represent a small displacement toward the main directions which they represent. The minor modification may be of a level difference or a directional difference. In **2a** the arm is slightly above the standard side middle situation in the direction of side high. In **2b** it is slightly in the direction of side low; these are illustrated in **2c**. In **2d** the modification is slightly toward forward diagonal middle; in **2e** slightly toward backward diagonal middle. These are illustrated in **2f**.

2.2. The modification of the direction may be two-dimensional, for example, the small displacement may be upward and slightly forward of the sideward middle point, i.e. toward the forward diagonal high direction, shown in **2g**, or the point may be slightly forward and downward, i.e toward the forward diagonal low direction, as in **2h**.

2.3. As can be seen, the pins indicate a position slightly towards an adjacent main direction, they cannot refer to a direction which is farther away. It is important to note that these pins are *judged from the fixed end of the limb*, i.e. the shoulder. If only the lower arm moves, the directional reference is to the elbow. The gesture moves directly to the modified point in space, as illustrated in **2i**, in which the arm ends slightly below standard side middle; in **2j** it ends slightly above forward middle.

2.4. The need for the small linking bow arises from the frequent use of pins to show relationship. In **2k** a couple is standing side by side with arms opened sideward. The above pin states that A's right arm is just above B's left arm and thus has a different meaning from the pin used with the small linking bow in **2a**. In **2l** a simple statement is made for three dancers. Dancers Y and Z have their left arms in front of their neighbor (X and Y), while X and Y's right arms are behind their neighbor (Y and Z).

2.5. While performance of these minor intermediate points is not always precise, the distance from the main direction is approximately 7.5°. Modifications indicated by pins also apply to intermediate directions.

Proximal Analysis

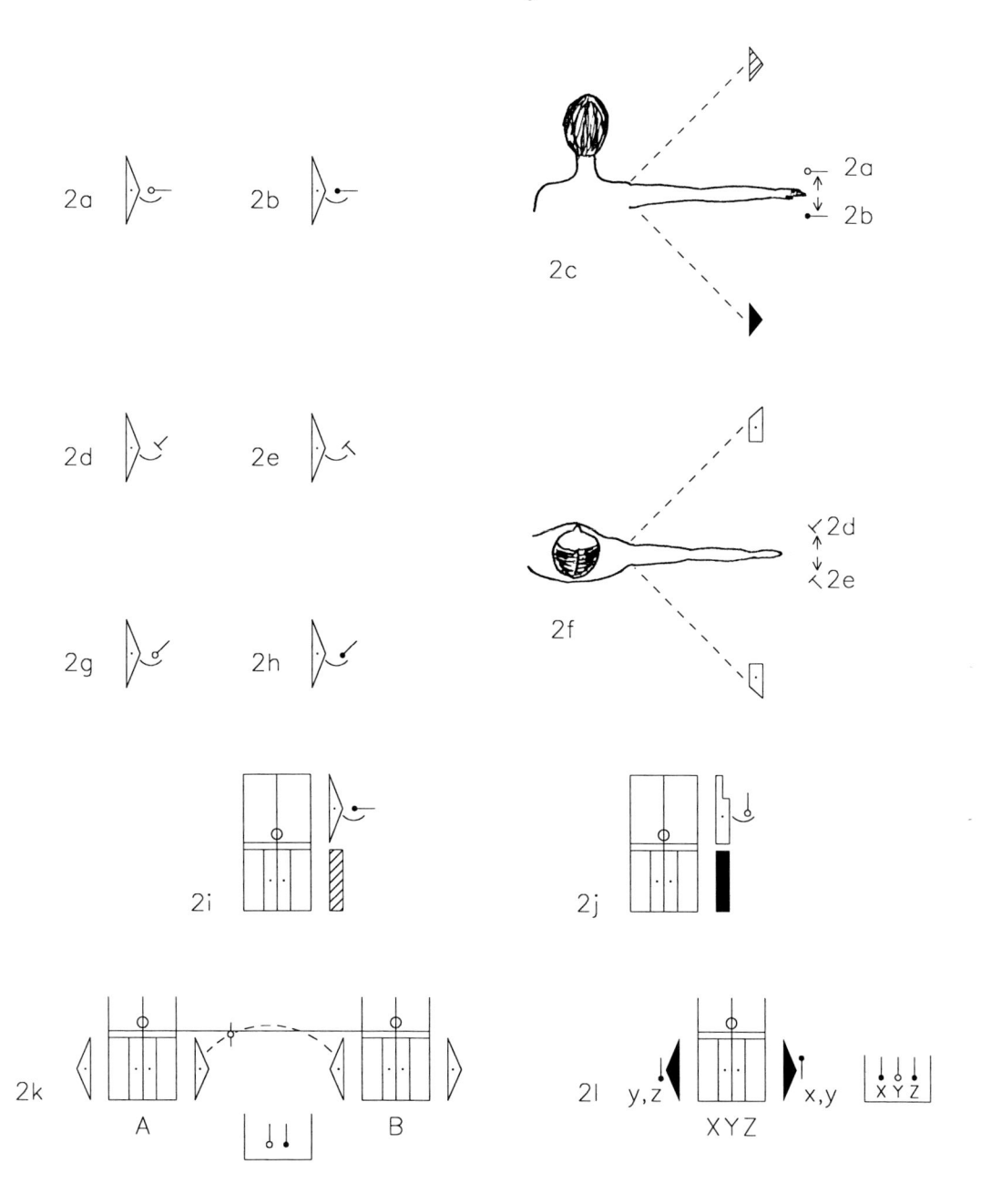

2a 2b

2c

2d 2e

2f

2g 2h

2i 2j

2k A B 2l y,z XYZ x,y X Y Z

II PATHS FOR GESTURES - STANDARD ANALYSIS

3 Peripheral and Central Paths

3.1. In moving from one point to another the limbs can take many paths. These may be peripheral paths, central paths, or one of the many intermediate paths. We deal first with the larger distinctions with examples for the right arm.

3.2. **Peripheral Path.** Ex. **3a** shows an arm movement passing through directional points which are 90° apart, the result is a peripheral circle. From each point to the next it is expected that a quarter circle arc will be followed.

3.3. **Central Path.** Passing through the center point for the arm (the shoulder being place middle) is shown in **3b** the path forming an angle. The extremity of the arm follows this path, the elbow bending and, depending on the rotational state of the arm, displacing sideward (inward rotation) or downward (outward rotation). In **3c** the central path is from forward middle to backward middle, the hand passing near the shoulder without actually touching.

3.4. **Standard Path.** For the standard performance of paths between points around the body, the distance between the 26 cardinal directional points (place middle being omitted) is designated as follows: a 1st degree distance is to an adjacent (neighboring) point (a 45° displacement), as illustrated in **3d**. The diametrically opposite point (180°) is termed the 4th degree point. Between these lie the 2nd (a 90° displacement) and 3rd (a 135° displacement) degree points.

3.5. Because of the anatomical structure of the joints of the body, all movement is circular, the path of the extremity takes the shape of a curve or arc. This is expected in a 1st degree distance, **3e** (seen from above) and also for a 2nd degree which produces a quarter circle, **3f**. It is now the standard rule that 3rd degree paths are also performed on the natural peripheral curvè, passing through the intermediate points unless otherwise indicated, **3g**.[5]

3.6. **Aimed Destination.**[6] For transition to a 4th degree point (the extreme opposite) the standard performance is a comfortable, non-emphasized movement, the arm bending and the hand passing fairly close to the shoulder, **3h**, but not as close as in **3c**. To achieve this path, which is termed the 'aimed destination', the elbow flexes, leading the arm to the opposite direction; toward the end of the movement the wrist flexes to keep the hand on this unemphasized path. Neither of these actions of flexing should be stressed.

Peripheral and Central Paths

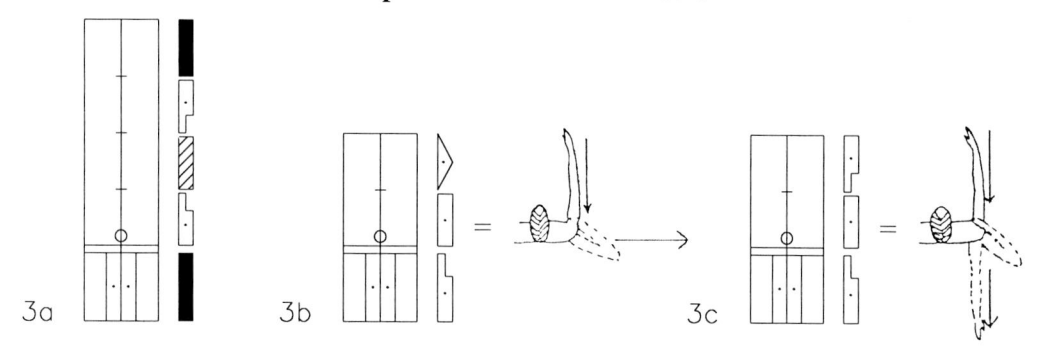

3a 3b 3c

Standard Path

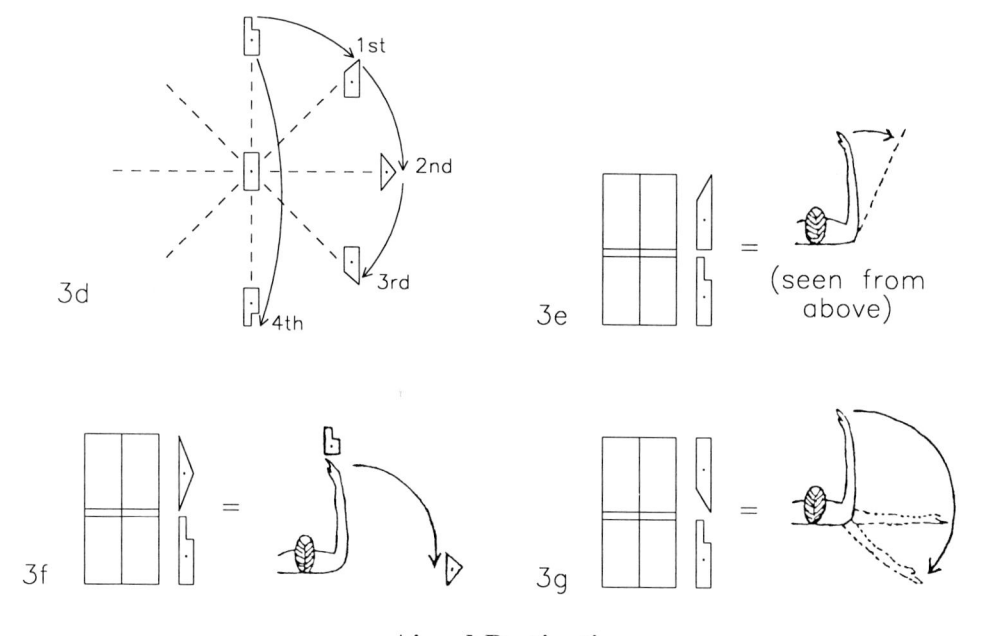

3d 3e (seen from above)

3f 3g

Aimed Destination

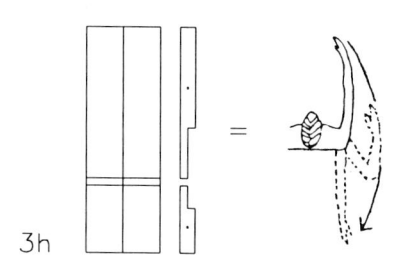

3h

4 Indication of Aimed Destination, Straight or Peripheral Path for Gestures

4.1. **Aimed Destination.** As explained in 3.6, the unemphasized path to a 4th degree point is to move in a simple, comfortable way, allowing the arm to bend, with no emphasis on the path itself. The term for this kind of performance is 'aimed destination'. When performing this kind of arm gesture, emphasis is not on the pathway, rather the reverse, one is aiming to arrive at the designated point, the manner of performance is not the focus. This is in contrast to the established standard peripheral path for 1st, 2nd and 3rd degree destinational points for which the arm is usually normally extended (see 3.5 and illustrations for **3e**, **3f** and **3g**).

4.2. An aimed destination to a 3rd degree point is indicated by a direction sign (the destination) linked to the end of a duration line (which shows the timing) by a small vertical destination bow, **4a**. In this example the movement is from forward middle to the right back diagonal middle point. For comparison, the standard path to a 3rd degree point, **3g**, is repeated here. Another example is given in **4b** where the arms move to different 3rd degree points.

4.3. **Passing Flexion.** Because performance of aimed destination movements involve some arm flexion, it would seem that statement could be made in terms of passing flexion. Ex. **4c** shows the flexion as a passing state, the timing of this flexion (where it starts and finishes) being indicated by the start and end of the vertical bow. This timing can vary, of course. Ex. **4d** shows a different use of the flexion sign to approximate the path between 3rd degree points. In the description given here, timing is specific. The writer must choose the movement description which is the more appropriate. Such flexion details may be important for a particular analysis, but they do not serve the need for a simple statement of a 'aimed destination' spatial performance.

4.4. **Inward Path Indication**. If the peripheral path is not to be followed, an inward path toward place middle can be shown, as in **4e**. In this example the arm does not reach the place middle, this would be written as in **4f**. The inward path might also be a minor deviation from the line of the path of the movement toward a particular direction, as in **4g**. In **4e** and **4g** the performer is made aware of the modification thus the shape of the path is being featured. In contrast, for an aimed destination, nothing is stated about the shape of the path.

Advanced Labanotation

Aimed Destination

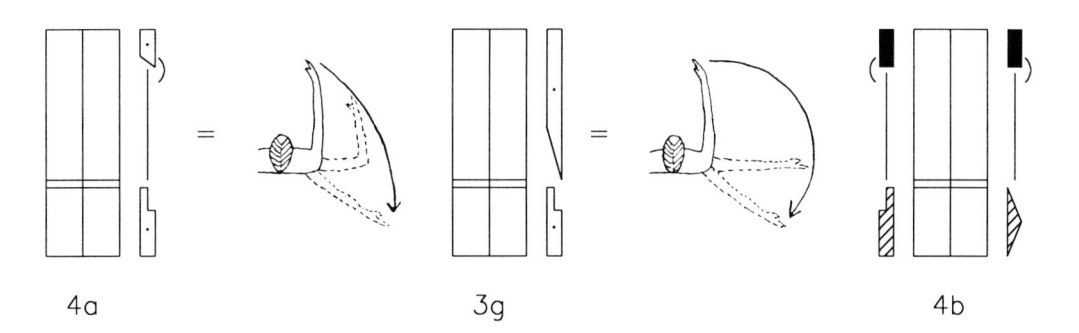

4a   3g   4b

Passing Flexion

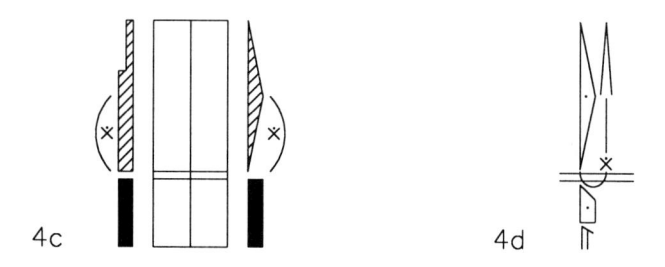

4c   4d

Inward Path Indication

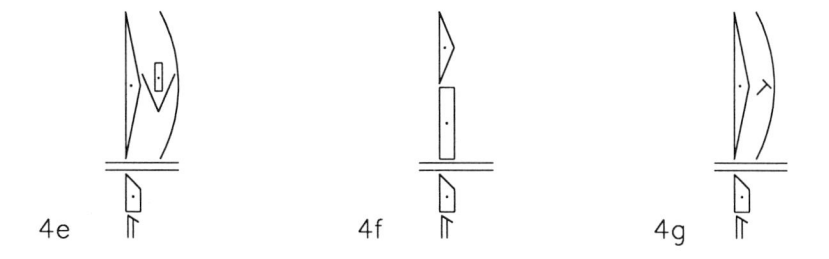

4e   4f   4g

4.5. **Straight Path.** In performing a straight path the extremity, the finger tips will follow a straight line. The path of **4h** is illustrated in **4i**. Ex. **4j** shows a straight path in another setting, the hand must pass fairly near the head to achieve this movement. A straight path to a 4th degree point, as in **4k**, is close in performance to **4l**, but in the former the focus is on the path whereas in the latter it is on the central point, passing close to the shoulder joint.

4.6. The movement (motion) which takes place in **4m** is forward horizontal, as also is the destination. Emphasis on the straight path nature of **4m** can be indicated by adding the straight path sign, as in **4n**. Without the path sign the performer may not be aware of the path of the extremity of the arm as it moves. In most instances the path of the gesture is not on a straight line. Indication of straight paths is valuable in mime gestures, as illustrated in **4o**. This gesture could be one of wiping a surface in front of you, or, if performed slowly, feeling a wall.

4.7. **Peripheral Path.** If there is a need to stress the peripheral curve between 3rd degree points, it can be shown as in **4p** or **4q**. These have the disadvantage of giving specific timing which may not be desired. Such timing is discussed in Section 5.

Advanced Labanotation

Straight Path

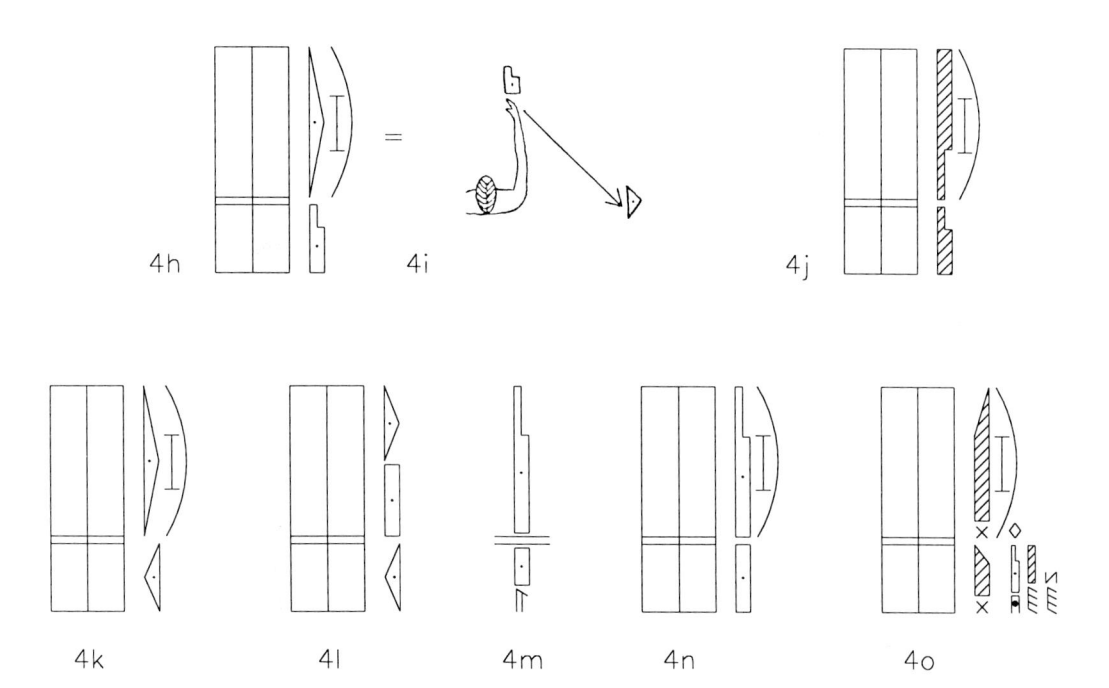

4h 4i 4j

4k 4l 4m 4n 4o

Peripheral Path

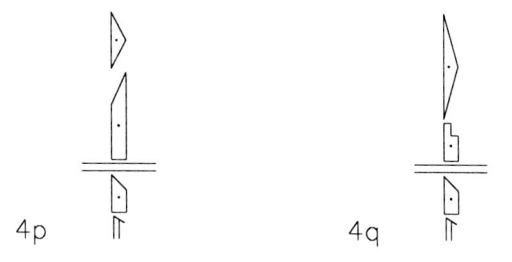

4p 4q

5 Timing for Third Degree Pathway

5.1. For 3rd degree peripheral paths, timing may dictate that a direction passed through needs to be stated. The performance of **5a** is evenly spaced over the three counts. In **5b** the side middle point passed through is stated. The timing here is still even. But in **5c** two counts are taken to arrive at the diagonal forward point and hence a swifter movement to the back diagonal.

5.2. When a change of level occurs on a third degree pathway, the statement of the direction passed through can affect both timing and the path itself. In **5d** the gesture starts forward high and ends at the right back diagonal middle point. Note the difference in the shape of the path when a side middle direction is passed through, as in **5e**, or a side high direction is used, **5f**. Further variations on this path are given in **5g** and **5h**, the difference lying in the spatial pathway as well as the timing. The last two, **5g** and **5h**, could also have the timing of **5b**.

5.3. **Empty Direction Symbol for Pathway.**[7] To show a smooth spatial transition from starting point to destination, the device of an empty direction symbol can be used. In **5i** the side symbol is given no level, the arm will follow the natural intermediate level for that path. The direction passed through in **5j** is the forward diagonal, no level is indicated, the arm will lower gradually on its way to the destination.

Timing for Third Degree Pathway

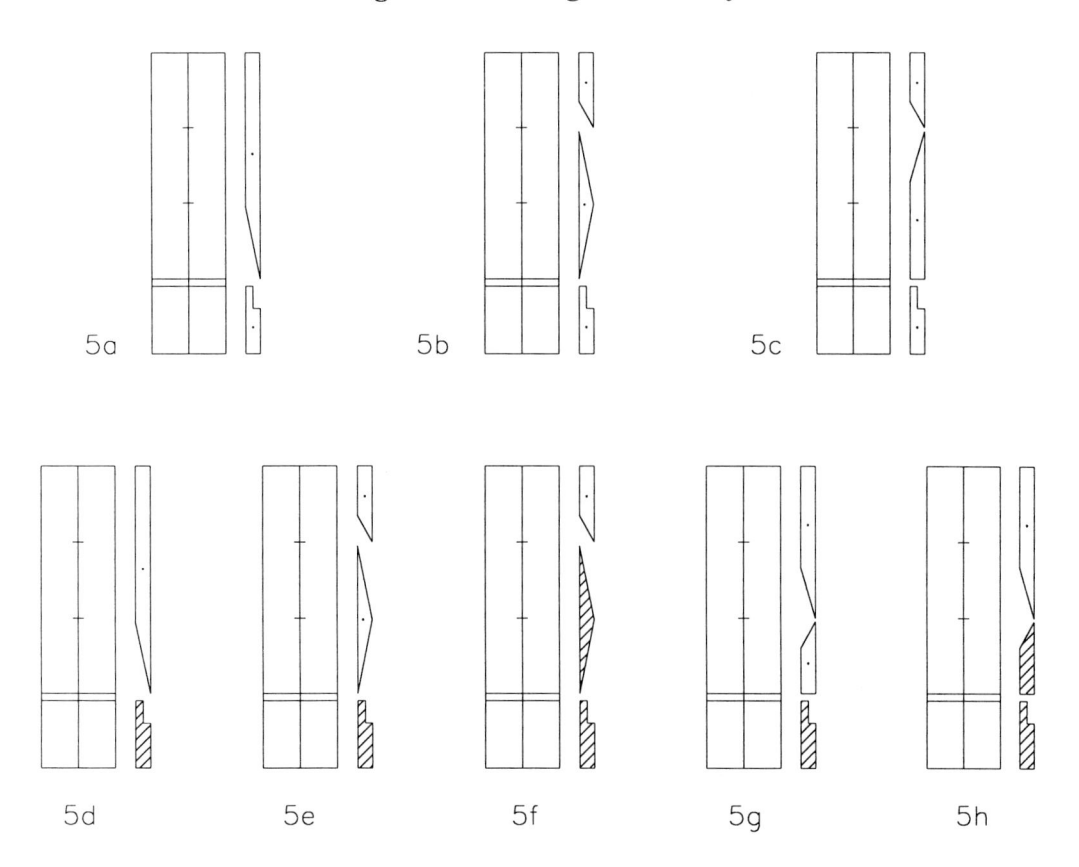

5a 5b 5c

5d 5e 5f 5g 5h

Empty Direction Symbol for Pathway

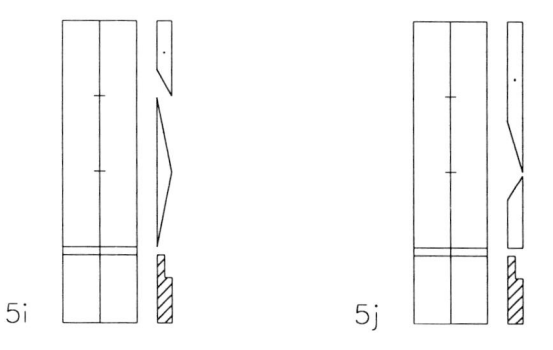

5i 5j

6 General Indication of Spatially Central or Peripheral Paths

6.1.   **Spatially Central or Peripheral Paths.**[8] Not all paths for gestures need to be specifically spelled out. For movement exploration and to indicate the sense of a movement, the intention and expression of making use of the periphery, or of a gesture passing centrally, are valuable. For such use exactness in performance is generally not required.

6.2.   The signs for spatially central and for spatially peripheral[9] are derived from the diamond shape representing space, spatial aspects, **6a**. A small 'tick' extending inward, as in **6b**, represents spatially central; when the 'tick' extends outward, **6c**, the idea of spatially peripheral is expressed. These signs are abbreviated to the more practical signs of **6d** and **6e** for placement within a column, bow, etc. As indicated, the signs may be reversed.

6.3.   A half-arrow is added and the tick extended when the movement is going from central to peripheral, **6f**; the half-arrow is reversed to show a movement from peripheral to central, **6g**.

6.4.   These signs are applied to gestural paths to indicate the manner of performance. In **6h** the arm moves from left forward high diagonal to right backward low diagonal. The standard performance to this 4th degree point is for the extremity of the arm to pass near the torso. But here the movement is stated to be peripheral, thus it will make an arc, the exact placement of this arc is not indicated. This performance is also true for **6i**. Moving from place high to place low on a peripheral path can have many interpretations.

6.5.   In contrast in **6j** the simple quarter circle path to a 2nd degree point is not followed, instead the arm moves spatially inward on its way to side low; exact performance is not expected, freedom of interpretation is allowed. The path of **6k** is to a 3rd degree point, the standard peripheral arc performance is not used, instead, the central indication states that a central path is to be followed.

6.6.   **Degree of Curve.** The following examples give a comparison between performances of a 4th degree path, here illustrated with the right arm moving from place low to place high. Ex. **6l** shows the specific indication of a straight path between these points, illustrated in **6m**. The standard, understood performance of **6n**, a slight curve (see 3.6), is illustrated in **6o**. The slight

Advanced Labanotation 17

sideward deviation of **6p** would produce approximately the result of **6q**. By adding a spatially large sign (see Section 11), the deviation is greater, **6r** and **6s**. The peripheral arc of **6t**, illustrated in **6u**, could be performed as **6v** or **6w**. The statement of **6t** leaves placement (location) of this arc open.

Spatially Central or Peripheral Paths

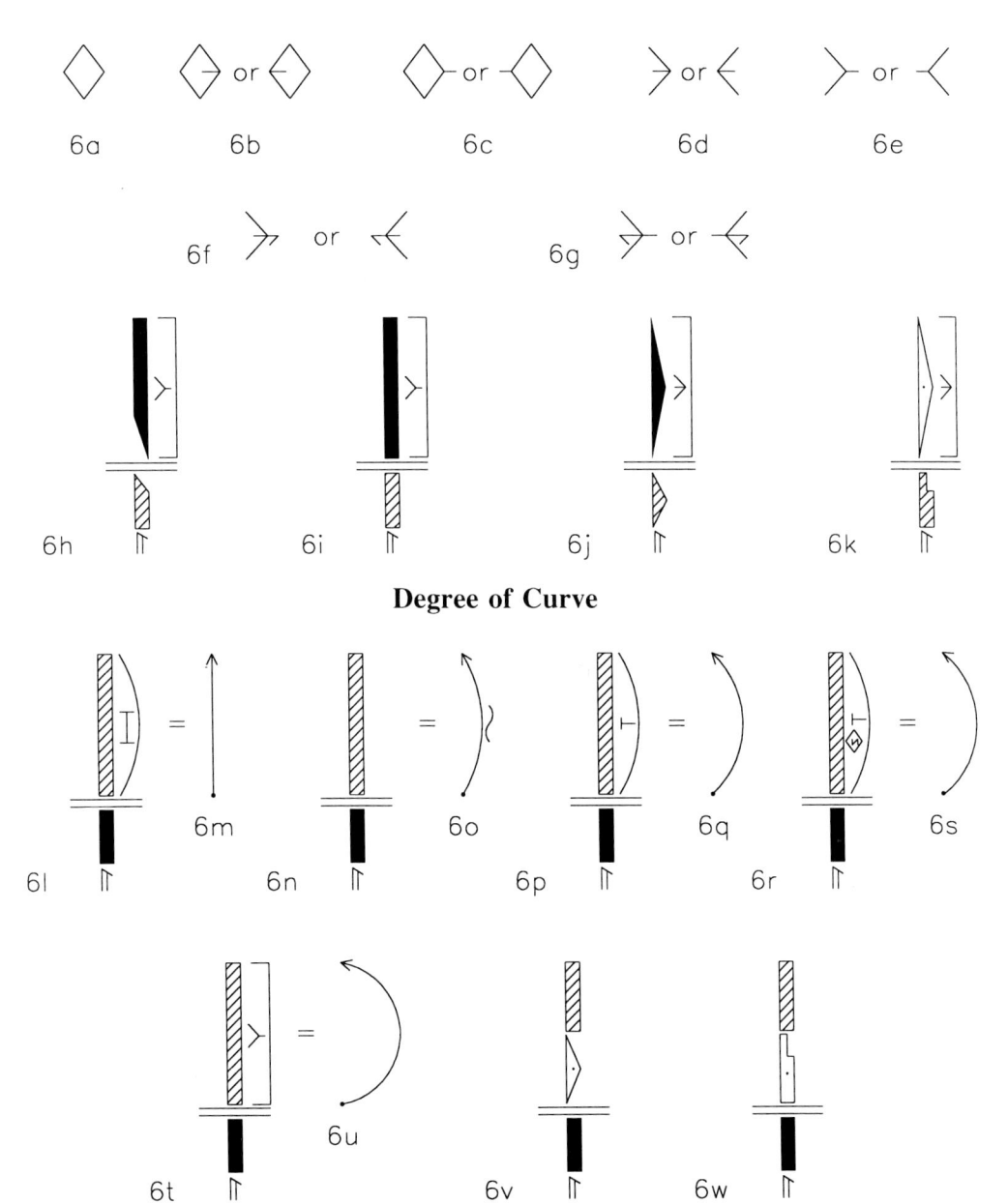

Degree of Curve

7 Sharp or Rounded Corners for Gestures

7.1. In **7a** a triangular pattern is described. The arm moves from point to point on standard paths, illustrated in **7b**. When performing such paths in space, it is possible, and may be desirable, to smooth the angular transitions so that the corners are rounded. It is also possible to accentuate, exaggerate the sharpness of the corners, and such performance may be desired. Use of a vertical phrasing bow, as in **7c**, gives the message of a fluent performance; this, however, does not make any statement about the shape of the transitions from one destination and the progression to the next.[10]

7.2. The two different performances of the basic space pattern can be indicated by signs based on the diamond of **7d**, the sign representing spatial aspects. To indicate a spatially rounded performance of the stated movement, the sign of **7e** is used, the curved arc being combined with the diamond shape. For an angular performance, an angular shape is combined with the diamond, **7f**.[11]

7.3. In **7g** the sharp corners are shown to be rounded, producing a softer outline, illustrated in **7h**. In **7i** the same basic pattern is shown to be performed with visibly sharp transitions, as in **7j**. Another even sharper angle is given in **7k**, illustrated in **7l**. The transition angle is stated in **7m** to be rounded, shown in **7n**.

Advanced Labanotation

Sharp or Rounded Corners for Gestures

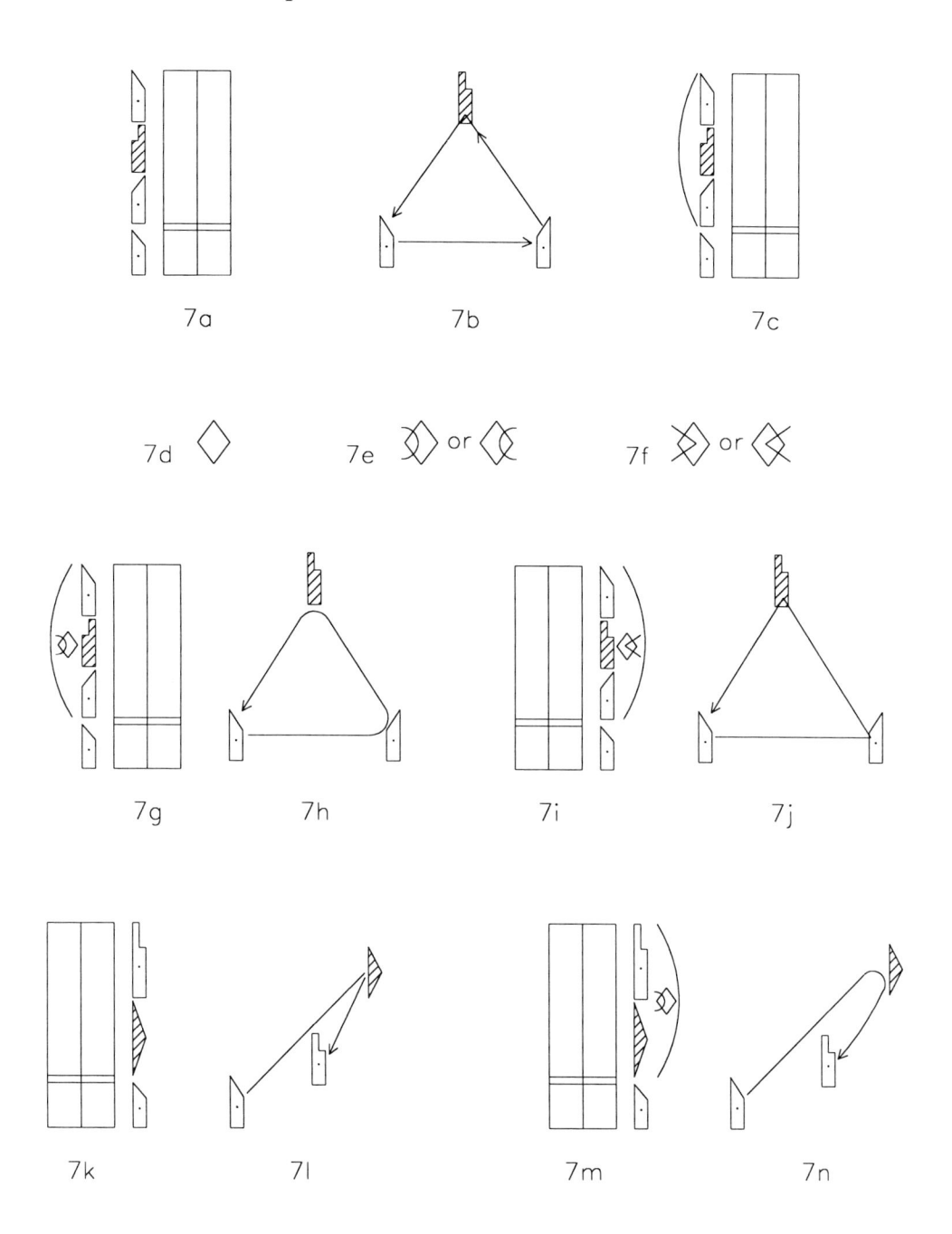

7a 7b 7c

7d 7e 7f

7g 7h 7i 7j

7k 7l 7m 7n

8 Retrace Path

8.1. A simple device often used in exercises as well as in choreography is that of retracing a path, a 'there and back' pattern. The indication for retracing the path, useful for fairly simple movements, is particularly practical for complex gestural paths. The body remembers the path and it is not difficult physically to reverse and retrace that path.

8.2. The shorthand device used, a double ended arrow, **8a**, is derived from the use of this arrow on floor plans to show the performer retraces the path, **8b**. Note that it is the *movement* that has just been performed which is repeated in reverse, not the symbols.

8.3. In **8c** the path of the leg gesture is to be retraced; on the return the leg will rise to forward middle on its way to touch the floor at the right side, and then slide on the toe to the starting position, i.e. the forward low toe contact with the floor. In **8d** this retracing has been spelled out.

8.4. In **8e** the flowing arm design will retrace the same path after a slight pause. This example has been fully written out in **8f**.

8.5. The flowery hand design of **8g**, which might occur as part of a gentleman's bow, is reversed, ending close to the body, as at the start.

Retrace Path

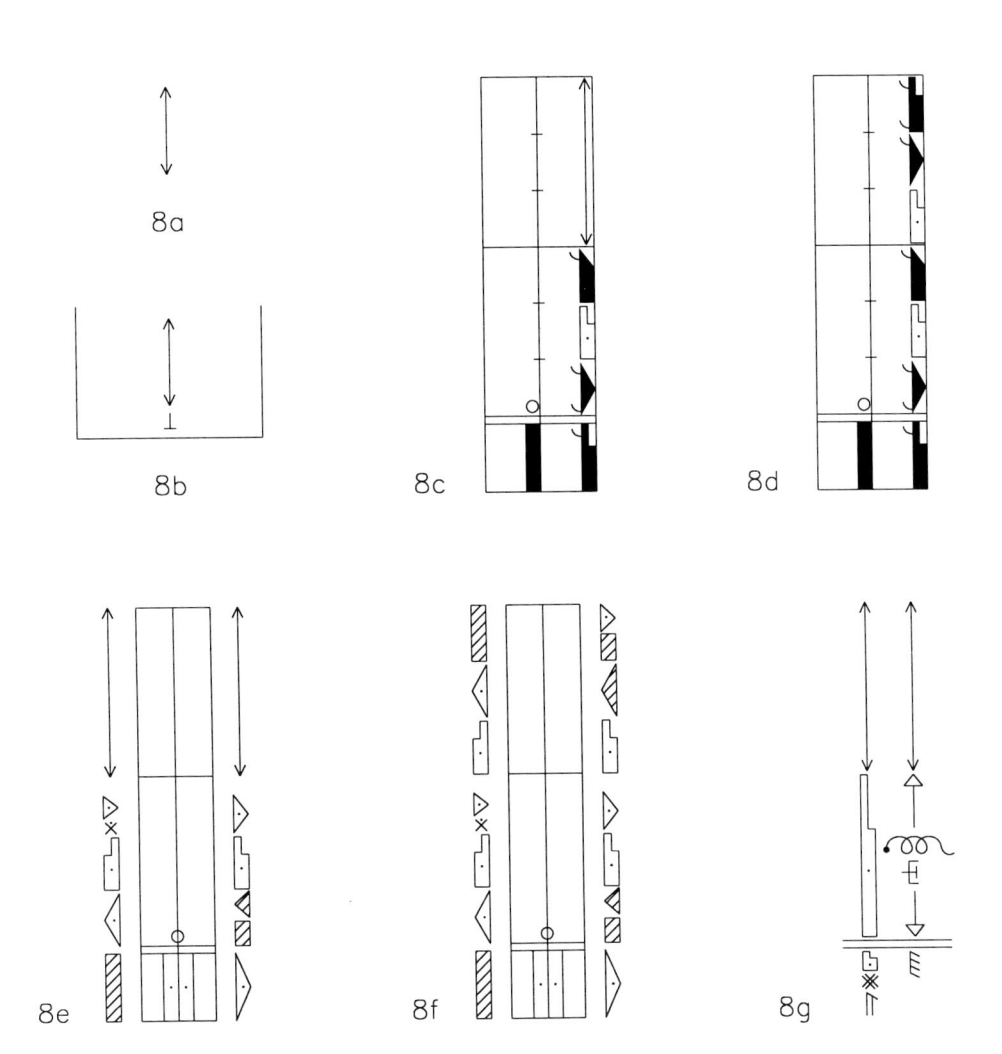

8a

8b

8c

8d

8e

8f

8g

III DEVIATIONS FROM THE PATH OF A GESTURE

9 Analysis of Deviations

9.1. Deviations are slight detours from the normal course of a path, this may be the path of a gesture or a path across the floor. Deviation from the standard performance of a gestural path in space is discussed here. Deviations from a path across the floor are presented in Part IV.

9.2. A deviation may be thought of as an outside influence pulling the limb or part of the body off its normal, standard course. This influence, like a magnet, is strong enough to cause a detour, an indirect way, but not strong enough to prevent the ultimate destination being reached.

9.3. As a basic example to be explored, we take a path in front of the body where it is easy to see and experience the variations. Ex. **9a** indicates an arm gesture moving from left forward diagonal middle to right forward diagonal middle. The path of this gesture naturally follows the standard horizontal curve; in the illustration of **9b** it is drawn as a straight line, as if from 'shoulder-view'.

9.4. From any standard path there is a sphere of possible deviations, as **9c** illustrates. While many deviations are basically two-dimensional, they may be three-dimensional.

9.5. **Single Deviations.** For a single deviation, the direction of the deviation is judged from the *center point* on the line of movement, **9d**. From this center point, the cross of axis directions radiate out, providing what can be imagined as 'magnets' which pull the limb off the standard course, thus causing the deviation.

9.6. The direction of the deviation is shown by the appropriate pin placed within a vertical bow. Ex. **9e** states an upward deviation, as illustrated in **9f**; **9g** shows the same basic movement, but performed with a downward deviation before ending at the right forward middle point, as illustrated in **9h**.

9.7. The vertical bow indicates a passing state, in this case a change in direction which gradually comes into effect and then gradually disappears. By the end of the bow the deviation is over, it has disappeared, the limb ends in the standard direction, as though no deviation had occurred.

Advanced Labanotation

Analysis of Deviations

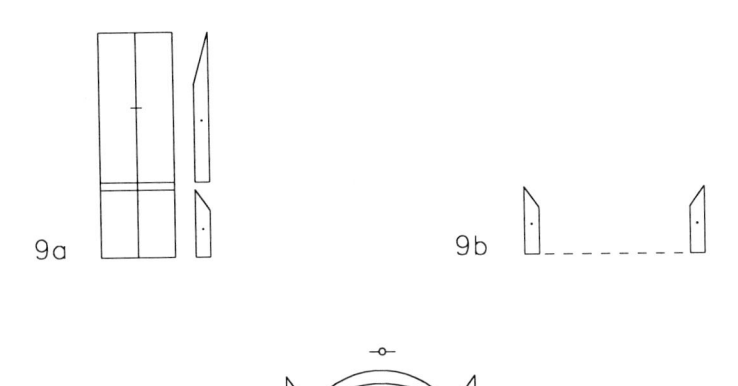

9a

9b

9c

Single Deviations

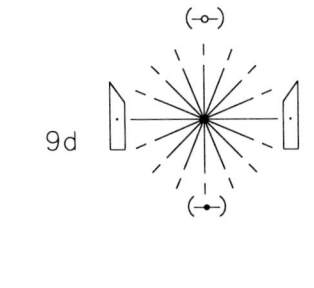

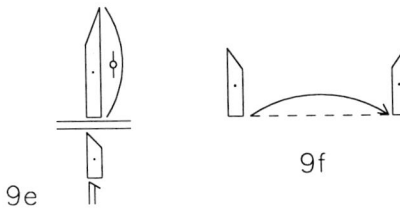

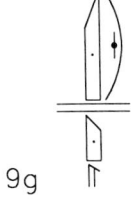

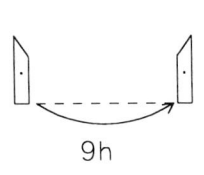

9d

9e 9f 9g 9h

9.8. Single Symmetrical Deviations. For the chosen basic movement of **9a**, upward or downward deviations are the most likely since they are easy and comfortable to perform. No change in how the arm is held need occur. In deviating over forward, as in **9i**, the arm must extend or an inclusion of the upper body should take place, since the deviation is further away from the body, beyond the established line of the movement. In **9j** the deviation is backward, toward the body, and so the arm will flex slightly.

9.9. Ex. **9k** shows a forward-upward deviation, a mixture of **9e** and **9i**, so a slight extension will be needed, just as in **9l** a slight flexion will be needed for the backward-downward deviation.

9.10. Compound Symmetrical Deviations. More than one deviation may take place on a single path. Ex. **9m** shows an upward and a downward deviation evenly spread over the established path. Between the deviations the limb returns to the basic path. This may also be written within one bow, as in **9n**. The path is illustrated in **9o**.

9.11. Each such multiple deviation for a single gesture has its own imagined local center of directions. Ex. **9p** illustrates the two centers of direction required by the double deviation of **9o**. The path of **9q**, which has three even deviations, illustrated in **9r** will require the three imagined centers of **9s**.

Advanced Labanotation

Single Symmetrical Deviations

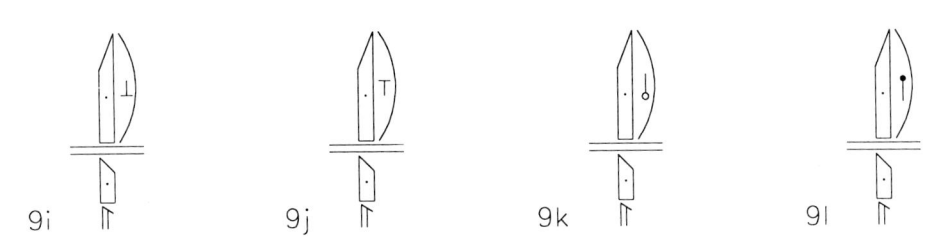

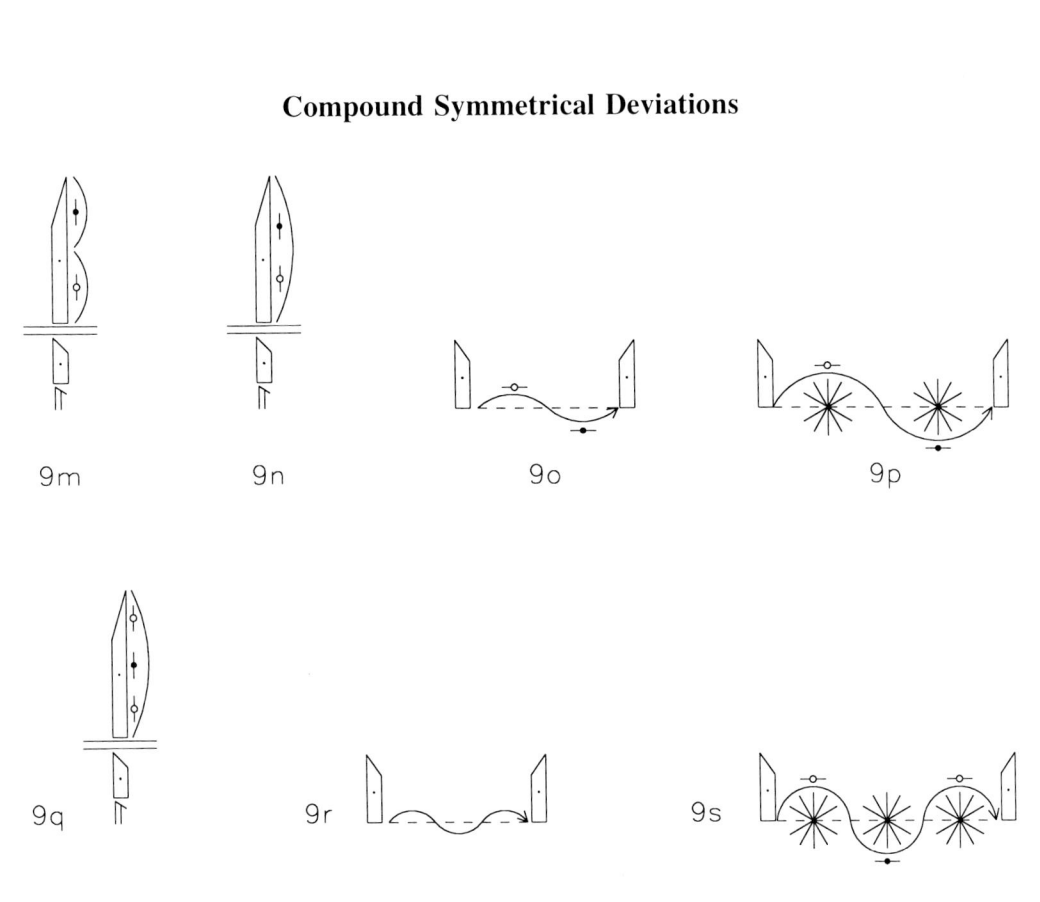

9i 9j 9k 9l

Compound Symmetrical Deviations

9m 9n 9o 9p

9q 9r 9s

10 Other Kinds of Deviations

10.1. **Asymmetrical Deviations.** All the deviations we have dealt with so far have had 'magnets' placed at right angles to the line of the movement thus producing an even curve. A direction, 'magnet', which is at a lesser angle, will produce an unevenly shaped, an assymmetrical pathway. The side high deviation of **10a**, illustrated in **10b**, will exert a greater influence at the start of the movement, since the limb is closer to that direction and less of an influence as the arm moves toward its destination.

10.2. The reverse is true of **10c**, illustrated in **10d**, where the pull of the deviation is weak at the start and stronger at the end. Similar unevenly shaped deviation paths occur on this path when there are diagonal 'pulls', as in **10e**. On two-dimensional paper **10b** and **10f** appear alike, but **10f** moves diagonally forward with a slight extension.

10.3. **Non-Centered Deviations.** A deviation can occur at the start of a path, before the end of the path or somewhere during the movement. Where and when the deviation starts and ends is shown by the start and end of the bow. Ex. **10g** shows an upward movement, a 'bulge' at the start of the gestural path, once completed, the limb follows the standard path, illustrated in **10h**.

10.4. Ex. **10i** shows the same temporary upward curve to occur in the middle of the path, as in **10j**. In **10k** this curve occurs only near the end of the path, illustrated in **10l**.

Advanced Labanotation

Asymmetrical Deviations

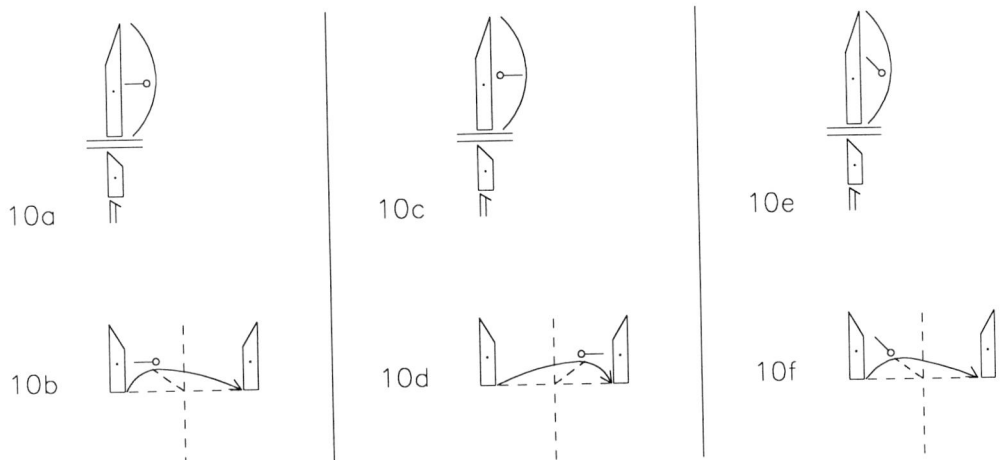

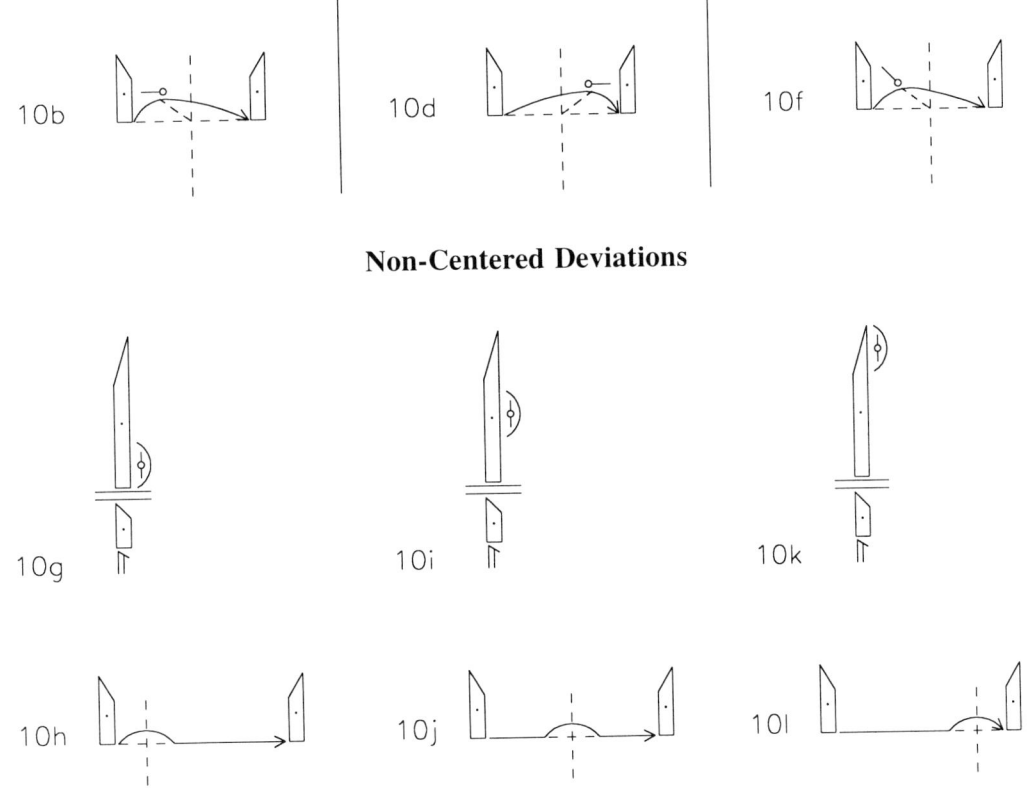

10a

10b

10c

10d

10e

10f

Non-Centered Deviations

10g

10h

10i

10j

10k

10l

10.5. **Regressive (Jagged) Deviations.** A pin indicating the opposite direction to that of the main path indicates a momentary regression, as in a zig-zag. Ex. **10m**, with illustration in **10n**, shows two such regressive 'jags' on the path. No clear timing is indicated in **10m**; in contrast, timing is shown more specifically in **10o**.

10.6. **Loops.** Loops can also be shown with pins, though this may soon reach the stage where the movement is best described through Design Drawing.[12] Note in the examples below some of the possibilities in writing loops on such a path. Each example is followed by a Design Drawing equivalent of the pin indications.

10.7. Ex. **10p**, illustrated in **10q**, shows a loop in the middle of the path, a loop which rises upward. This same pattern is shown through Design Drawing in **10r** for which the surface is shown to be forward middle, i.e. directly in front.

10.8. In **10s**, illustrated in **10t**, a downward deviation occurs at the start, then an upward loop at the middle and another downward deviation before arrival at the destination. Ex. **10u** is the Design Drawing equivalent. The pattern of **10v**, illustrated in **10w**, shows one downward loop occurring soon after the start and another soon after the center part of the path. Note use of the repeat sign here to avoid writing the pins again. Ex. **10x** shows the Design Drawing equivalent.

Advanced Labanotation

Regressive (Jagged) Deviations

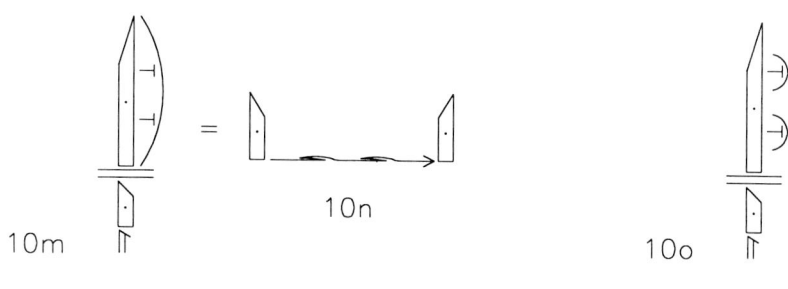

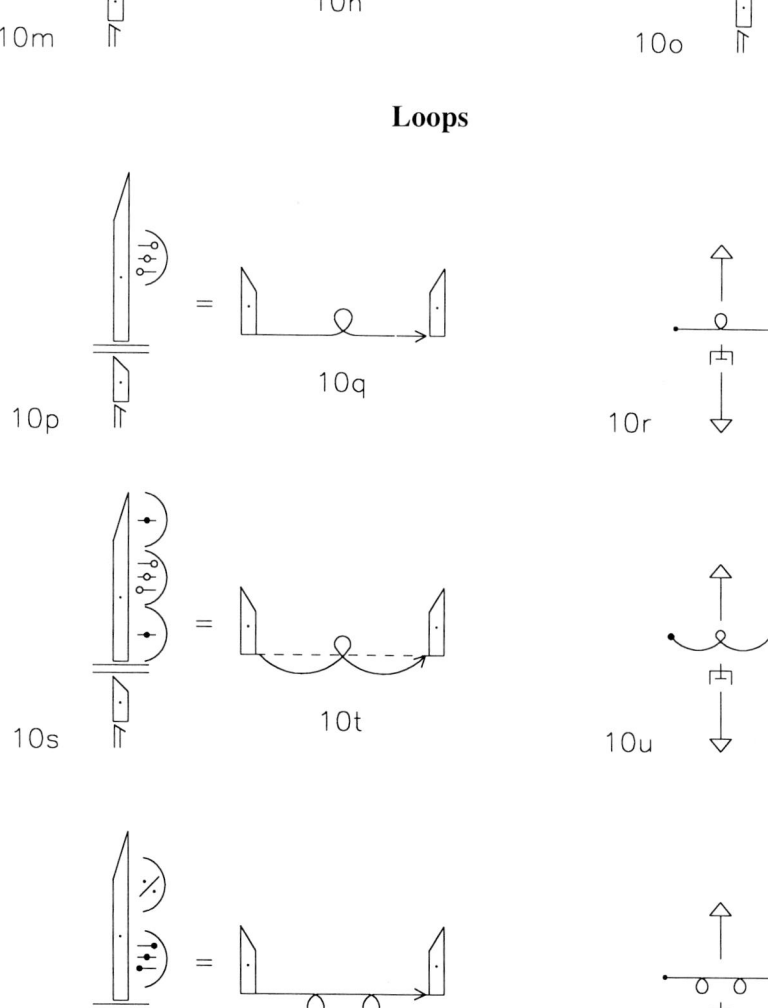

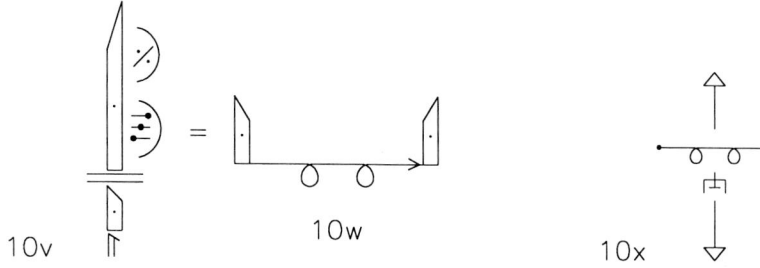

10m 10n 10o

Loops

10p 10q 10r

10s 10t 10u

10v 10w 10x

10.9. Reference to Standard Directions. In certain contexts it is easier to view the direction of a deviation from a gestural path in terms of movement toward a major Standard Directional point. The size of such deviation is not larger unless an indication of size is included.[13] Such reference to a direction is a different analysis from the use of pins which relate to the cross of directions centered on a path of the movement, the standard analysis for gestural deviations.

10.10. In **10y** the arm deviates backward of the rising path as it moves to side high. The path and the pin are interpreted from the usual Standard Directions.[14] A slightly different intention is to deviate toward the left backward low direction. If this description is wanted, a small version of the appropriate direction symbol is used, **10z**. As it is not a pin, the system of reference is clearly that of the Standard Cross, direction being judged from the proximal joint. Deviation toward a major direction may be easier to determine than the appropriate pin which relates to the center of the line of movement.

10.11. It should be noted that the paths of **10y** and **10z** are not identical, the curve of **10z** being slightly lopsided, the 'bulge' coming earlier on the path. For general use an empty direction symbol may be appropriate, **10aa**, the exact shape of the curve not being important.

10.12. A similar example is given for deviation from a horizontal path. In **10ab**, in relation to the center of the line of movement, there is a 'pull' to the left front high diagonal; a symmetrical curve results. If, however, the starting point is place low, **10ac**, this asymmetrical deviation is not so easy to determine, the performer can relate more readily to **10ad**, but must remember that the diagonal middle direction is not reached, the curve does not pass through it.[15]

10.13. **System of Reference Based on the Path.**[16] The standard analysis for deviations on a path, such as **10ae**, already explored, can be rotated to serve examples which have a change of level, as in **10af**. Symmetrical deviations can still be visualized as being 'above' or 'below' the stated line, as though the line were horizontal. For this the key of **10ag** is used; it states the spatial cross of directions centered on the placement of the path.[17] For placement within the deviation bow, the key is simplified to **10ah**. In **10ai** the deviation is 'upward'; in **10aj** it is 'downward'; these can relate to the illustration of **10af**.

10.14. Ex. **10ak** is comparable, the arm moves from right side high to left forward diagonal low. In **10al** the local centered deviation is 'above', as seen from the slanted line; in **10am** the deviation is 'below'. In these the key has been placed in a bracket or it may be placed alongside and tied with a bow to the deviation indication, as illustrated.

Advanced Labanotation 31

10.15. With the range of possible directional movements, the observer chooses that description which seems immediately obvious, the one which most clearly describes the event, even if it means a switch of key within one score.

Reference to Standard Directions

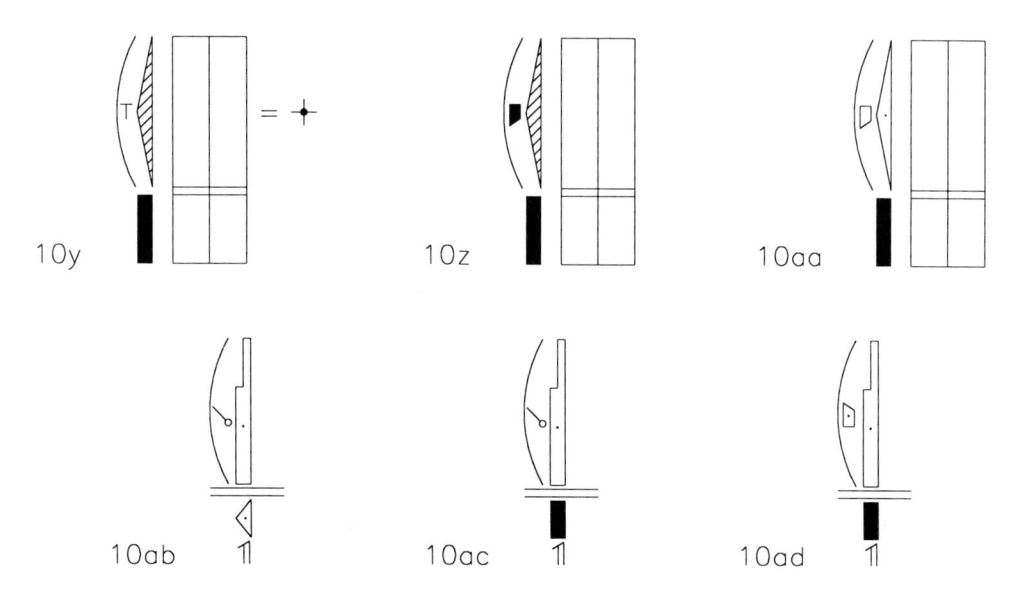

10y   10z   10aa

10ab   10ac   10ad

System of Reference Based on the Path

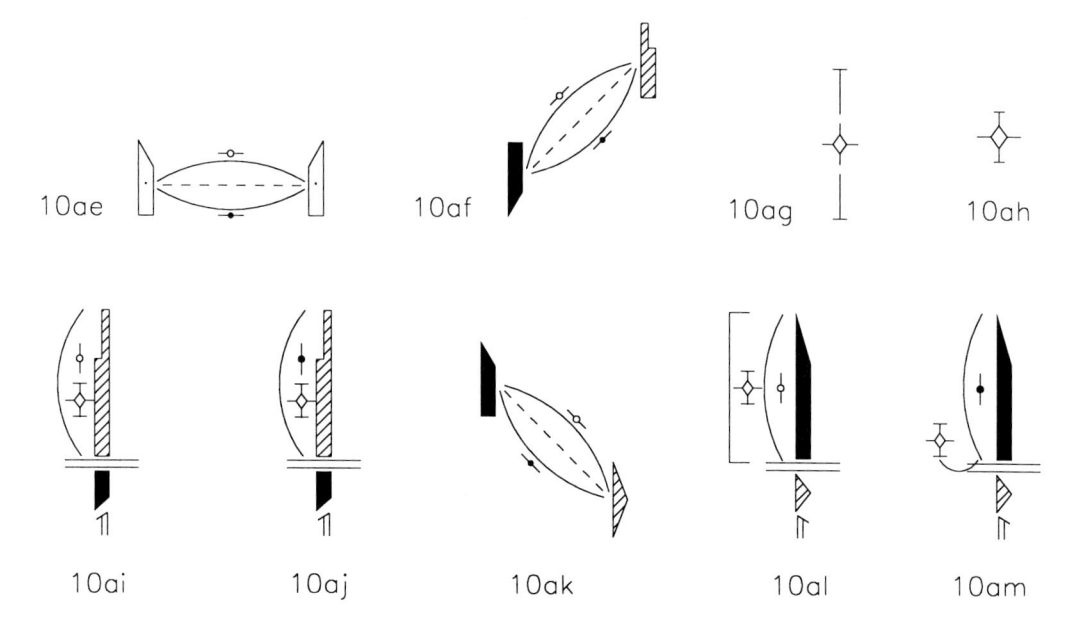

10ae   10af   10ag   10ah

10ai   10aj   10ak   10al   10am

11 Size of Deviation from Path of Gesture

11.1. It is often not important or desirable to pin down an exact size or degree for a deviation, but where the choreographer wishes to be precise or a stylistic detail is not faithfully represented without greater precision, a range in size can be shown. As a general rule no deviation written as such should become large enough to pass through another major direction. Once that sized curve is reached, the *major* direction passed through should be written rather than a deviation. Ex. **11a** shows an average, upward deviation, unspecified in size.

11.2. If desired, the relative size of deviation can be shown. The spatial size (displacement) is shown by placing the appropriate indication in a diamond thus stating clearly that reference is to spatial aspects, **11b**. This size statement is then placed within the curved deviation bow, **11c;** here a large upward deviation is described. (See also Ex. **6r**) If the X were placed by itself with the deviation pin in the bow, **11d**, an action of flexion would be described.

11.3. Ex. **11e** indicates the scale as generally applied to deviations from a gestural path, here illustrated for the upward deviation of **11a**. Ex. **11f** shows the scale in profile, 22.5° being an extra large deviation, shown by the triple wide sign. For these indications the addition of dots to show intermediate degrees is not commonly used. Note that these diagrams are not mathematically precise, they are intended to convey the idea of scale for movements which, in dance, are not usually precise.

11.4. Note that this scale for deviations from the path of gesture is larger than that for displacements from a point (described in Section 22), the reason being that a slight movement away from an established point, such as a tiny up and down displacement, can easily be seen, whereas a comparable displacement from the path of a gesture is barely visible. Hence the difference between the scale which defines the size of deviation from a path and the scale defining the size of displacement from a point. For most purposes size need not be precisely measured, but an indication can be given to convey the intention, the general idea. Here the possibilities, the range, the limits have been explored for the instances where such specific description is needed.

Size of Deviation from Path of Gesture

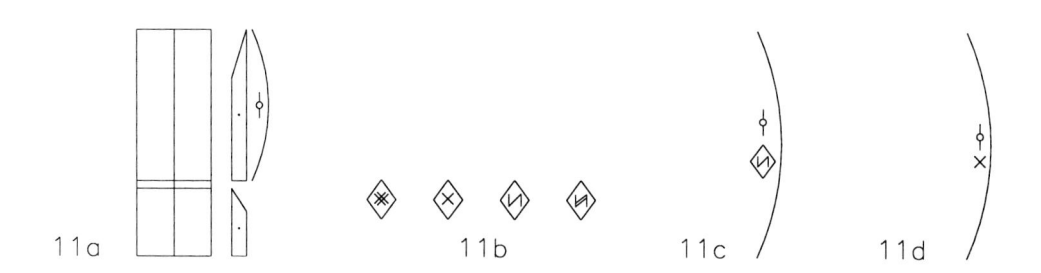

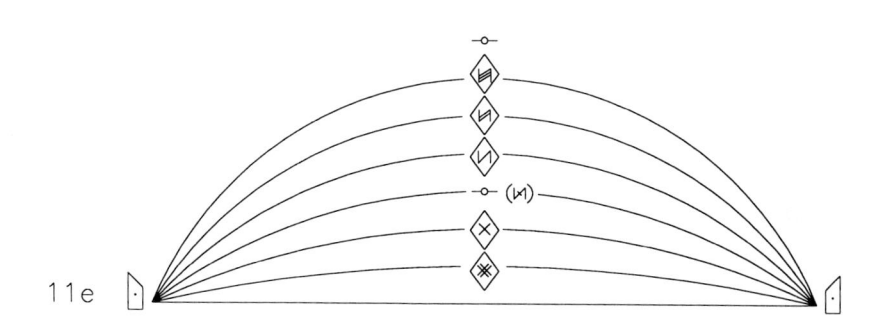

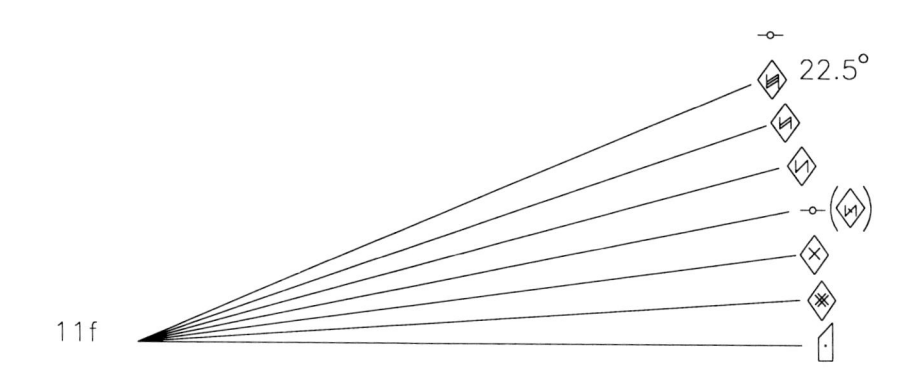

11a

11b

11c

11d

11e

11f   22.5°

IV MODIFICATION OF PATH ACROSS THE FLOOR

12 Veering off Normal Path

12.1. A path stated by the direction of the steps in the support column may deviate slightly toward another direction. In the following exploration we progress from a very slight to a marked modification of a forward path toward the right front diagonal direction. The basic path is written in **12a** and the resulting floor plan in **12b**. The displacement pins in **12c** produce a slightly wide gait but this difference does not affect the basic path of **12b**.

12.2. A minor deviation in the path is produced by the steps of **12d**, illustrated in **12e**, each step being displaced slightly to the right of the normal forward line. The deviated path is shown in **12f** and marked d) in diagram **12g**. A slightly greater deviation would be the result of **12h**, in which each step is a 1/3 way deviation from forward to the right diagonal, illustrated in **12i**. This produces the path of **12j**. This path is marked h) ($^1/_3$) in the diagram of **12g**.

12.3. The next degree in showing the veering from the forward path toward right diagonal, is to place the diagonal direction in a straight path sign alongside the steps to be modified. This produces the halfway deviation of **12k**, illustrated in **12l**. This path is marked k) ($^1/_2$) in the diagram of **12g**.

12.4. The veering away from forward is sometimes thought of as a sideward displacement and written as **12m**. This is not a good description, the movement should be written as a diagonal path, **12n**, illustrated in the floor plan of **12o**. With sideward displacement in mind, a more appropriate description is that of **12p** which states a deviation toward sideward, a description in terms of motion, a digression which is usually experienced and not specifically measured. (For the toward sign, see Section 25.) Another motion description could be that of **12q**, the arrow within the sideward symbol designating that, from where you are, a sideward motion should take place. (For Direction of Progression see Section 24.) No degree of veering is stated for examples **12p** and **12q**.

12.5. Any displacement further to the diagonal than **12k**, should be described as diagonal steps veering toward forward. For such a diagonal path, all the degrees of deviation explored here for the forward path can be applied.

Veering off Normal Path

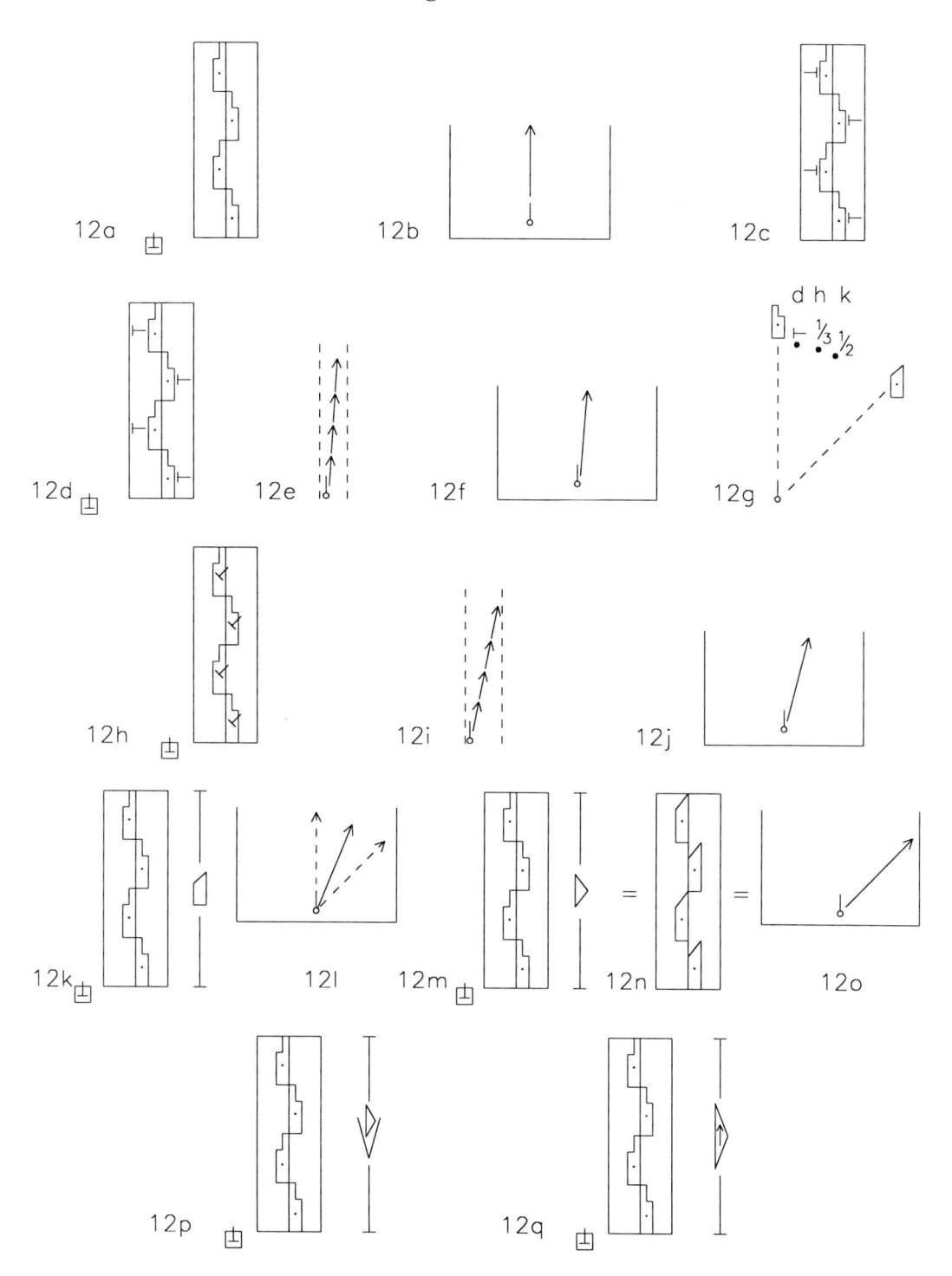

Spatial Variations

12.6. **Distance in Modification of Path.** As with length of step, signs modifying distance for paths are understood to be space measurement signs. The overall path of **12r** should be very short; the number of steps may not be known. Ex. **12s** gives the more precise statement that each step is very small. Here use is made of the Motif sign for steps. Placement can also be in a bracket, as in **12t**.

12.7. Degrees of deviation can be written with space measurement signs as in **12u**, a double narrow sign showing slight displacement; a narrow sign, **12v**, allowing a bit more deviation; and the wide sign of **12w** allowing even more. The small vertical bow linking the two signs here is necessary because, if it were omitted, such space measurement indications could refer to the size of the steps.

12.8. The degree of deviation from the basic path can also be indicated by an intermediate direction. In **12x** the displacement will be one quarter-way toward the right diagonal, that is, half of **12k** (and its floor plan **12l**), because of the double statement of forward. This quarter-way path is illustrated in **12y**

12.9. The aim of the path may be to arrive at a designated stage area, such a statement of arrival is written as in **12z**.

12.10. An area in the room may act as a 'magnet', drawing the performer off the stated path toward that area. In **12aa** it is the downstage right corner of the room (stage). Depending where on stage the performer is located, such movement toward this corner will vary. In **12ab** the performer starts near the upstage right corner, the resulting path will veer only slightly sideward; in **12ac** the performer is more downstage and hence the pull toward the same corner in the room will produce a more sideward displacement. (For the toward sign see Section 25.)

12.11. **Modification of Circular Path.** Modification of a circular path may be in the amount of change of Front (turning) or the shape of the circle. Ex. **12ad** shows the degree to be more or less one full circle. Such an indication may occur in a group dance or when some leeway is allowed and exact change of Front is not important.

12.12. A more common need is to indicate some freedom in the shape of the circle, for this the ad lib. sign is placed at the start of the circling sign, **12ae**. The shape of the full circle may, for example, result in **12af** or in **12ag**. If it is important, reference to the floor plan can be shown with the indication of **12ah** placed next to the staff, the message being "See floor plan."[18]

Advanced Labanotation

Distance in Modification of Path

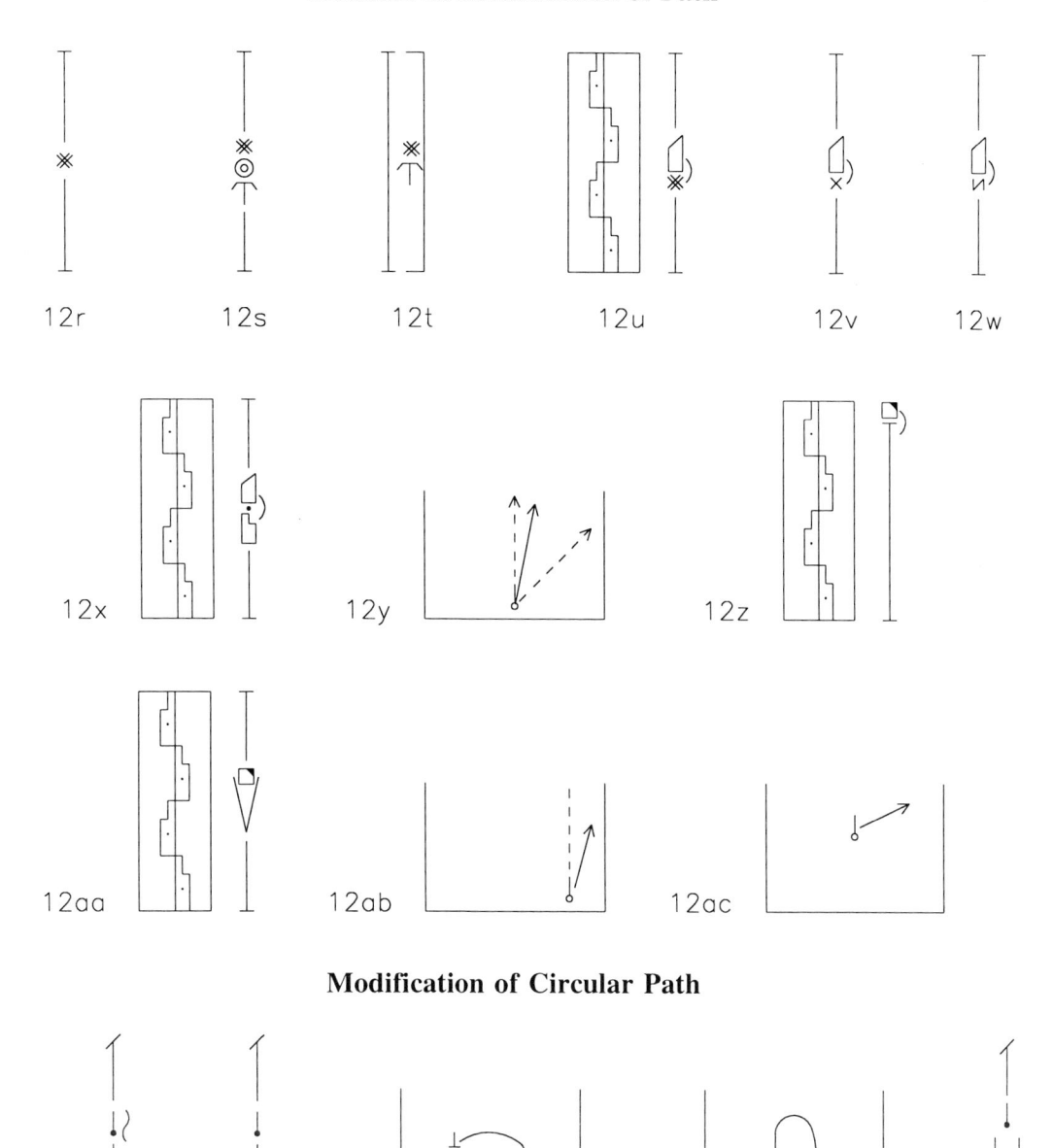

12r   12s   12t   12u   12v   12w

12x   12y   12z

12aa   12ab   12ac

Modification of Circular Path

12ad   12ae   12af   12ag   12ah

13 Detour to Avoid a Person or Object

13.1. As we know from walking down a crowded street, only a slight deviation from a straight path is needed to avoid a person or obstacle. It may be enough to state on which side one passes as in **13a**, where the partner (or other person, indicated by P) is on the performer's right when passing.

13.2. If a slight swerve is needed or is choreographically important, it can be indicated as a deviation written in a path sign. In **13b** the steps are forward and the deviation to avoid someone or something is to the performer's left, illustrated in **13c**. In **13d** the steps are sideward and the deviation is forward, therefore you will pass in front of the person or obstacle, as shown in **13e**.

13.3. **Timing of Detour.** The timing of the deviation can be indicated by the length of the bow. In **13f** there is a more gradual veering off course and return to course.

13.4. When passing a partner, there is often no change of Front, though a slight body twist may occur as in **13g**, where the chest twists slightly left, then returns to normal. In some folk dances the body turn is often toward the person being passed, a more gracious version, shown in **13h**.

13.5. The deviations of **13f** and **13g** can also be written by adding a deviation bow to the path sign, as in **13i** and **13j** respectively. The length of the bow indicates the timing, the duration of the deviation. The performers must coordinate spatially in order to pass at the appropriate moment.

13.6. The previous examples state when the deviation occurs but not the location, this can be shown on a floor plan, as in **13k**.

Advanced Labanotation

Detour to Avoid a Person or Object

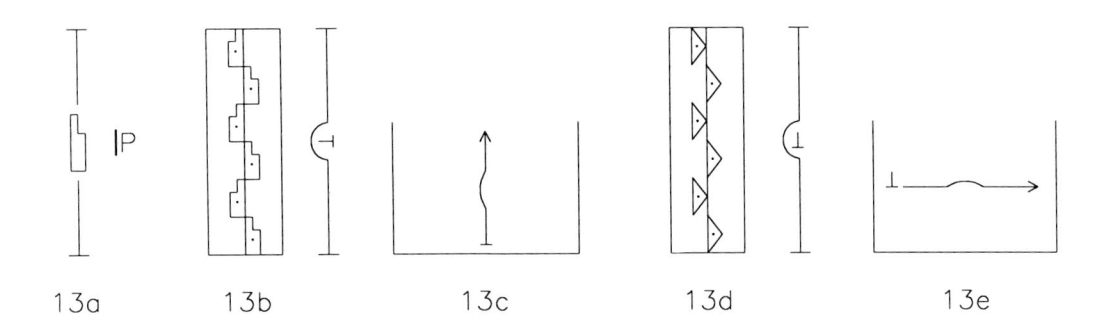

13a   13b   13c   13d   13e

Timing of Detour

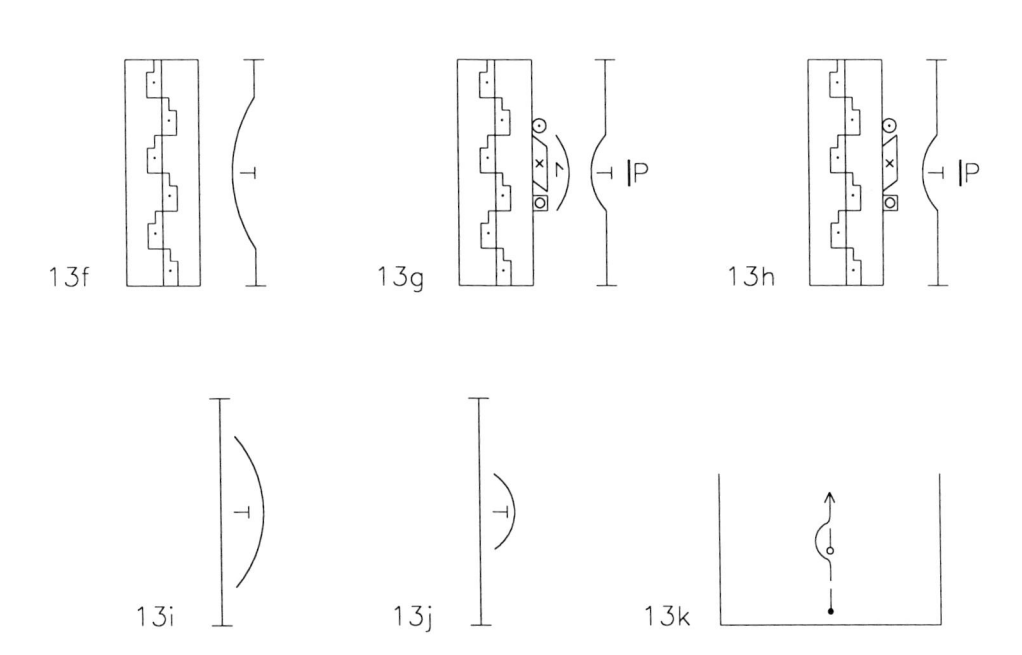

13f   13g   13h

13i   13j   13k

14 Displacement for Step Patterns in Place - Choice of Description

14.1. Many dances employ a repeated step pattern which often is performed without traveling, it stays 'on the spot'. The step may have a very slight to and fro movement, but basically the performer does not move through the room. However, in many instances, specific traveling may take place. Such traveling may be described in three ways: a) direction judged from the Standard Directions, b) from the Constant Directions, or c) as moving toward a particular part of the stage. Notice the differences between the following examples.

14.2. In **14a** the gradual traveling is sideward; each dancer will travel to his or her right side. Because in the floor plan here they are all facing different directions, the paths will be into different directions, as illustrated in **14b**. In **14c** the direction traveled is given in terms of the Constant Directions Key, thus the group in a circle will gradually move toward the Constant Right direction. No matter where the dancers are facing, they will travel on parallel paths, **14d**.

14.3. **Toward, Away From an Area.** In **14e** the instruction is to travel toward the stage right center area, thus each path of the dancers spread around the stage will start to converge toward that focal area, **14f**, but the area will not be reached.[19] (For area signs see Section 44.)

14.4. A group can also move away from a particular stage area. In **14g** the four performers, each of whom is facing a different direction, gradually travel away from the downstage center area, their paths being illustrated in **14h**.

14.5. **Reaching a Destination.** Such gradual traveling can also be shown to have the aim of arriving at a particular destination. In **14i** the circle of performers, who start in the upstage left stage area, end in the downstage right area, illustrated in **14j**. Arriving center stage is stated for **14k**, each dancer adjusting the step direction to produce that result, illustrated in **14l**. Note use in these floor plans of the wedges (the open wedge for a female, the black one for a male) to indicate ending location and resulting direction faced.

Advanced Labanotation

Displacement for Step Patterns in Place

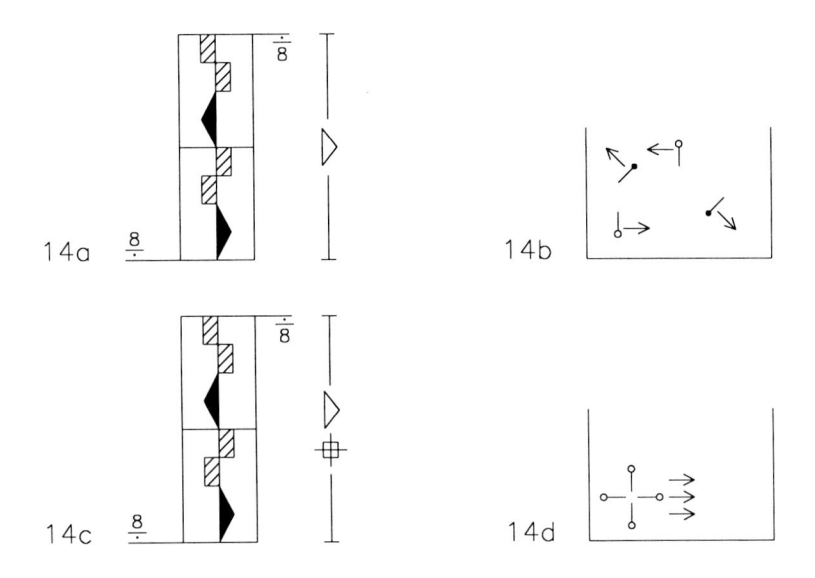

14a 14b

14c 14d

Toward, Away From an Area

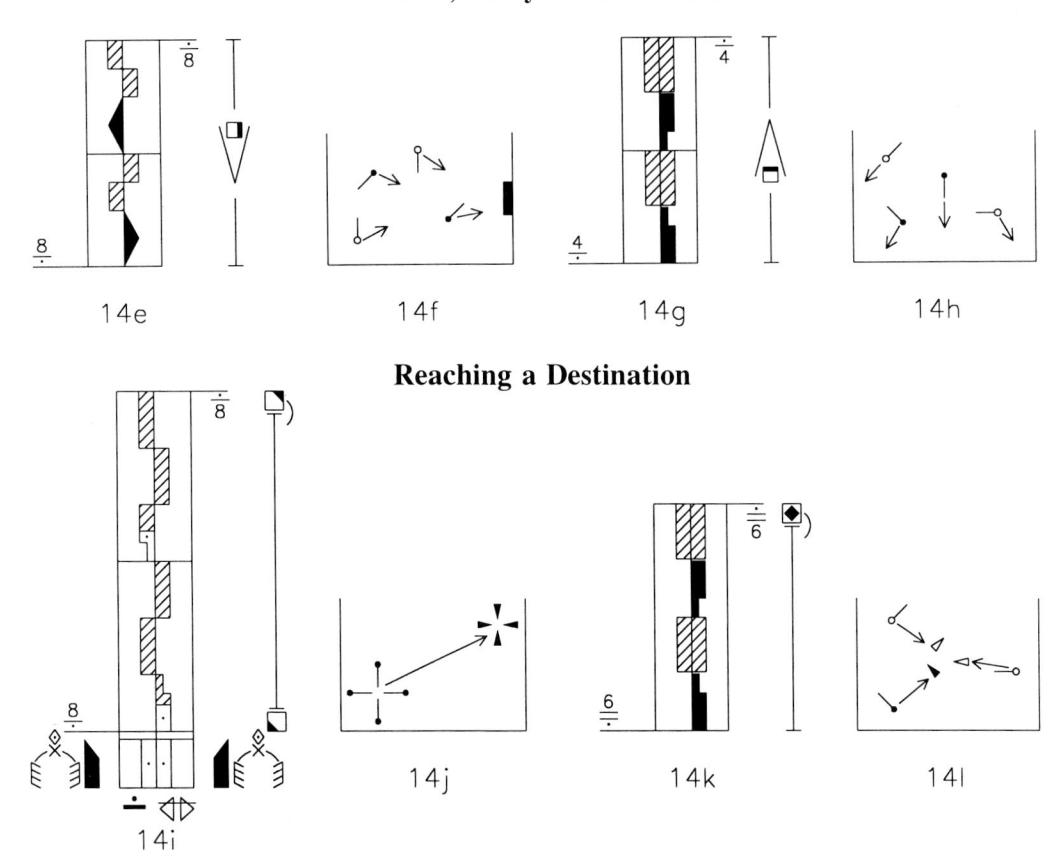

14e 14f 14g 14h

Reaching a Destination

14i 14j 14k 14l

15 Displacement Paths Combined with Turning or Circling

15.1. The examples **14a-14l** can also occur while turning or gradually moving on a circular path. Again the choices of key, Standard, Constant, or toward an area (focal point), produce different results.

15.2. **Displacement Paths Combined with Turning.** The lilting step of **15a** does not travel, there is only gradual turning. Ex. **15b**, illustrated in the floor plan of **15c**, shows revolving on a straight path, the direction of travel being taken from the dancer's Front at the start. For each person the path is different, as shown in **15c**.

15.3. Ex. **15d** also gives revolving on a straight path, but here the path is side right according to the Constant Key, thus all paths are parallel, as shown in **15e**. However, each dancer ends facing in his/her own direction.

15.4. **Displacement Paths Combined with Circling.** Ex. **15f** shows displacements on a circular path.[20] The to-and-fro motif gradually moves on a $1/4$ counterclockwise circular path. To achieve this the steps to the right will be slightly larger, those to the left slightly smaller, the overall result being shown in the plan of **15g**.

15.5. Ex. **15h** describes a circle of people revolving counterclockwise while traveling as a group into the Constant right back diagonal direction, the circle traveling two step lengths (see 38.1), illustrated in **15i**.[21] Each person in **15j** travels to the right on a $1/4$ counterclockwise circular path, as illustrated in **15k**.

Advanced Labanotation

Displacement Paths Combined with Turning

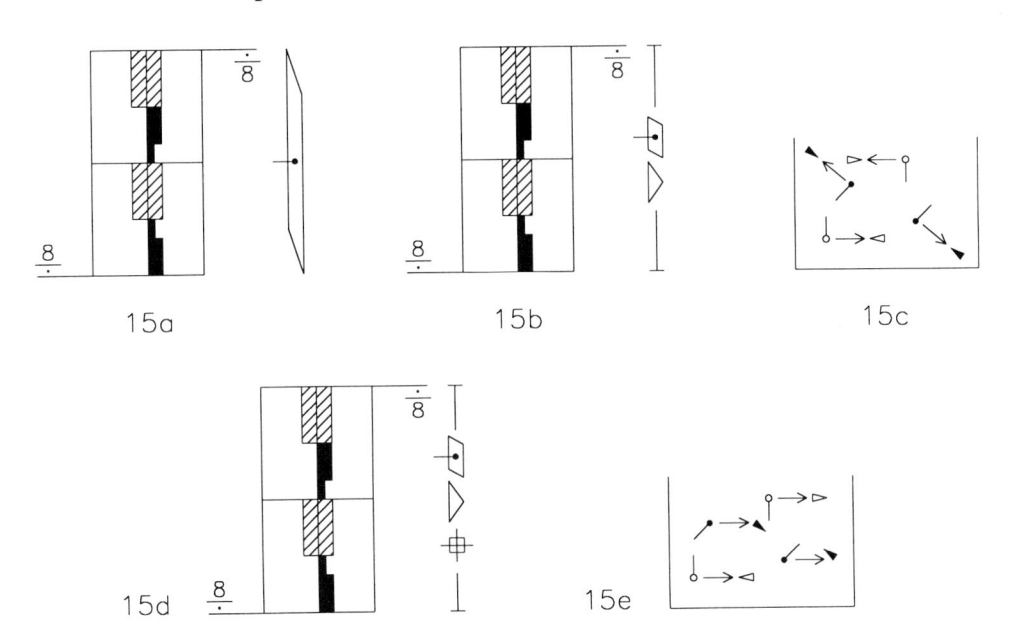

15a

15b

15c

15d

15e

Displacement Paths Combined with Circling

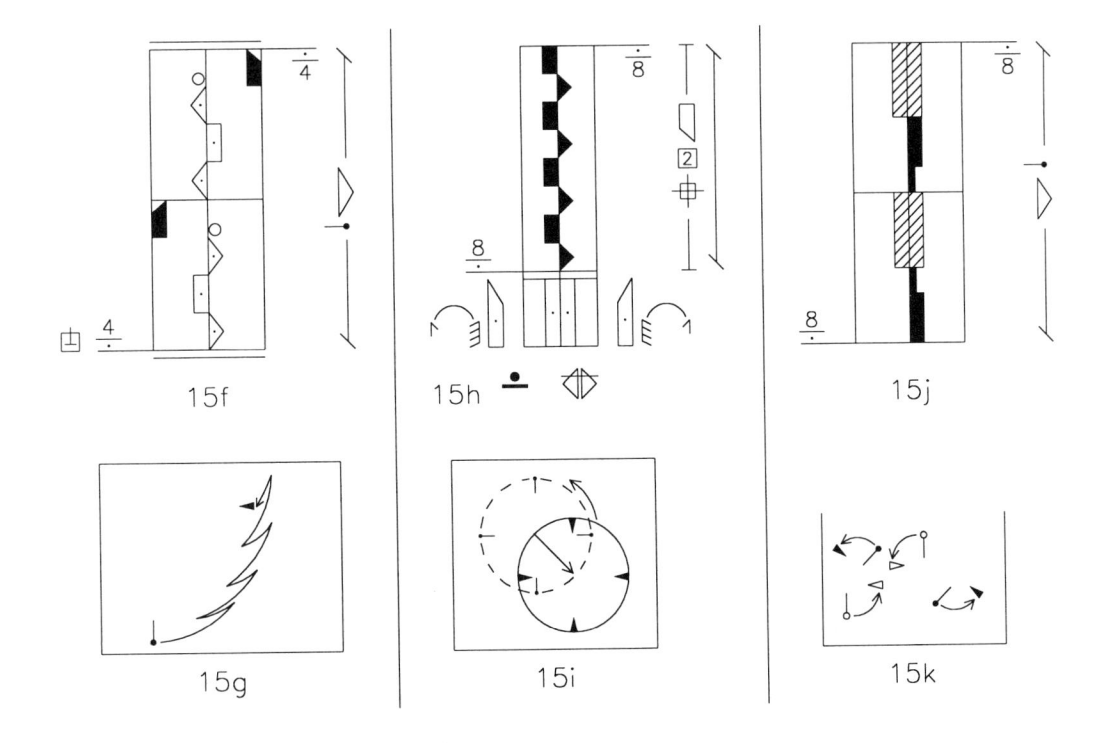

15f

15g

15h

15i

15j

15k

15.6. In **15l** a circular path is to be achieved, and yet the traveling as a whole is to be into the same Constant direction. To achieve this, a quarter circle arc is stepped ending toward Stage Right in relation to where each dancer started, **15m**. If a ½ circle were written, the arc would be larger (for direction in a circular path according to Constant Directions see 15.8-10).

15.7. For **15l** one must imagine the ¼ circle as in **15n**, and then place the ending wedge directly to Constant Right of the starting position as in **15o**, thus showing the aim. The ¼ circle arc must then be moved (here toward upstage), so that the ending position is spatially correct and one has also achieved the ¼ circle arc, **15p**.

15.8. When reference for travel is to a Constant Direction, as in **15l**, directions change in relation to the dancer as s/he turns. Because such a direction cannot produce a circular path, the direction becomes the aim of the circular path, therefore the circling must deviate ('bulge') away from this line, as in **15m**. The larger the degree of circling, the larger the deviation. These same facts apply to traveling described in relation to a part of the room.

15.9. Traveling while circling may have the aim of moving toward a part of the room or stage. The waltz-like steps of **15q** should perform ¼ circle counterclockwise and at the same time approach the center front area. In the floor plan diagram of **15r** the aim for each individual is shown here by the dotted line for explanatory purposes. A ¼ circle path must be performed ending at this destination. A comparable example, **15s**, shows four performers moving away from the center front area, again on a ¼ counterclockwise circle, illustrated in **15t**.[22]

15.10. In **15u**, illustrated in **15v**, a half circle is accomplished. The performer starts near the upstage center area and ends near the downstage center area. Again the dotted line on the floor plan indicates the aim of the ½ circle. In this way any circling which needs to have the direction of traveling indicated through Constant Directions or Room Area indications can be plotted, the dancer can determine how the circle will lie in relation to the aim.

Displacement Paths Combined with Circling

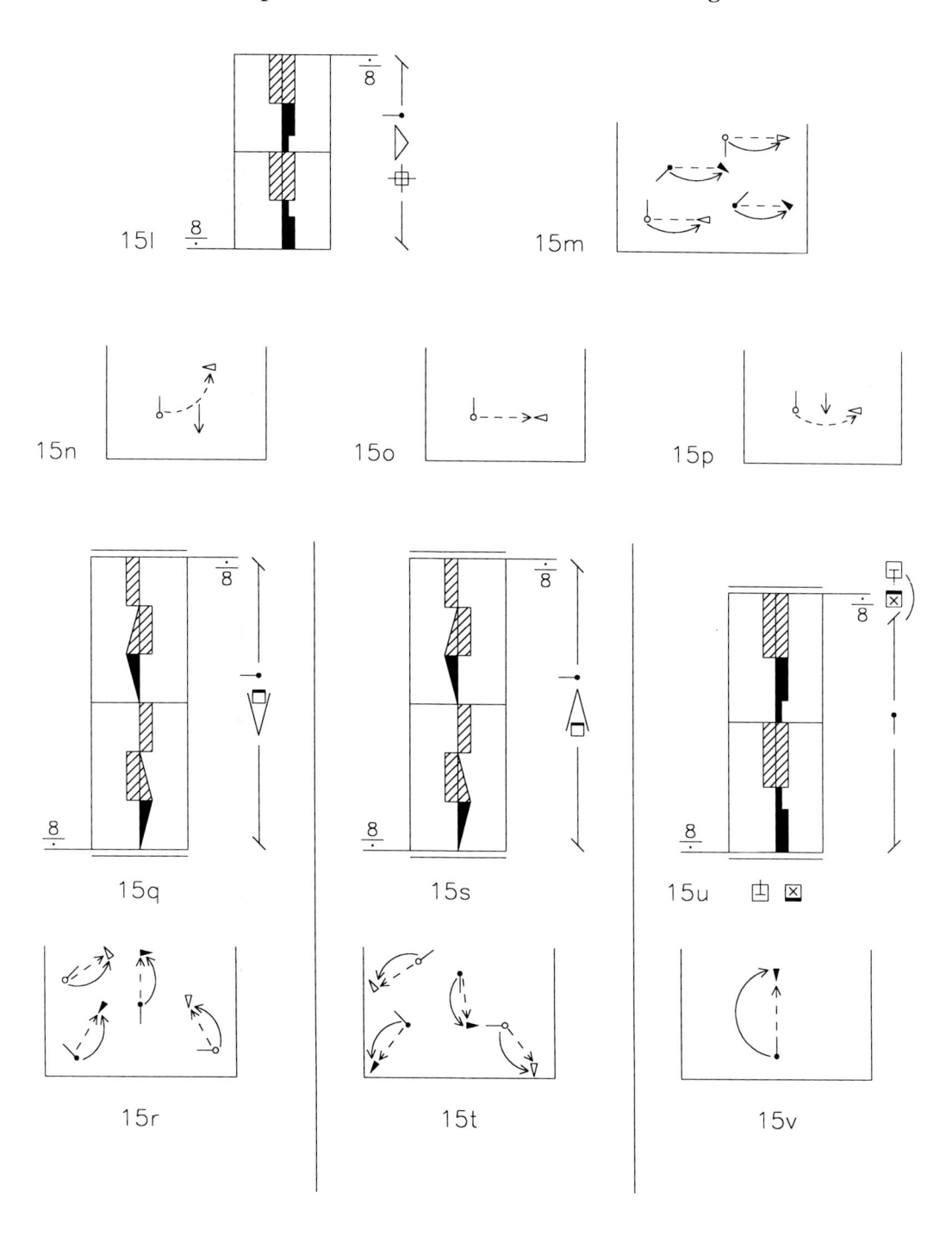

15l 15m

15n 15o 15p

15q 15s 15u

15r 15t 15v

V MINOR MOVEMENTS

16 Displacements from a Point

16.1. Minor movements away from an established point are often to and fro movements which may be frequently repeated, as when waving the hand; they may also be small circular movements. Displacements may be of shoulders, head, or other part of the body. Here they are explored for the arm; the original and more commonly used description for such displacements will be given first. Minor movements may also be described from Polar Analysis, using Polar Pins (see Section 23).

16.2. **The Distal Center.** For displacements from a standard directional point, the description of the movement (direction and level) refers to that point at which the extremity of the limb is situated, the Distal Center.[23] At this Distal Center there is a cross of axes comparable to the central cross of axes in the body, using the same Standard System of Reference, unless another system of reference is indicated. It can be compared to the main kinesphere of the body, each distal center having its own small kinesphere. It thus includes all the possible directions for displacement around that center.

16.3. **Distal Analysis**. The drawings of **16a** and **16b** illustrate the globe of directions around the extremity of the arm, shown here in two locations. This center serves for minor displacements of the whole arm moving in one piece, the lower arm, the hand, the fingers. The Distal Center located at the right elbow, **16c**, is the center for upper arm movements (designated by the elbow), when the arm is bent. The center at the wrist serves for minor lower arm movements when the wrist is bent, **16d**. Each finger has its own Distal Center, **16e**.

16.4. **Distal Displacements**. Such minor movements are indicated with pins which state the direction and level of the displacement. The following are commonly met examples, each easily understood. In **16f** the arms make slight downward and upward movements repeatedly, illustrated in **16g**. The minor displacements of the extremity in **16h**, shown in **16i**, are forward and backward. With the arms forward in **16j**, the hands make small sideward movements, illustrated in **16k**. In these examples the displacements are at right angles to the shaft of the limb, thus no key is needed to understand the notation. The performer is aware of the displacement of the extremity of the arms. With the whole arm moving one is aware of the finger tips moving above or below, forward or backward, etc., of the established point, the distal point at the extremity of the arm.

Advanced Labanotation

Distal Analysis

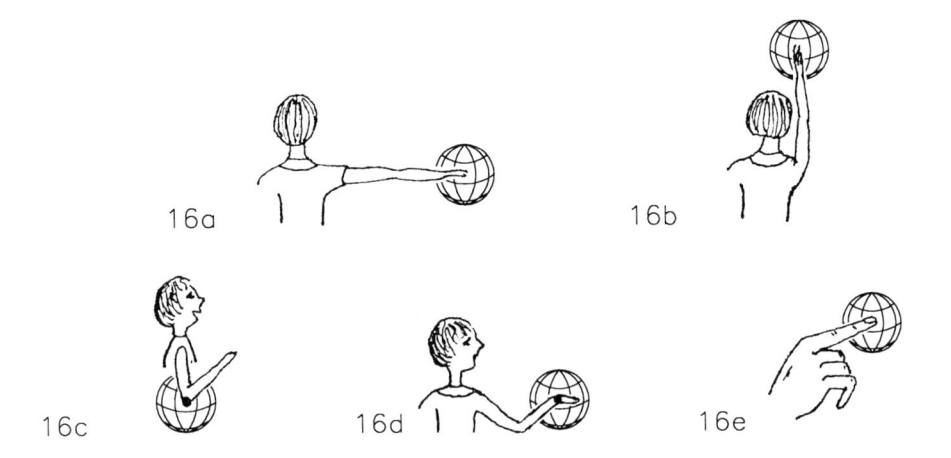

16a

16b

16c

16d

16e

Distal Displacements

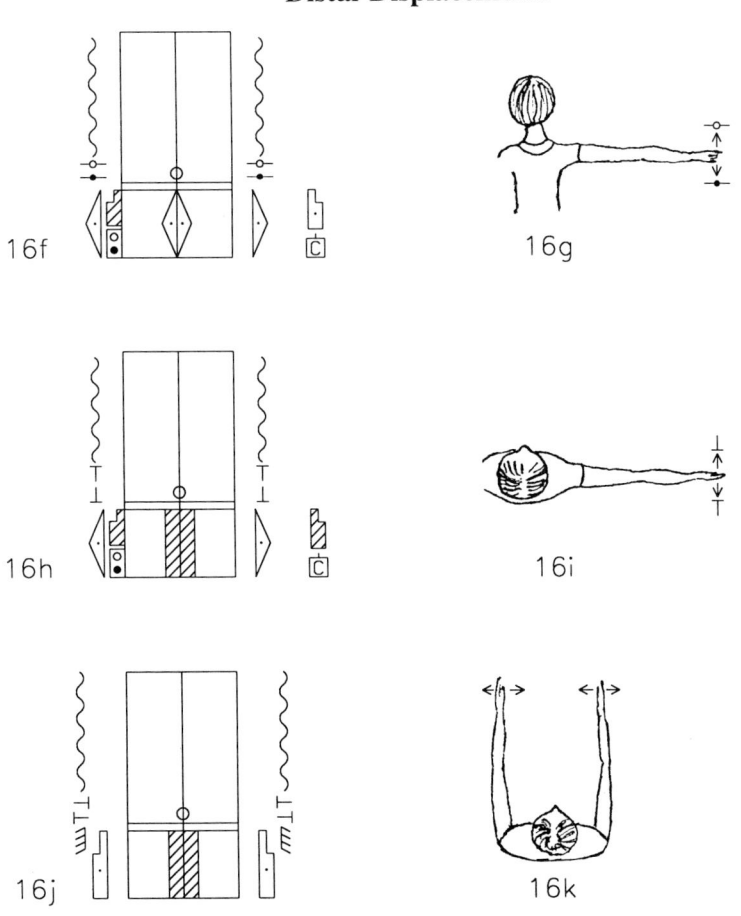

16f

16g

16h

16i

16j

16k

16.5. The Proximal Center. The following examples illustrate the alternate analysis which focuses on the proximal joint (the fixed end) of the moving limb, that is, describing the displacement as judged from the proximal joint: the shoulder for the whole arm, the wrist for the hand. (See Section 2.)

16.6. Proximal Analysis. The small to and fro (side to side) head movements of **16l** are very small inclinations (tilts). Because these movements are experienced as minor tilts, the Proximal Analysis is commonly used.[24] It has been observed that Distal Analysis, i.e. the displacement of the top of the head, **16m**, is not how the performer tends to think of or experience this head movement. A similar experience occurs with **16n**, very small head nods which are mentally linked to minor head tilts, movements from the base of the neck, rather than description of the minor displacements of the top of the head, **16o**.

16.7. Distal Center Key. Although Distal Center Analysis was that originally established and has been the most commonly used description, Proximal Center Analysis officially became the standard.[25] As a result Distal Analysis requires a key, **16p**, based on the Standard System of Reference, indicating a cross of axes beyond the base. When the key is not used, all distal center pins must have a small stroke added to indicate that this key is being used, as in **16m** and **16o**.[26]

16.8. Comparison between Distal and Proximal Analyses. In the following examples the same movement is written first with Distal Analysis, then with Proximal Analysis. With the right arm sideward, palm facing down, the hand makes a small down and up movement, **16q**. The fact that this movement has been described verbally as down and up makes clear its analysis. Nevertheless, a small stroke has been added to the pin indicating that the movement is judged from the cross of axes at the Distal Center. In **16r** the description of the same movement is from Proximal Center. Similarly in **16s** the hand moves slightly forward, then backward (Distal Analysis), the same being shown in **16t** from Proximal Analysis, the movement being toward the diagonal middle directions. With the arm up in **16u** the extremity moves slightly from side to side, written here with Distal reference; the Proximal description, **16v**, shows movement toward the two side high directions.

16.9. An interesting variation shows small three-dimensional displacements. With the right arm diagonal middle, **16w**, the extremity moves at a right angle to this direction; in Distal terms to high left forward diagonal and low right backward diagonal; in Proximal terms, **16x**, it is toward forward high and then side low. It is up to the individual to choose which description is easier to understand and quicker to read.

Advanced Labanotation

Proximal Analysis

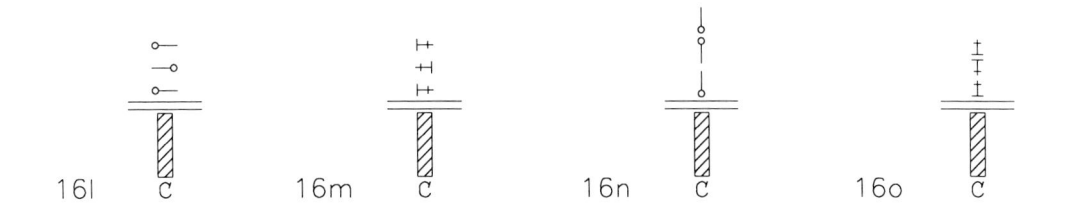

16l 16m 16n 16o

Distal Center Key

16p

Comparison between Distal and Proximal Analyses

Distal	Proximal	Distal	Proximal
16q	16r	16s	16t
16u	16v	16w	16x

16.10. **Distal Analysis.** Two slightly different elbow displacements are now given, actions that occur in jazz as well as in the dance of certain cultures such as African and Caribbean. With the arms sagittaly up in **16y**, the elbows displace sideward (outward), the accent being on the outward movement. With the arms in a similar lateral placement, **16z**, the elbows have an accent forward. Note that Distal Analysis is used in both these examples, the tick being placed on the pin shaft in **16y** while in **16z** the key is placed in a bracket next to the notation. This key can be stated at the start of a score to show that all such minor movements will automatically be interpreted as distal and thus eliminating the need for a small stroke across each pin.

16.11. **Use of Specific Directional Keys.** Minor movements can be shown to relate to the Body Key, as in **16aa**. Here the torso is tilted and the arms are described as sideward from the Body System of Reference. The directions for the minor up and down displacements are understood to relate also to this key. By stating the Body Key more explicitly for the arms, as in **16ab**, there is no doubt about the interpretation of the minor displacements which follow. Whatever the key for the arms, it is understood that palm facings and other hand indications will refer to the same key unless otherwise stated.

16.12. The Stance Key is used in **16ac**. The performer basically faces Front, but with the chest twisted, the forward-backward directions for the arms relate to the stance front, as do the accented sideward hand displacements.

16.13. Starting in 2nd position in **16ad**, with the chest twisted to the left, the sequence which follows is read from the Constant Cross. The performer then tilts the chest backward high (physically sideward left) while the arms 'extend' forward to the audience, the right high, the left middle level. The arms then have a small sideward separating movement.

16.14. **Cancellation of Minor Displacements.** A minor displacement will remain in the stated situation unless it is cancelled. In **16ae**, at the end of the three sideward proximal displacements, the extremity ends toward left side high. The general cancellation sign (inverted V) is used in **16af** to cancel the last displacement. Use of the 'center' pin for the proximal description to bring it back to the stated direction is shown in **16ag**. The distal displacements of **16ah**, comparable to **16ad**, can be cancelled by the general cancellation sign, **16ai**, or a return to center, **16aj**.

Advanced Labanotation

Distal Analysis

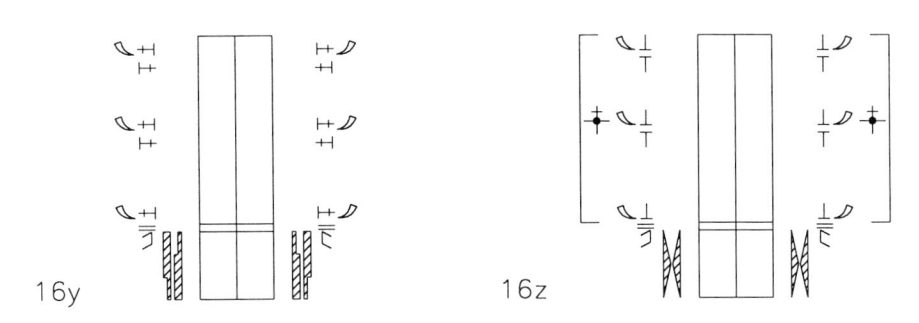

16y   16z

Use of Specific Directional Keys

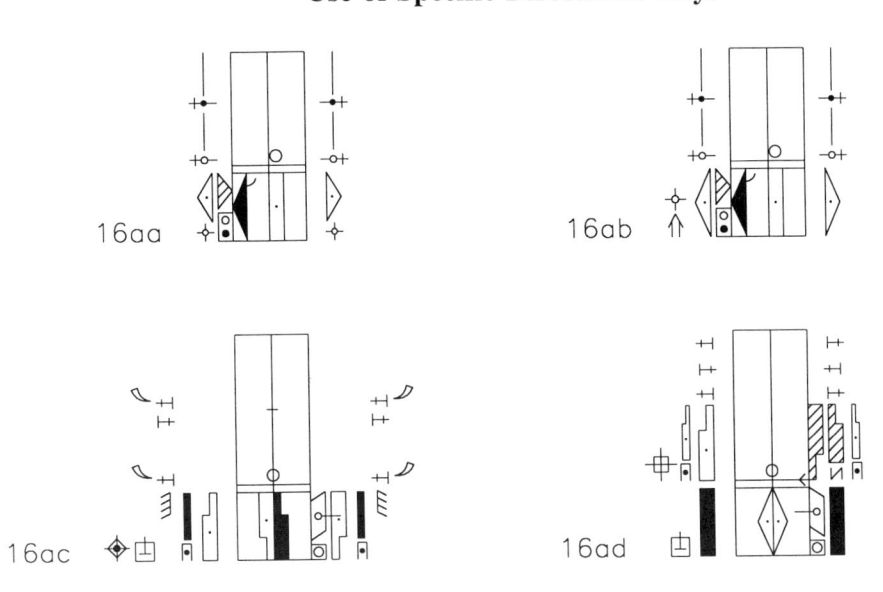

16aa   16ab

16ac   16ad

Cancellation of Minor Displacements

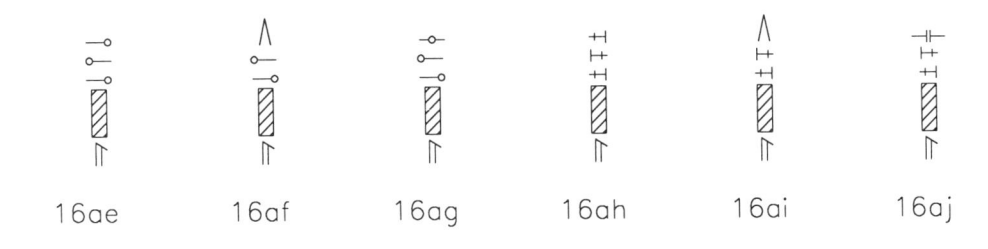

16ae   16af   16ag   16ah   16ai   16aj

Spatial Variations

16.15. **Direction of Relationship.** Pins are used with relationship signs to indicate the direction from which a relationship - near, contact, grasping, etc. - comes. (See Advanced Labanotation Handling of Objects, Props.) The following is introduced here to clarify a point which is not always readily understood. In **16ak** the arm starts forward middle, from there it makes a small displacement upward, above where it was. The arm starts in the same place in **16al**, the hand then touches a post, the relationship being that the hand is above the post when contact occurs. To achieve this relationship, the arm has to move *slightly down*. One is not necessarily aware of this fact, but it takes place. The pin states the direction *from which the contact came*.

16.16. The next example follows this same comparison but moves to another direction. The arm is again forward in **16am** and the first action is to move slightly to the right. With the same starting placement in **16an**, the hand contacts the post from the right. This means a small movement from the right toward the left, must have occured for the contact to take place.

16.17. **Size of Distal and Proximal Displacements.** While exactness in size of displacement may be hard to achieve physically, a guideline is needed. The third-way intermediate point of **16ao** is 15° above side middle. For the next three examples which start at the side middle point, the distance of displacement is 7.5°. For the movement to side middle in **16ap**, distal analysis is used for the slight rise; **16aq** is the same but using the proximal analysis. Ex. **16ar** is identical to **16aq** but performed as one movement, so that the arrival is at the same point as the finish of **16ap** and **16aq**.

16.18. The signs for spatially smaller, **16as**, spatially much smaller, **16at**, spatially larger, **16au**, and spatially much larger, **16av**, may be added in a bracket to give a range of variation in size which is sensed, intended, but not measured.

16.19. Displacement from a point, particularly when repeated in a to-and-fro pattern, can be quite small and yet quite visible. In contrast, a deviation from the path of a gesture, as described in 11.4, must be comparatively larger to be clearly visible. Thus **16aw** and **11a** (repeated here as **16ax**) are not normally comparable in size.

16.20. **Types of Movement.** *Peripheral displacements* occur within a small circle of which the shaft of the limb is the axis. These movements require only a small movement in the proximal joint. *'Spoke-like' displacements*, from center to periphery or vice versa, require the limb to flex slightly or extend along the line established by the shaft of the limb (its longitudinal axis).[27]

Advanced Labanotation

Direction of Relationship

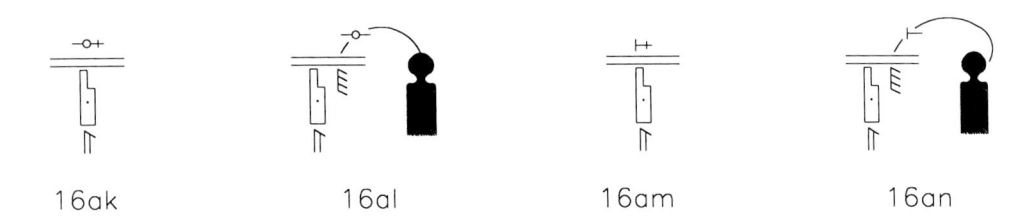

16ak   16al   16am   16an

Size of Distal and Proximal Displacements

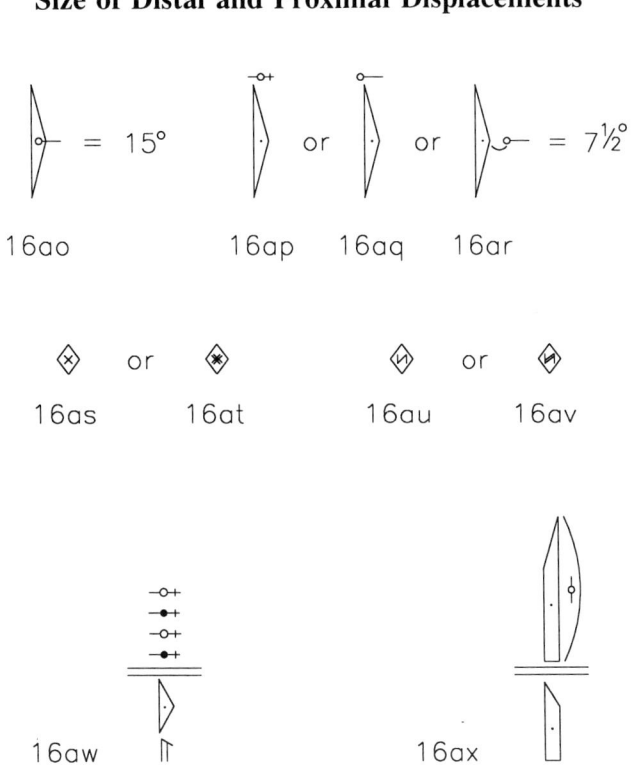

16ao   = 15°   16ap or 16aq or 16ar   = 7½°

16as or 16at   16au or 16av

16aw   16ax

17 Vibrating Actions

17.1. The minor displacements explored so far often occur rapidly as in vibrating movements, comparable to *tremolo* sounds in music. Two pins suffice to indicate the direction of the vibrations, these are followed by a wavy line with small curves, **17a**. In this example the hand vibrates down and up continuously. The hand vibrates sideways on a level with the top of the head, **17b**. In **17c** the hand starts near the heart (note the double in-between pin showing the left side of the front of the chest) and vibrates backward and forward, fluttering as though expressing intense love.

17.2. The palm is near the cheek in **17d**, the minor movement causes it to touch the cheek and then move away; this action like a butterfly's wing close to the face, is repeated rapidly, no specific number of times. This action could also be described as a contact followed by a release occuring rapidly, as in **17e**, the spatial event is similar but the manner of performance is subtlely changed.

17.3. Standing in a small 2nd position, knees bent, **17f** shows the knees to be 'knocking', trembling, as if in fright. Instead of the small ticks on the pins (strictly required or Distal description), the Distal Center Key is shown alongside in an addition bracket. An expressive repeated gesture saying "No, no!" is given in **17g**. With the palms forward, the hands rapidly move outward and then inward as though wiping the thought away.

17.4. The vibrating pattern of **17h** shows a horizontal forward-backward displacement. If the torso is off the vertical, as in **17i**, the same physical forward-backward hand displacement now needs pins for forward high-backward low. Easier to read is **17j** in which the Body Key is stated next to the pins.

17.5. While we are aware of the hands being slightly displaced in these examples, it is the wrist articulation which makes the hand movements possible. In **17g** it is very slight lateral wrist flexion which takes place. If the lower arm is to vibrate, the articulation occurs in the elbow, with possible passivity in the upper arm. It is not the joint action which is written, but rather the spatial patterns of the part being featured.

17.6. **Cancellation of Vibrations**. With such swift repetitions no final displacement situation is stated, the movement is understood to peter out, i.e. return to the original situation. In **17k**, however, an ending state is given.

Vibrating Actions

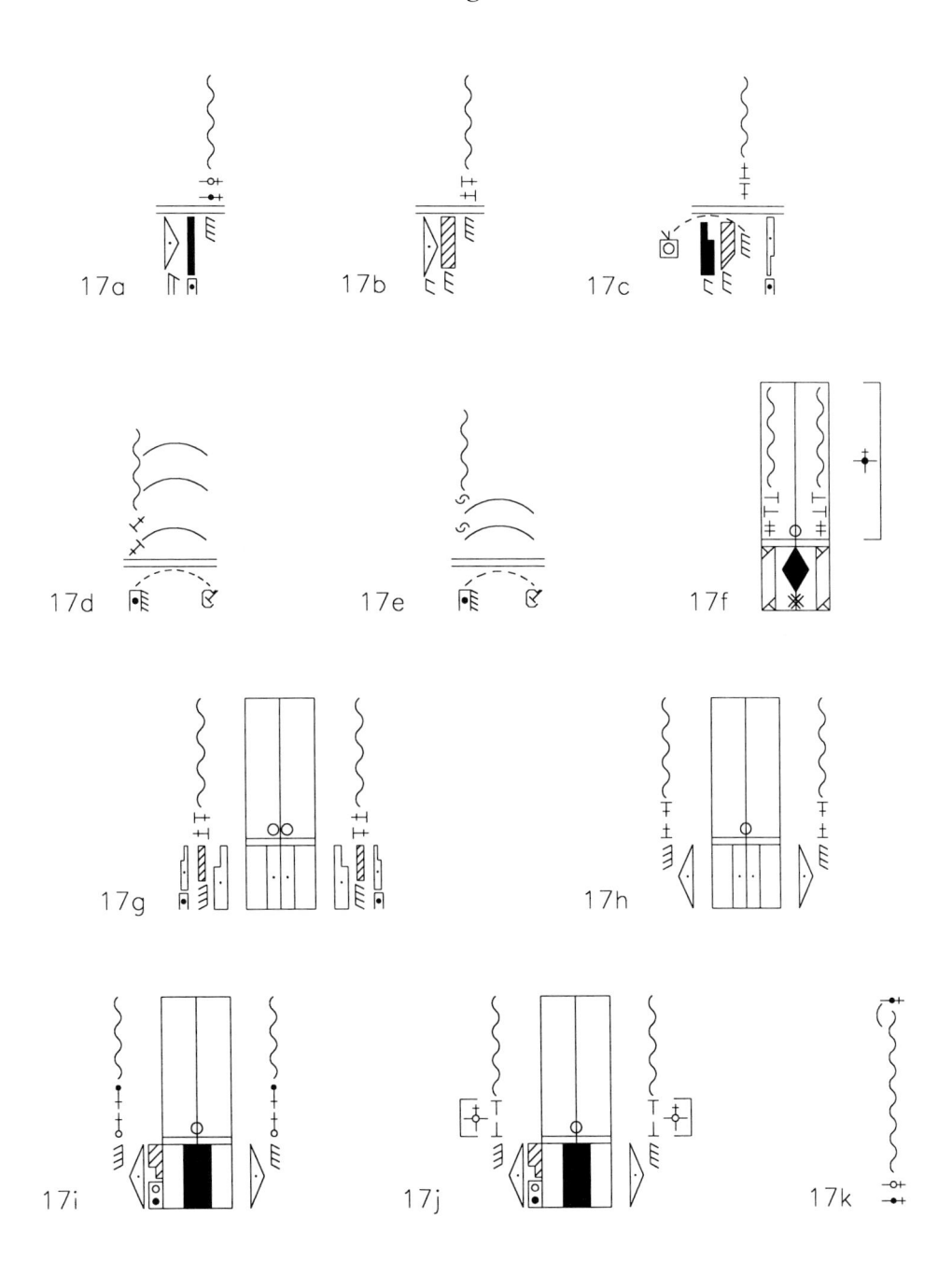

17a

17b

17c

17d

17e

17f

17g

17h

17i

17j

17k

18 Minor Circling Movements

18.1. A small circular movement can be written with a series of pins. The directions for these pins are judged, as usual, from the performer's Standard Key unless a Constant or Body Key is indicated. Often such circular movements are fairly quick. Ex. **18a** shows a starting position with the right leg bent, the toe touching the floor. From this position the extremity, the toe, makes a quick circular pattern sliding the toe on the floor. The circle starts by deviating backward and ends again at the side. In this case the floor controls the displacements, resulting in a Distal Center description. In this case the Distal key need not be stated. In **18b** this same circular pattern is performed more slowly and a vertical phrasing bow is used to indicate the unity of the action. This bow is not a passing state bow because there is no main movement from the path of which a deviation needs to take place. The timing for each displacement can, of course, be shown as in **18c**, a duration line following each pin. This usage does not provide the same sense of phrasing.

18.2. The lower leg (the extremity) makes a small circle in **18d**. This circle is comparable in miniature to the larger lower leg circle of **18e**, it is therefore judged from the proximal point. The circular movement for the right index finger in **18f**, identified as distal displacements, is specifically shown to end up. Ex. **18g** shows the same movement written with proximal pins. It can be seen from these two examples that the pins themselves reveal whether a distal or proximal reference is being used. The hand circle of **18h** ends forward.

18.3. **Intermediate Placements of Limb.** When a limb is in an intermediate direction, as in the next two examples, the question arises as to exactly which pins to use. How precise do the pins need to be? In **18i** the series of pins spells out a circle, the lower leg executing a small circle of this kind. Another example is **18j**, again a small lower leg circle.[28] Note that Polar Pins, discussed in Section 23, do not pose a problem when applied to intermediate direction placements.

Advanced Labanotation

Minor Circling Movements

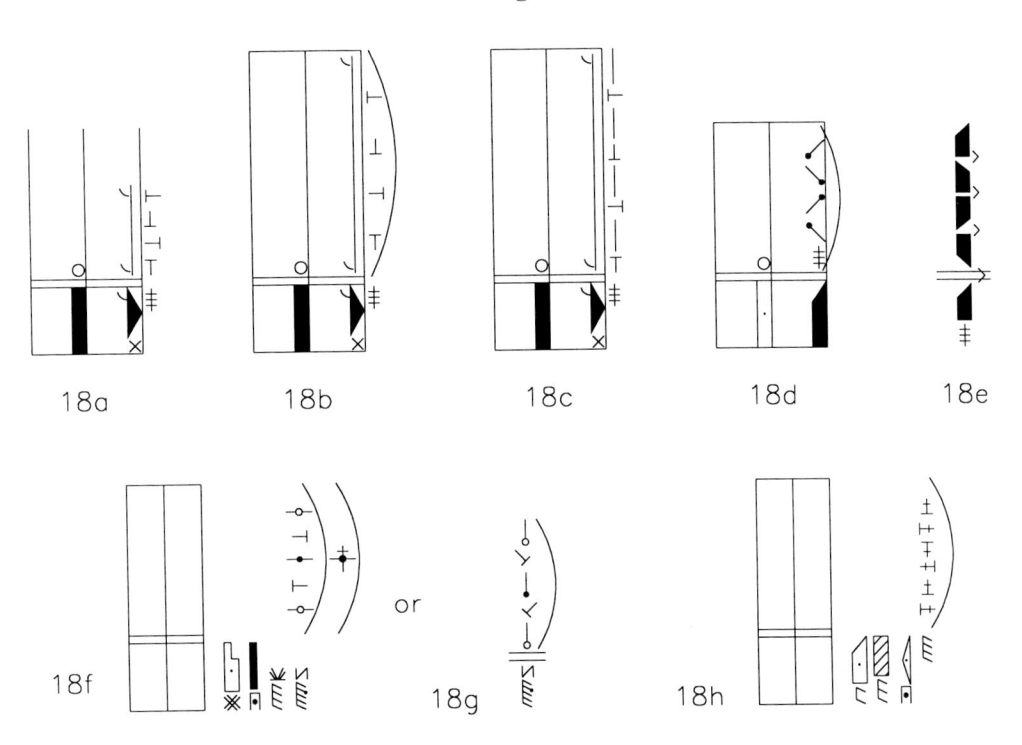

18a 18b 18c 18d 18e

18f 18g 18h

Intermediate Placements of Limb

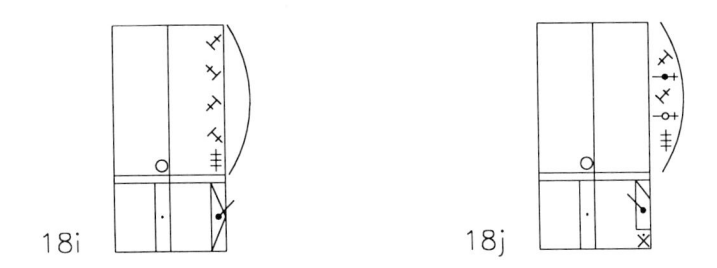

18i 18j

18.4. **Size of Transitional Arm Deviations.** In the arm pattern of **18k**, the arms 'swing' from one side to the other, the right arm following an unemphasized circular path to end crossed behind the back. The notation in this example gives the directions through which the arms should pass. These transitional directions are modified by the signs of **18l** meaning lack of emphasis, an unemphasized performance. This modification may well result in less than fully articulated directional movements.

18.5. By using pins instead of direction symbols in **18m**, the spatial size of the transition is diminished. The size can be augmented by adding the spatially larger sign, as in **18n**, it remains, however, smaller than **18k**.

18.6. The device of placing small direction symbols but with no level in the vertical deviation bow, as in **18o**, provides a greater awareness of the directions without fully using them, as was the case in **18k**. In **18o** there is a result lesser than **18k**. Not given here is any indication of a swinging quality for the movements.

Size of Transitional Arm Deviations

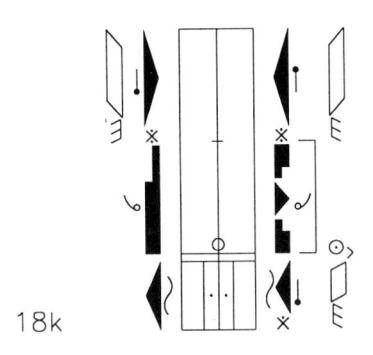

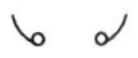

18k

18l

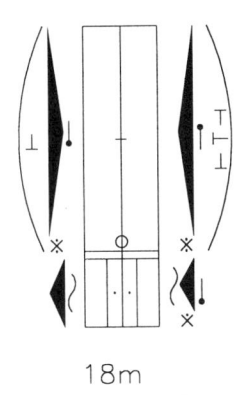

18m 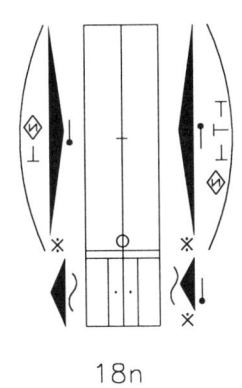 18n 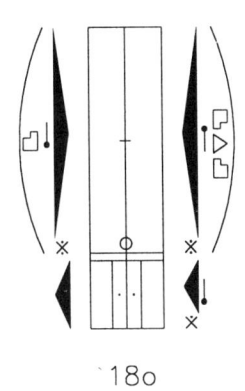 18o

19 Minor Shifting Actions

19.1. Minor movements are usually very small tilts in that the extremity travels farther than the part near the base (as happens in tilting the torso, or lifting an arm). However, minor movements may also be shifts, comparable to major shifting actions, but on a small scale. The chest is shown to shift forward in **19a**: this same 'equal' sign, ' = ', is placed on the pin to show a very small such action, **19b**.[29]

19.2. What is the point of reference for these shifting actions? *The point of reference for such shifts, larger or smaller, is the normal centered situation (place) for that part of the body.* Thus in **19c** the head shifts forward of its normal situation (place), it then shifts sideward of the normal place situation, and then backward of the normal place situation. In the same way the minor movements of **19d** follow the same pattern but at a much smaller scale. The diagram of **19e** illustrates these four movements.[30]

19.3. The difference between displacement of the extremity and shifting of a body section needs to be observed. In **19f** the extremity of the hand, the finger tips, displace from side to side, as illustrated in **19g**. This is achieved by small lateral wrist flexions; in the abstract drawing of **19h** the circle at the base represents the wrist. In contrast, **19i** shows small lateral shifts of the hand, as illustrated in **19j**, the whole unit of the hand being displaced sideward through accomodating articulation in wrist and lower arm. This passive lower arm reaction, spelled out in **19k**, is understood to occur and need not be indicated.

Advanced Labanotation

Minor Shifting Actions

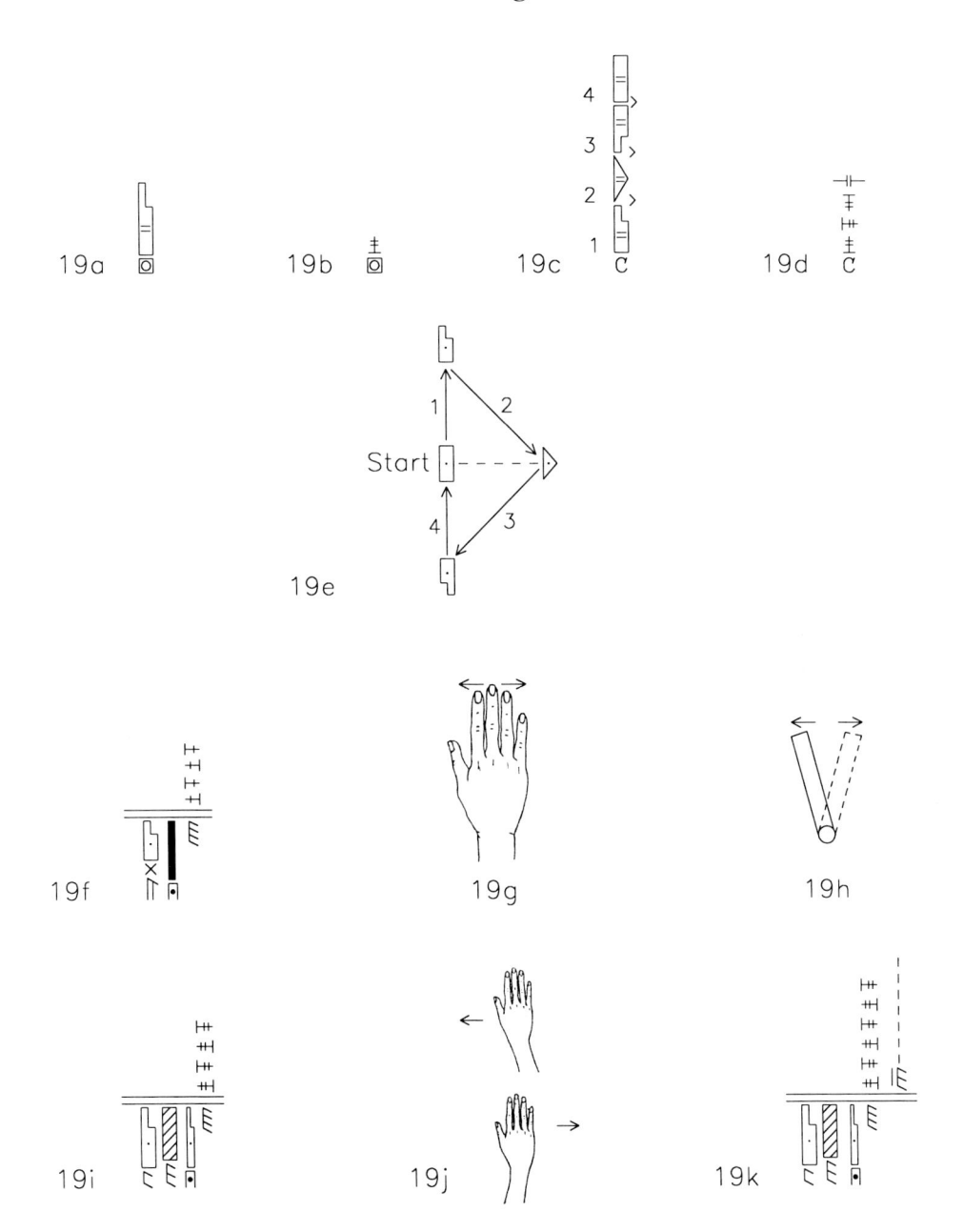

19a

19b

19c

19d

19e

19f

19g

19h

19i

19j

19k

20 Deviations for Successions

20.1. The following material is discussed more extensively in the Advanced Labanotation issue *Sequential Movements*. We repeat it here briefly for a complete account of Spatial Deviations.

20.2. Successions, sequential movements, which occur without a change of situation for the limb or torso, require a minor displacement in one direction or another. This minor displacement is indicated with a pin. Ex. **20a** shows a succession in the torso, a body 'ripple'over forward; in **20b** it is over the right. In each case the base of the torso (the pelvis) will make a small motion into the direction of the pin and the rest of the torso will follow sequentially, each part in turn ending in its normal alignment. In **20c** the arm has a succession over backward; it is via down in **20d**, i.e. in the direction of the little-finger-edge, and so on. Note that in each of these the displacement is gone by the end of the vertical bow, this bow having the effect of a passing event for a directional displacement.

20.3. **Overlapping Successions.** Ex. **20e** shows two overlapping successions for the right arm. The successions are augmented by occurring in two opposite directions, the first downward succession being followed by another deviation upward. Note the use in this example of an arm sign to identify the additional column to the right. Such addition is generally seen as not needed when there are no other indications present which would require clarification.

20.4. **Retained Displacement.** By placing the deviation in a bow it is clear that, when the movement is finished, this displacement has disappeared. In **20f** the pin for the direction of the succession is not placed in a bow and so the arm will finish slightly above side middle.

Advanced Labanotation

Deviations for Successions

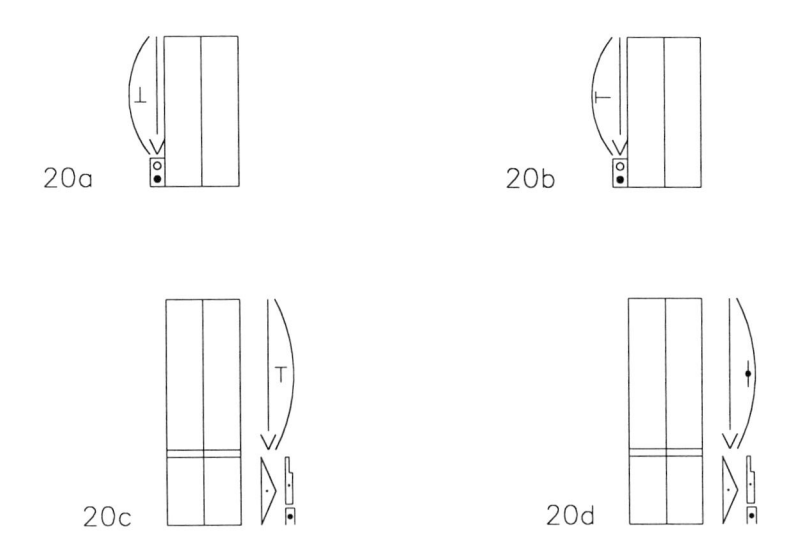

20a

20b

20c

20d

Overlapping Successions

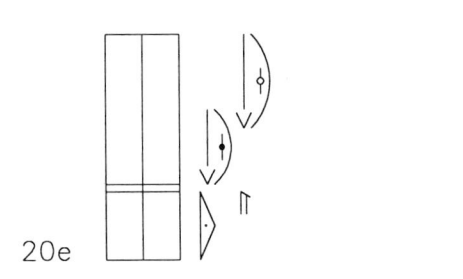

Retained Displacement

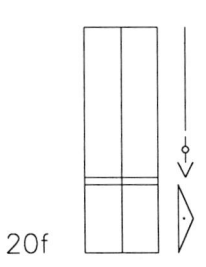

20e

20f

21 Timing

21.1. **Indication of Duration.** Duration is shown by a vertical duration line following the pin, **21a**. The length of this line indicates the length of time taken to complete the movement. The phrasing bow, which links separated pins to express the unity of the series of pins, also indicates duration and produces a smooth performance. Thus in **21b** there will be a sustained transition between the pins, the duration of the overall movement being the same as **21a**.[31]

21.2. Ex. **21c** shows a motion toward a displacement. The length of the toward sign indicates the duration of the movement.[32] (See Section 25 for the difference between reaching a destination and motion toward a destination.) Because movements indicated by pins are small displacements, there may be little difference between motion toward such a displacement and arrival at the stated displacement.

21.3. **Indication of Speed.** When a movement described with pins needs to be very fast and the pins cannot be drawn small enough, the sign for much speed is placed next to the movement in an additional bracket. In **21d** a circle is shown for the hand with the indication for much speed shown next to it.[33] This is followed by repeat signs placed close together to indicate continuation of the movements with speed. Equally, an enlargement of the notation can be placed alongside the movement staff and linked to it; within the staff a simplified version will be indicated.

21.4. **Momentary Displacement.** A passing nod of the head (momentary displacement) is shown in **21e**; the slower nod is followed by two quicker ones. The bow indicates that each is just a passing, temporary departure from the normal placement. The length of the bow gives the timing of the movement and the return to normal placement, both of these being of equal duration.

21.5. Uneven timing for a movement, such as **21e**, can be shown as in the next two examples. A slower nod of the head is given in **21f**, followed by a sudden return to normal. In contrast, in **21g** the nod is accented and the return to normal is slower.

21.6. **Emphasis on Destination.** The timing device of **21h**, an action stroke linked with the destination[34] provides the advantage of showing an accent at the moment of arrival at the displacement.

Timing

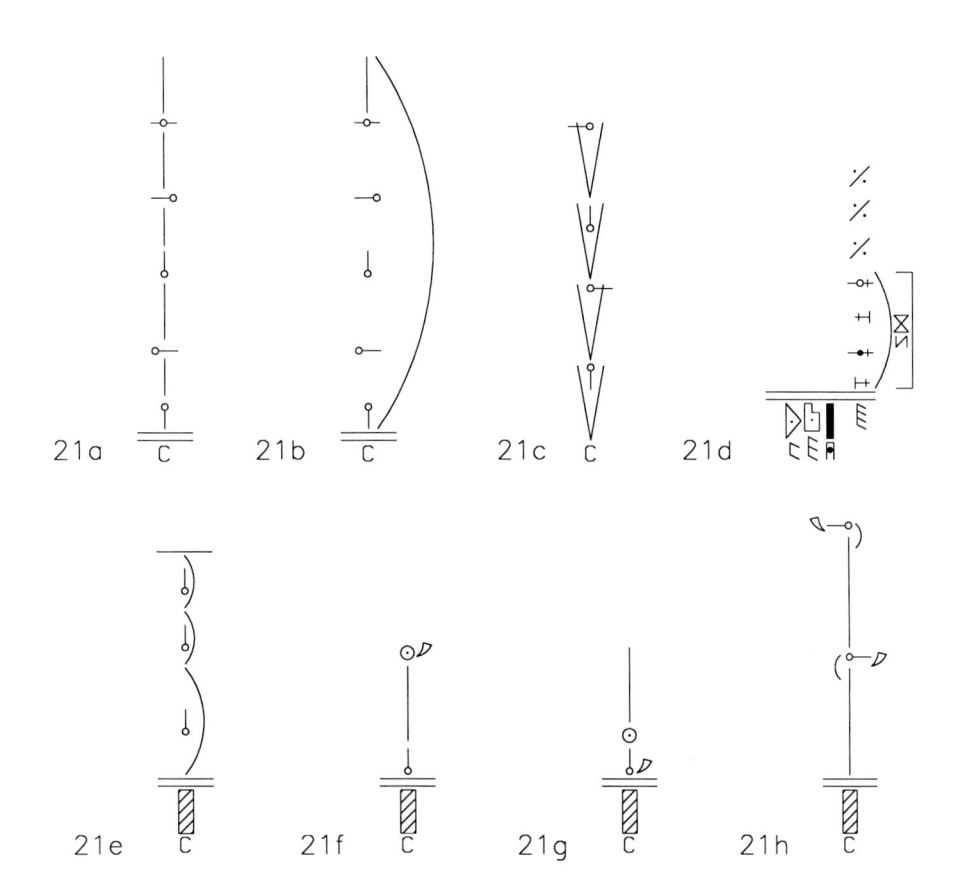

21a   21b   21c   21d

21e   21f   21g   21h

22 Size of Displacement

22.1. A small displacement from an established location is clearly visible, whereas a displacement of a similar size from the path of a gesture can barely be seen. For this reason the scale of displacements from a point is smaller than the scale established in 11.3 (**11f**) for deviations from a path. While it is often desirable to leave exact performance of deviations, of displacements, to the individual, for many pantomimic gestures it is important to give indication of size. The space measurement signs of **22a**, **22b**, **22c** and **22d** placed within a diamond, as in **22e**, **22f**, **22g** and **22h** indicate that the movement is to be performed on a smaller or larger scale than written.

22.2. These signs are placed in an addition bracket next to the material they modify. In **22i** the arm circle is to be performed much smaller than the direction symbols indicate. In **22j** the hand circle written with pins (which usually indicate small movements) are to be performed much larger than the pins suggest.

22.3. The following sizes have been established for displacements. *General Rule:* using the right side middle direction as the established point, **22k** shows a movement to standard points 45° below and then 45° above right side middle; **22l** a movement 22.5° (halfway) below and then 22.5° (halfway) above right side middle. The third way points of **22m** and **22n** show 15° below and 15° above the side middle point (all third-way points). (See Section 1 for intermediate directions.) The displacements of **22o**, fall within the range of 7.5° (deviations).

22.4. Ex. **22p** illustrates the range of degrees found practical for displacements. The scale for Distal Analysis is stated as follows:

22q = a 2.5° rise, combined with pin
22r = a 5° rise, combined with pin
22s = a 7.5° rise, use of an unmodified above pin.
22t = a 10° rise, combined with pin
22u = a 12.5° rise, combined with pin
22v = a 15° rise; note that a third-way displacement toward side high no longer lies in the range of description with a pin and a space measurement sign, it is shown as in **22v**.

Size of Displacement

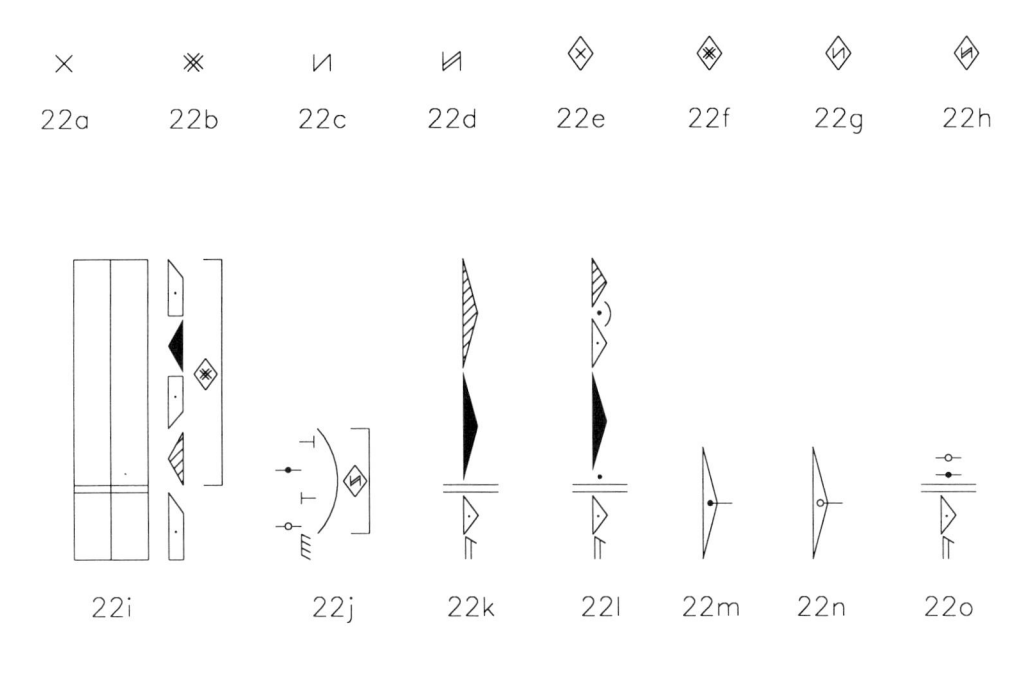

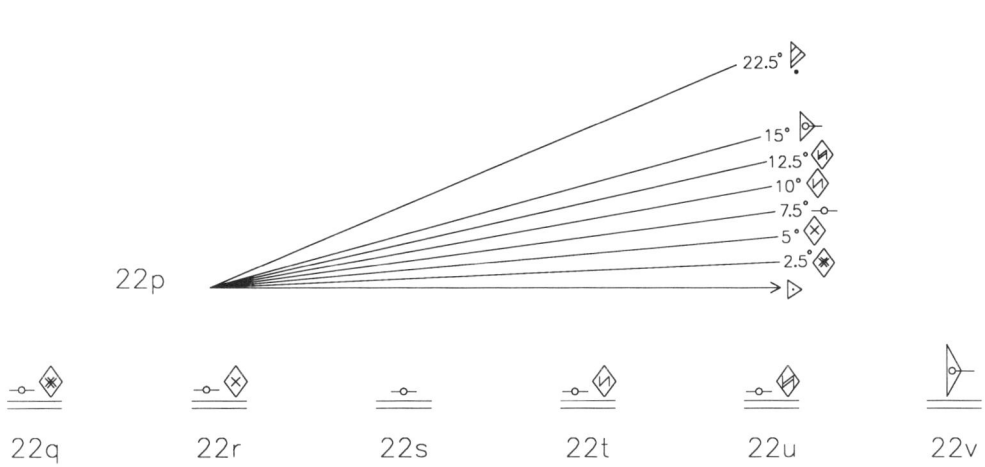

×	※	⋈	⋈	◇	◆	◇	◆
22a	22b	22c	22d	22e	22f	22g	22h

22i 22j 22k 22l 22m 22n 22o

22p
- 22.5°
- 15°
- 12.5°
- 10°
- 7.5°
- 5°
- 2.5°

22q 22r 22s 22t 22u 22v

22.5. **Clarification**. When the flexion or extension signs are placed below a pin and not in a diamond, as in the next two examples, they mean a slight arm flexion followed by an upward displacement, **22w**. Ex. **22x** means the arm extends prior to a slight downward displacement. With use of the diamond it is clear whether they are measurement signs and refer to distance or are flexions or extensions of the limb.

22.6. In ordinary examples, such as **22y**, the arm gestures forward and at the same time draws in closer to the center, the smaller distance causing a flexion, the two ideas of flexion and distance can be said to be served at the same time. The measurement signs within a diamond indicate distance and are placed next to the pin they modify. Ex. **22z** states a small distance below (5°), while **22aa** shows a 10° displacement forward.

Size of Displacement - Clarification

22w   22x   22y   22z   22aa

23 Polar Pins

23.1. **The Disadvantage of Proximal and Distal Pins.** Use of proximal and distal analysis to indicate minor deviations from a point (e.g. vibrations) was discussed in Section 16. When the body part is in an intermediate direction or while the limb is moving, these modes of analysis for displacements often become difficult to use and the correct choice of pin becomes hard to determine. In **23a** a 'down-up' movement of the arm in diagonal high direction, is given with proximal pins. In **23b** the same is given with the arm halfway between the diagonal and forward high directions. Here the pins become harder to read. Exs. **23c** and **23d** show the same movement judged from the distal center.[35] Third-way intermediate directions, as in **23e**, cannot be analysed with proximal or distal pins.

23.2. **The Idea of Polar Pins.**[36] Polar pins are comparable to the idea of the earth's poles, longitude and latitude. Because of gravity, in any situation we know where up and down are. We are aware of the 'rising' (upward motion) or 'sinking' (downward motion) in any movement. We are also attuned to knowing which direction is clockwise and which counterclockwise. In any situation we also know which direction is horizontally away from the center pole and which is toward the center pole (the 'spoke-like' movements).

23.3. Ex. **23f** illustrates the sphere around the body and the direction of rising movements; **23g** shows the direction of sinking movements. In **23h** the arrows indicate the clockwise direction, while **23i** shows the counterclockwise direction.

23.4. Ex. **23j** illustrates (bird's eye view) outward going 'spoke-like' movements, while **23k** shows inward 'spoke-like' movements. These 'spoke-like' actions are always horizontal, they can be compared to cross-sections of an orange, as in **23l**. Even near the top, the 'spokes' are always horizontal. In the drawing of **23m**, similar circles of such 'spokes' are shown around a vertical figure. From any direction the performer can determine an action which is horizontally moving toward the center pole, or horizontally away from it; any rising or sinking 'spoke-like' displacement is a combined form.

23.5. The vertical axis of the Polar System always remains vertical, it cannot be applied to the Body System of Reference. When the torso is tilted, as in **23n**, rising and sinking still relate to the vertical line of gravity. The image to bear in

Advanced Labanotation

mind for any placement of a minor polar pin movement, is of the polar sphere being closer to or further from the center of the body. Equally such a sphere can be imagined around the extremity of the limb involved, be it the knee or hand, the vertical 'pole' is centered at the proximal joint.

The Disadvantage of Proximal and Distal Pins

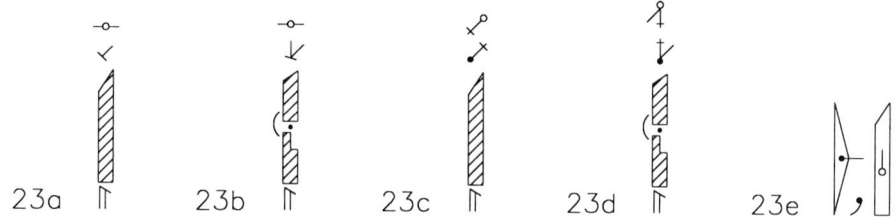

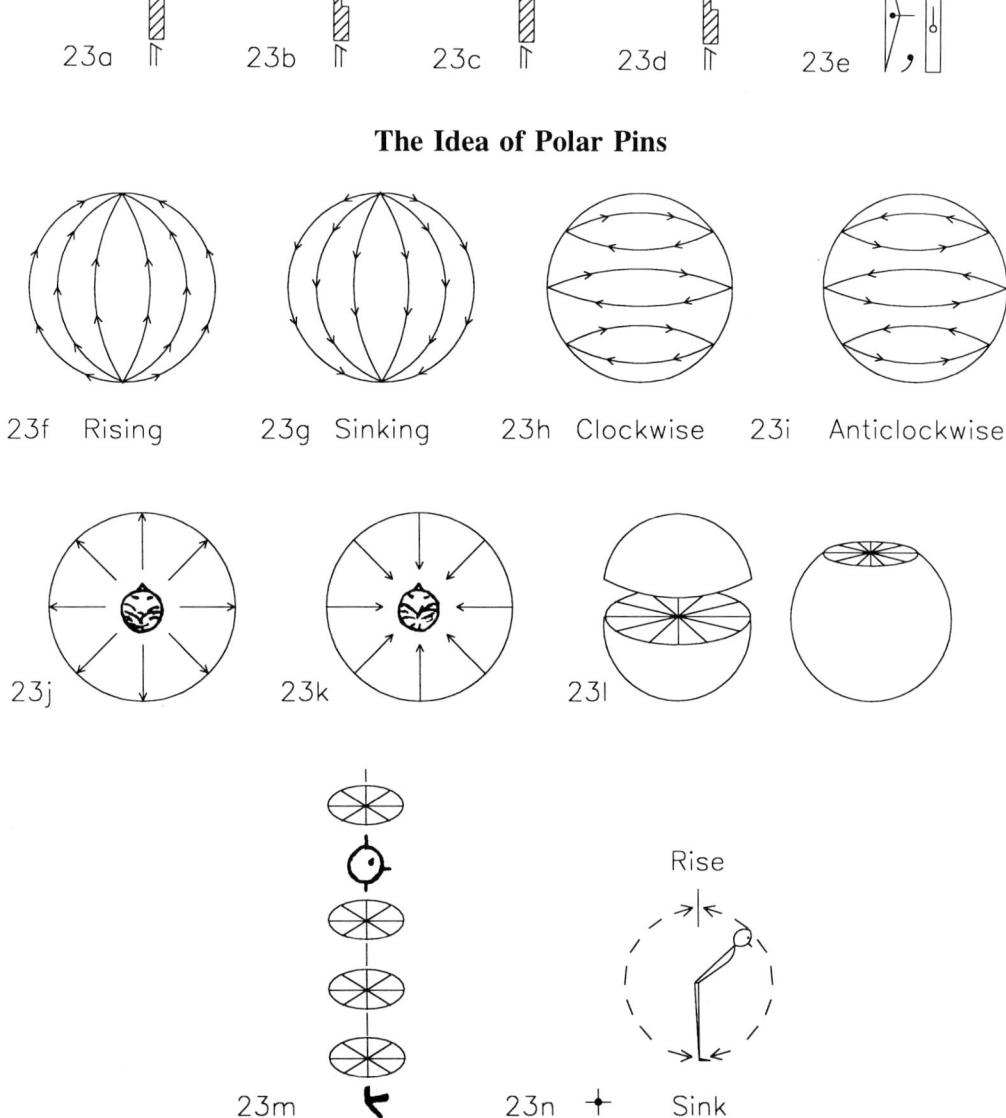

23a   23b   23c   23d   23e

The Idea of Polar Pins

23f Rising   23g Sinking   23h Clockwise   23i Anticlockwise

23j   23k   23l

23m   23n   Rise / Sink

23.6. **The Signs for Polar Pins.** Ex. **23o** shows the polar pins for rising and sinking; **23p** those for counterclockwise and clockwise, and **23q** for outward and inward horizontal displacements. When combined with rising or sinking or with horizontal circular movements, the arrows for outward and inward displacement must point **away** from the base of the sign for outward, as in **23aa**, and **toward** the base of the sign for inward, **23ab**. Ex. **23r** shows the center pins used for cancellation.[37]

23.7. Ex. **23s** shows the 'downward upward' (sinking, rising) movement of **23a** and **23c** written with polar pins. The movement of **23b** and **23d** given in **23t**, is clearly much easier to read. With polar pins, deviations from a third-way point can easily be indicated. Rising and sinking deviations from the position of **23e** are given in **23u** and **23v** with polar pins.

23.8. The pins are modified to show combined forms such as rising with counterclockwise displacement, **23w**; rising with clockwise displacement, **23x**; sinking with counterclockwise displacement, **23y**, and sinking with clockwise displacement, **23z**.

23.9. In combining these with spoke-like inward and outward movements, the visual relationship of the small arrow to the base of the polar pin is important and should be noted as this defines inward (toward the base of the pin) and outward (away from the base, i.e. toward the point). Ex. **23aa** shows the combined pins for rising outward and **23ab** for rising inward; the combined pin of **23ac** shows sinking outward and **23ad** shows sinking inward.

23.10. Counterclockwise outward displacement is shown in **23ae**; counterclockwise and inward is as **23af**. Similarly **23ag** shows clockwise and outward, with **23ah** showing clockwise and inward.

23.11. An example of the combined use of three of these possibilities is given in **23ai**, where, from a diagonal location, the right arm moves up, clockwise and outward, then down, anticlockwise and inward.

23.12. **Displacement from the Poles.** Because in the locations of the two poles (the vertically up and down points) there is no 'upward', no 'downward' and no horizontal displacement possible, displacements are best indicated with Standard System of Reference pins. With the arm straight up, or straight down, sideward displacements would be written as **23aj** for Proximal Analysis and **23ak** with Distal Analysis.

Advanced Labanotation

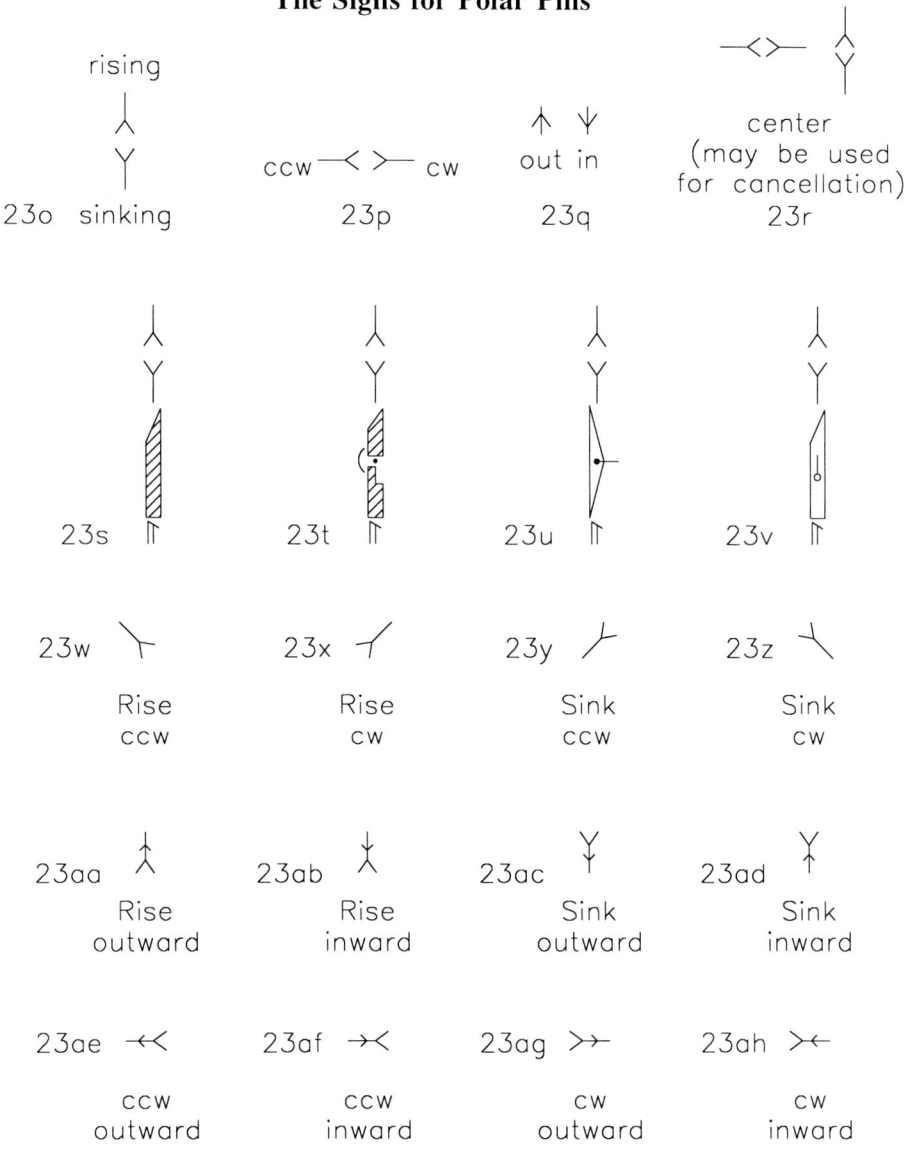

The Signs for Polar Pins

rising

23o sinking

23p ccw —<>— cw

23q out ↑ in ↓

23r center (may be used for cancellation)

23s   23t   23u   23v

23w Rise ccw

23x Rise cw

23y Sink ccw

23z Sink cw

23aa Rise outward

23ab Rise inward

23ac Sink outward

23ad Sink inward

23ae ccw outward

23af ccw inward

23ag cw outward

23ah cw inward

Displacement from the Poles

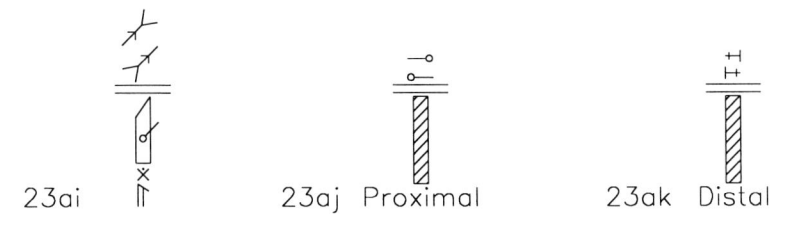

23ai

23aj Proximal

23ak Distal

23.13. **Analysis of Spoke-like Displacements.** Displacements which move on a spoke-like path in toward the center pole or away from this center, require some degree of flexion and extension in the facilitating body part. In **23al**, for the side to side action at the extremity of the arm (felt as being an action, a displacement, of the palm, but in fact one facilitated by the whole arm), the arm must extend slightly as the extremity (the palm/hand) moves to the right and flex slightly when moving to the left. Note that we are still dealing with very small movements.

23.14. The movement of **23al**, being in the lateral plane, can be written as **23am**, the palm displacing slightly to the right and left, facilitated, in fact, by passive arm accomodation, shown by the dotted line. The intent of the action is the palm displacement, hence the description being in those terms; although the arm must flex slightly, the focus is not on the arm movement. For a surface such as palm or face, a shifting action is automatically understood. If these pins were written for the hand, the shifting action would need to be indicated, **23an**; without the = sign for shifting, the hand would make a slight tilting movement, the extremity (the finger tips) moving laterally. (For minor shifting actions see Section 19.) The polar pin description for this sideward shift is **23ao**.

23.15. If the movement was intended to be experienced as a flexion-extension action, it could be written as **23ap**. Here there is a slightly lesser degree (the outward displacement) and then a slightly greater flexion for the inward action. Rather than stating degrees, the motion of approaching the state of being stretched followed by the motion toward becoming contracted could be written, as in **23aq**, but with the added indication that spatially the action should be very small.

23.16. In **23ar** the arm is again bent but now side high. This same displacement for the palm, **23as**, is written as before; if shown as a movement for the hand, **23at**, it would again be the same, as in **23an**. For polar description it is also the same because the displacement is horizontal, **23au**.

23.17. The hand is at a different angle in **23av**; an outward and inward shifting displacement for the palm would be **23aw**, for the hand **23ax**. To draw in on this same line using polar pins would be written as **23ay**, the displacement being rising and outward followed by sinking and inward. Described in terms of flexion the notation would be the same as **23ap** or **23aq**.

Advanced Labanotation

Analysis of Spoke-like Displacements

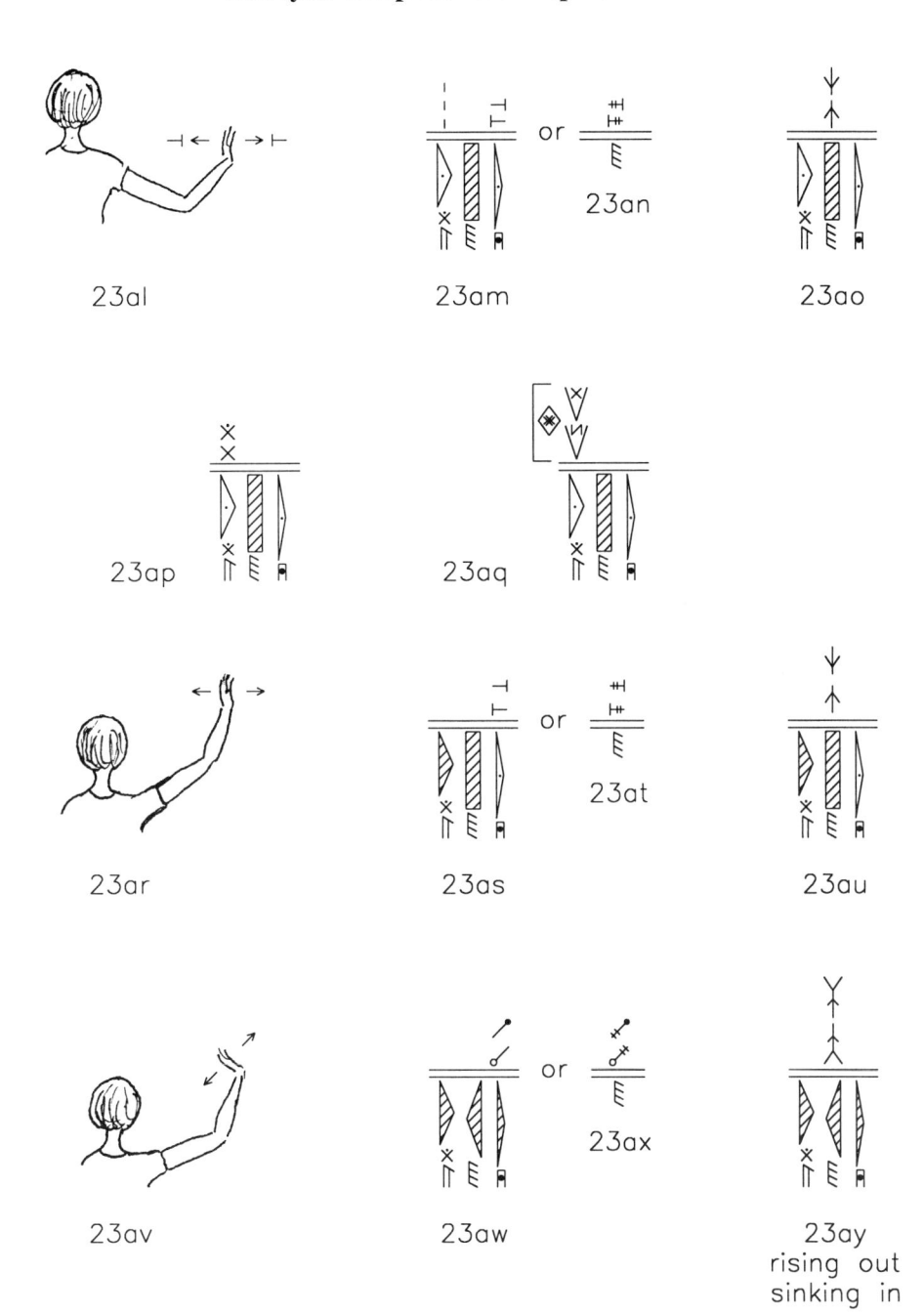

23al

23am

23an

23ao

23ap

23aq

23ar

23as

23at

23au

23av

23aw

23ax

23ay
rising out
sinking in

23.18. **To and Fro Polar Displacements.** Many minor displacements are a repeated departure in relation to a point, a 'toward' and 'away'. This may be fairly continuous or have a marked spatial or rhythmic pattern. In **23az** the arms move in opposition. This same pattern of minor vertical rising and sinking is repeated as the torso inclines and twists. The pattern continues in the same way because the rising and sinking motions can continue even though the torso has changed spatially.

23.19. An accented hand displacement rising clockwise is shown in **23ba**. It is followed by an unemphasised reverse path. This gesture repeats while the arm is moving to diagonal high, the chest twisting to augment the action. As the arm moves on to side high the direction of the accented displacement changes to sinking CW.

23.20. **Circular Displacements.** Circular displacements can also be shown with polar pins. Here we compare Proximal, Distal and Polar Analyses. Exs. **23bb**, **23bc** and **23bd** show a circular movement around the extremity of the forward pointing arm. One must keep in mind that Proximal and Distal displacements refer to the established starting point. The examples here are illustrated in **23be**, the path at first rising from the original point (marked 'x'). It continues by sinking clockwise, then sinking counterclockwise, followed by rising counterclockwise. Next to each of these displacements the two components are indicated separately in brackets. Polar pins show motion from where you are, your previous point of arrival, thus the second pin must be clockwise and sinking, the third counterclockwise and sinking, with the fourth being counterclockwise and rising.

23.21. In the sequence of **23bf** repeat signs have been used. The symmetrical circular pattern for the lower arm is repeated, then, with the change in arm location, it is repeated in reverse. The repeat sign always refers back to the notated example.

Advanced Labanotation

To and Fro Polar Displacements

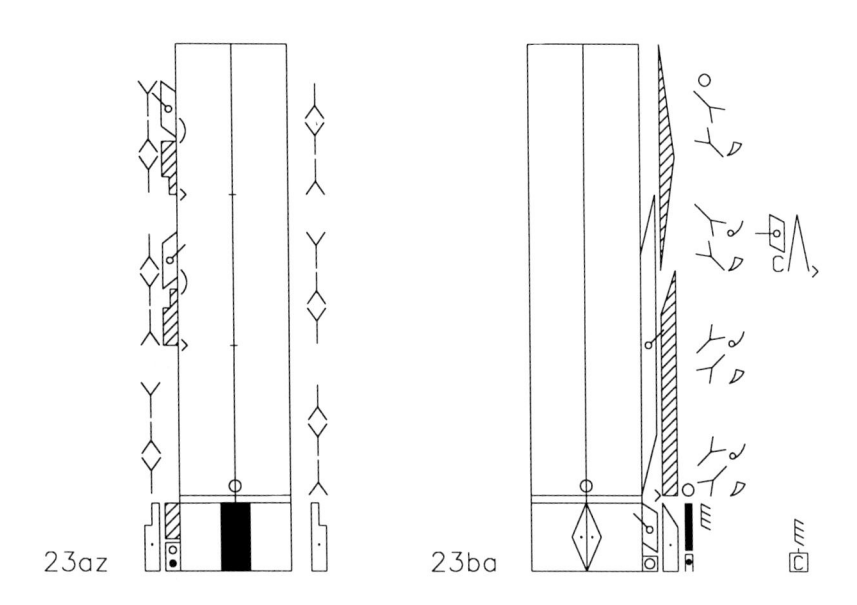

23az   23ba

Circular Displacements

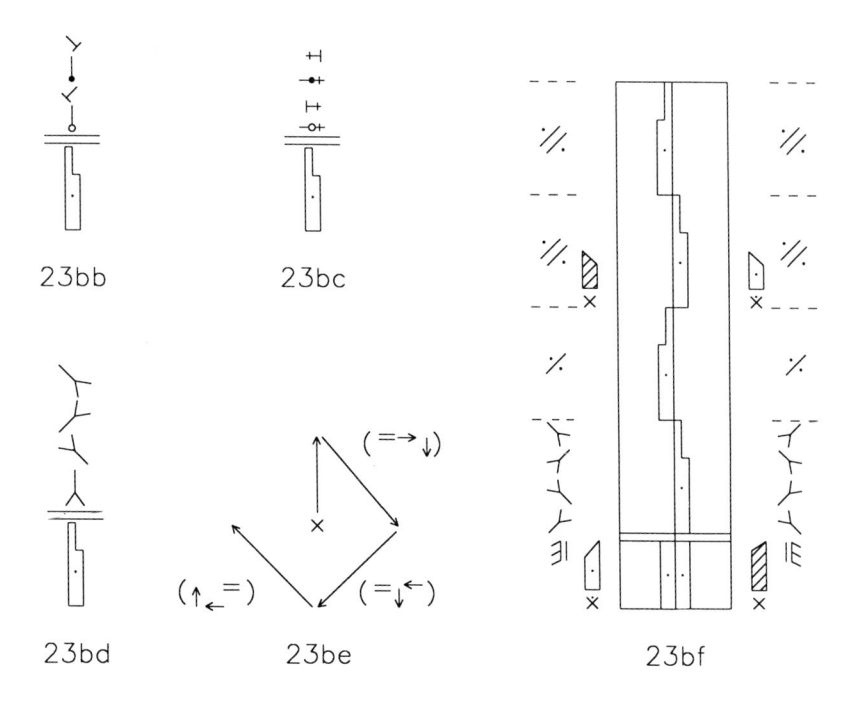

23bb   23bc

23bd   23be   23bf

VI MOTION VERSUS DESTINATION

24 Steps Versus Gestures, Direction of Progression, Shifting and Path Signs

The difference in interpretation between direction symbols in the support column and those in gesture columns was established early in the development of the Laban system.[38]

    24.1. **Direction in a Support Column.** When writing steps in the support column the symbols indicate *a motion into a certain direction from 'place'*. After each step the center of weight has arrived at a new place, the direction of the next step is judged from there. In **24a** the sideward step is sideward of where the forward step ended; the next step is forward of where the side step ended. The resulting path is illustrated in **24b**. The symbols do not represent a destination. Each step is a comfortable distance; even for one person, the step destination may differ slightly from one performance to another.

    24.2. **Direction in a Gesture Column.** When using direction symbols in the gesture column, they indicate *a destination for the free end of the limb, judged from the fixed end of the limb*. Whatever the starting position of, for example an arm, a forward middle direction symbol will always result in the same ending position in relation to the fixed end of this arm. This means that the path of (the extremity of) the limb will be different, if the starting position of the limb is different.

    24.3. Ex. **24c** shows the arm moving from forward middle to side middle. The peripheral path of the arm (the path of the hand), judged from the start, is diagonal right backward middle, shown in **24d**. In **24e** the arm comes from place high, when going to right side middle. The path of the hand here is right side low. It is clear that the direction symbol shows the destination and not the direction of the path traveled.

    24.4. **Direction of Progression.** One method, devised to indicate motion for gestures, expresses the same idea of progression, the direction of the motion, as is used for steps in the support column. To notate this *direction of the progression,* the symbol of an arrow is used. This is based on the idea of an arrow on a floor plan, **24f**, showing the direction of the movement.[39] At each point the movement picks up where the previous one left off, *the reference point for the next direction is the previous arrival point*. The arrow is placed within

Advanced Labanotation

the direction symbol. Logically it might be thought the arrow should point into the appropriate direction. However, the width of the direction symbols has dictated that, for whichever direction is being described, a forward pointing arrow is always used (as if a key). For the description of the direction of progression, each is a *motion*, there is no destination. Assuming that in **24g** each movement is of the same distance, the path indicated for the head will form a square, as illustrated in **24h** here each movement is numbered for clarity (compare this with **19e**). The path is comparable to the walking pattern of **24i**.

Direction in a Support Column

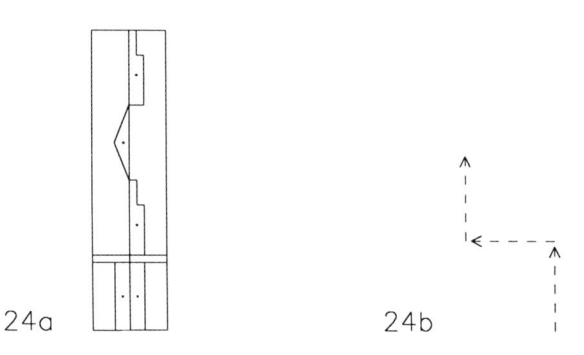

24a   24b

Direction in a Gesture Column

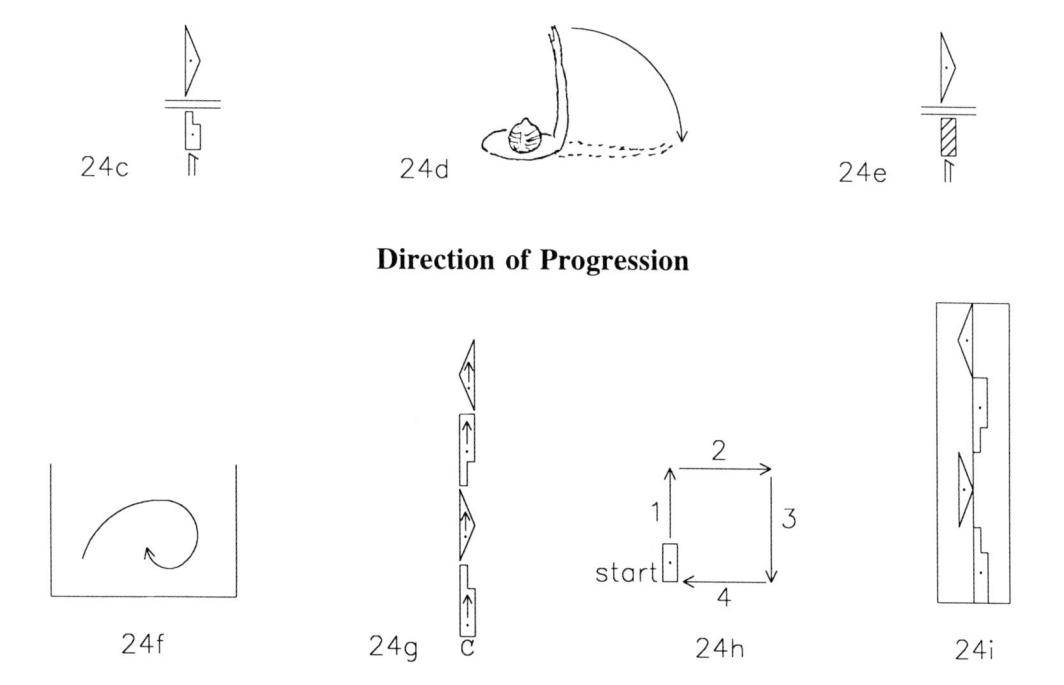

24c   24d   24e

Direction of Progression

24f   24g   24h   24i

24.5. In **24j** the right leg moves to the right at the same level, the resulting path being shown in **24k**; the right leg will end more or less diagonal right low. Arriving at a destination is not the point of the movement, the foot may have traveled sideward horizontal to push an object to the side. One can see that the same direction symbols judged normally, i.e. without the arrow as in **24l**, result in a very different movement, one for which the motion is one of rising, opening and moving backward, indicated in **24m**.

24.6. **Level.** When an arrow is written inside a middle level direction symbol, the dot may be placed before or after the arrow.[40] High and low level can be indicated around the arrow in a direction symbol. In **24n** the right arm moves diagonally right backward high, from wherever it was. The arm in **24o** starts diagonally left forward, it then moves upward, horizontally to the right, downward and horizontally to the left, as illustrated in **24p**.

24.7. **Minor Movements.** When using pins to indicate a minor direction of progression movement (comparable to the main direction symbols showing direction of progression), the arrow is placed at the end of the pin and the pin points into the appropriate direction. Ex. **24q** shows a small version of the displacement pattern of **24g**. A change in level can also be shown, as in **24r** which indicates a forward upward motion followed by backward downward, a shifting movement. If the same distance is used, the head returns to its normal position.

24.8. **Cancellation of Result of Previous Motion.** A back to normal sign will cancel the result of a previous motion, **24s**, or the normal situation for that part can be stated, **24t**. An ordinary direction symbol will cancel an arm, leg or torso gesture described previously as a direction of progression motion. These same cancellations are applied to minor direction of progression motions, **24u** and **24v**.

Advanced Labanotation

Direction of Progression (continued)

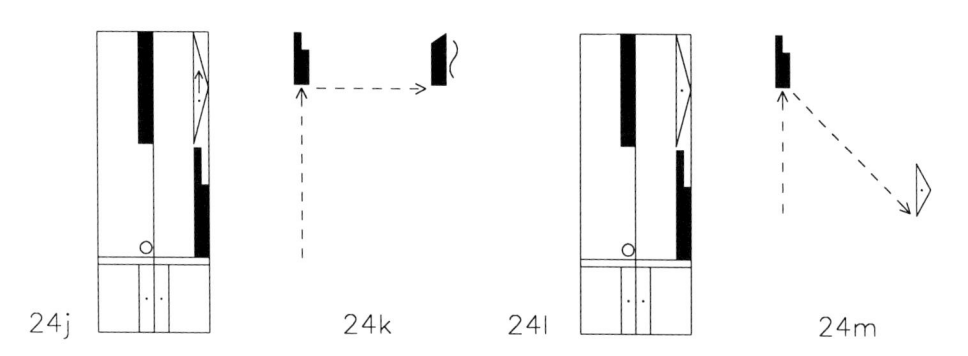

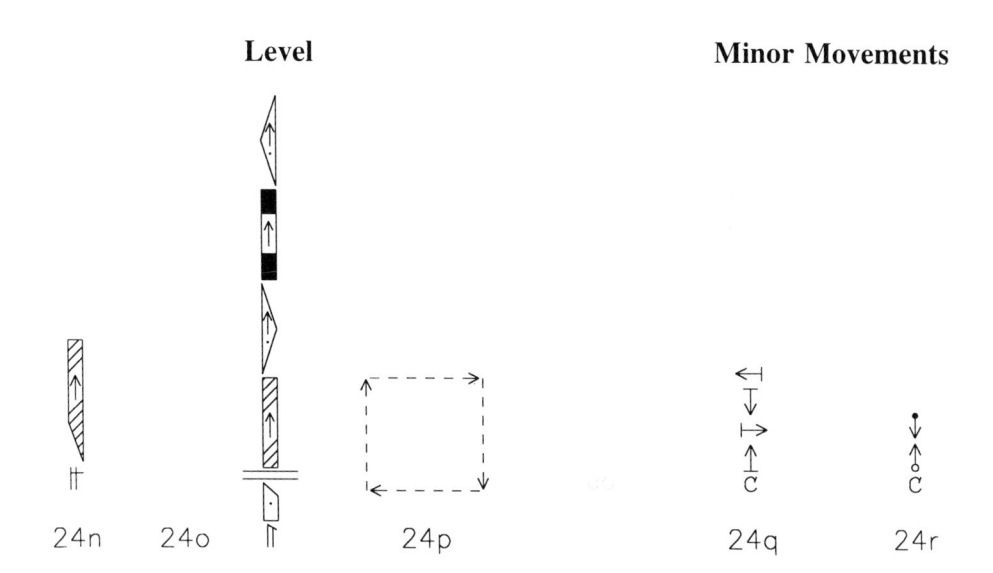

24j 24k 24l 24m

Level   Minor Movements

24n 24o 24p 24q 24r

Cancellation of Result of Previous Motion

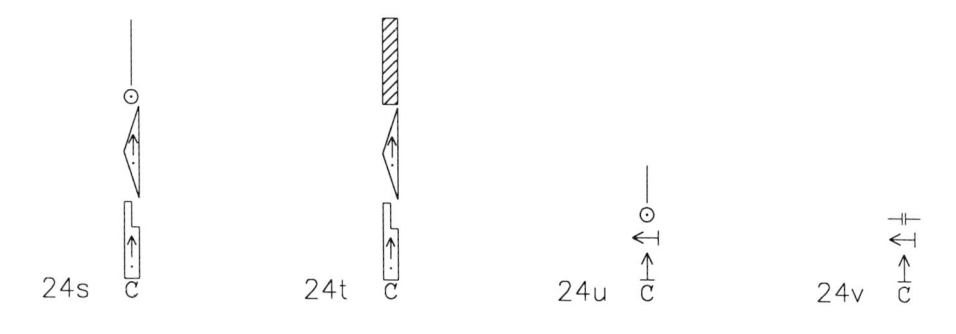

24s 24t 24u 24v

24.9. **Shifting.** One may think that for the head, **24g** or **24q**, repeated here, can also be written by indicating each movement as a shift, as in **24w**. However, for shifts the point of reference for directions is always the 'normal' state. Therefore shifts indicate destination in relation to that point, as illustrated in **24x**. Also, focus for shifting is on a specific anatomical action, while direction of progression movements do not specify shift, tilt or rotation. (For minor shifting actions see Section 19.)

24.10. **Motion Indicated by Path Sign.** Direction of Progression can also be indicated by showing the appropriate direction within a straight path sign, as in **24y**, which indicates virtually the same as **24z**. For quick movements such a path sign may become less easy to read, the ends of the path sign may look like horizontal pins (tacks), **24aa**. Using this path sign method, **24g** would be written as **24ab**.

24.11. Ex. **24ac** shows the arm performing a straight path in a right sideward direction, the extremity moving on a sideward line. Compare this with **24ad**, which describes a straight path with the destination to arrive at the Standard side middle destinational point. The movement of **24ad** is the same as **24ae**, the more usual statement of a straight line movement from forward to side (see Section 4 for indication of straight path for gestures).

Shifting

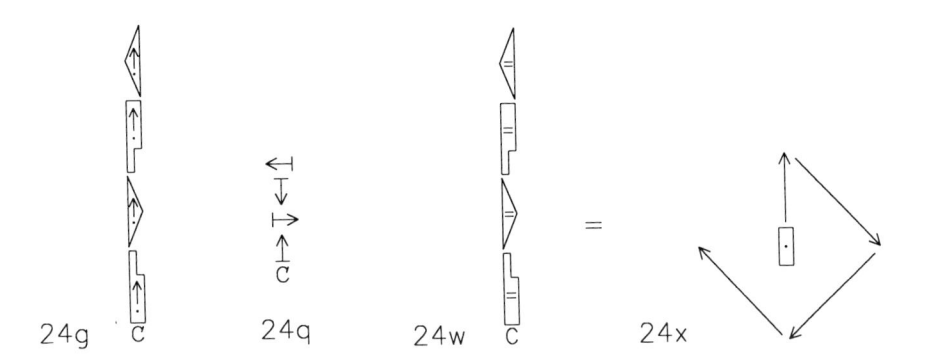

Motion Indicated by Path Sign

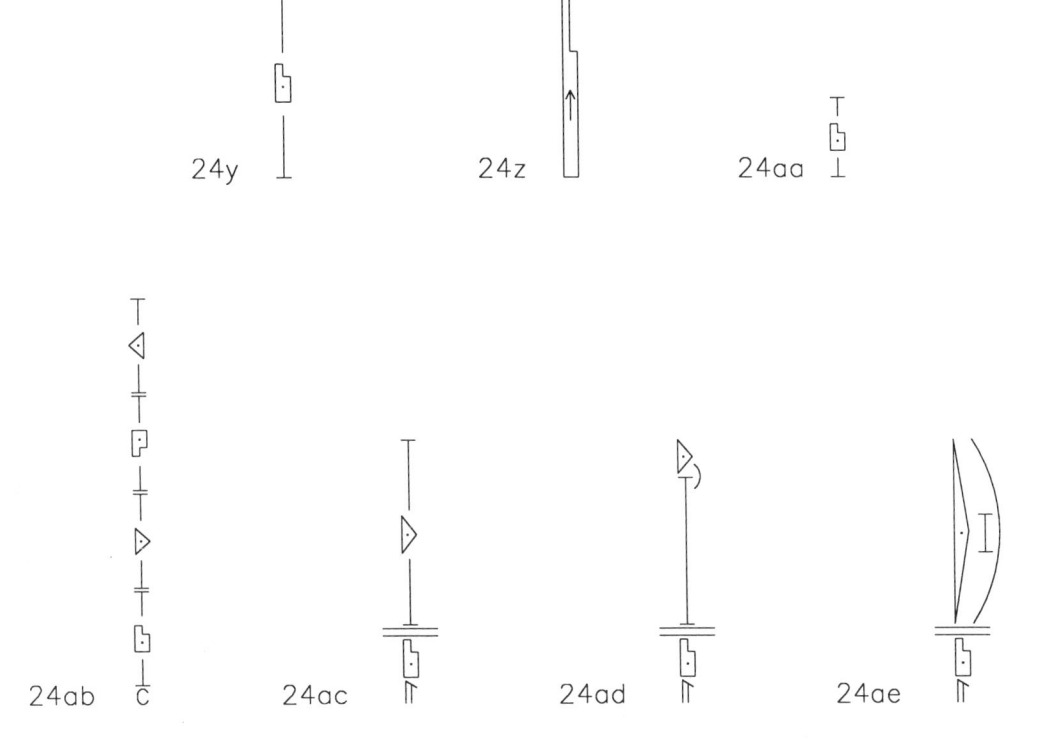

24.12. **Straight or Curved Direction of Progression.** There is, however, a difference between using the path sign, **24y** and the direction of progression arrow, **24z**, both repeated here. In the first there is an emphasis on the straightness of the path. Direction of progression shows a general direction, usually a straight path, but limitations of the body may cause the path to be slightly curved.

24.13. It is possible to indicate a deviation from a direction of progression path. In **24af** the arm deviates upward as it moves from the point forward middle on a horizontal path to the right. This same deviation may occur when the movement is described as a straight path, as in **24ag**.

24.14. **Flexion/Extension or Distance.** As stated in Sections 11 and 22, a contraction sign in front of a direction of progression sign for a gesture, as in **24ah**, indicates flexion of the limb. As the direction of progression is a form of path, such a sign could refer to distance traveled as is the case for steps which show the direction of progression; **24ai** indicates a short step. The same applies to extension signs (long steps). However, the distance for a gesture is best expressed through using statement of spatial size, as in **24aj**. Equally the sign for spatially small can be placed as a pre-sign before the direction symbol and linked to it with a small vetical bow, as in **24ak**.

24.15. To indicate flexion of the limb, the notation of **24al** states that the limb ends one degree contracted. Another description for this is that of **24am** in which the timing for the destinational state is given for the flexion. In this example the right arm starts extended diagonally right backward, the extremity then travels on a straight path forward horizontally, ending with the arm slightly bent. Because the arm must bend somewhat to achieve this path, the ending state of the limb being slightly bent is written as a destinational statement. Note the small horizontal bow linking this indication to the arm column.

Straight or Curved Direction of Progression

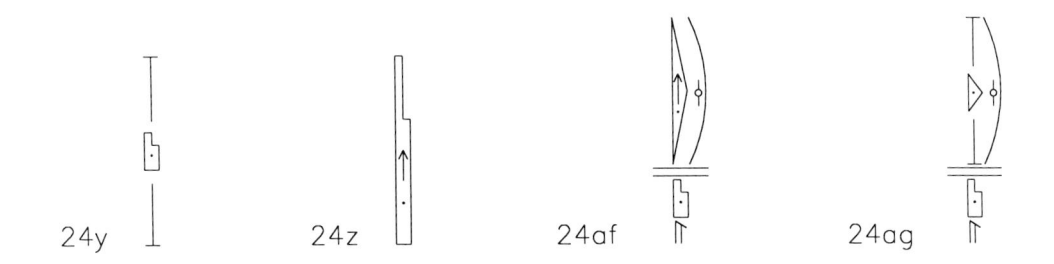

24y 24z 24af 24ag

Flexion/Extension or Distance

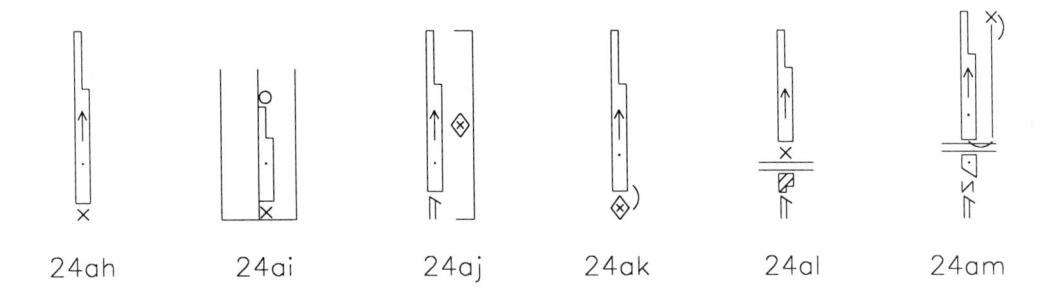

24ah 24ai 24aj 24ak 24al 24am

25 Toward, Away versus Destination

25.1. **Toward and Away.** Another form of movement which focuses on motion rather than destination is an action (a path for the whole body or a gesture) which moves toward or away from a person, object, part of the room or, for gestures, toward or away from a state. Ex. **25a** shows the toward and away signs.[41] For purposes of movement exploration, for which Motif Description (Motif Notation) is so suitable, less defined statements of movement are often needed. In structured notation an end result, here a destination, usually needs to be defined. However, Motif Description is more frequently met in choreographic scores of dances in which freedom of interpretation is desired.

25.2. The signs for toward and away may be used for the path of the whole body, as in **25b** which shows traveling toward a partner (P). In **25c** travel away from an object, a chair is shown. A path toward an area of the stage is expressed in **25d**; in **25e** the path is away from two men. Ex. **25f** shows a circular path moving toward the focal point, i.e. the center of the circle, thus producing an inward spiral path. Ex. **25g** shows an outward spiral path traveling away from the focal point.

25.3. Toward and away signs are also used in gesture columns. In **25h**, the hand approaches the face of P. Ex. **25i** shows that the hands move toward the knees. Note placement of both hands and both knees on one side of the staff; this often makes reading easier. The hand (arm) moves away from the left shoulder of P in **25j**. Ex. **25k** shows that the hands (arms) move away from the knees. In this symmetrical example the instruction is written on each side of the staff. In **25l** the arm suddenly moves away from a hot pan after touching it. (See 25.8 for use of the away sign as a cancellation.)

Advanced Labanotation

Toward and Away

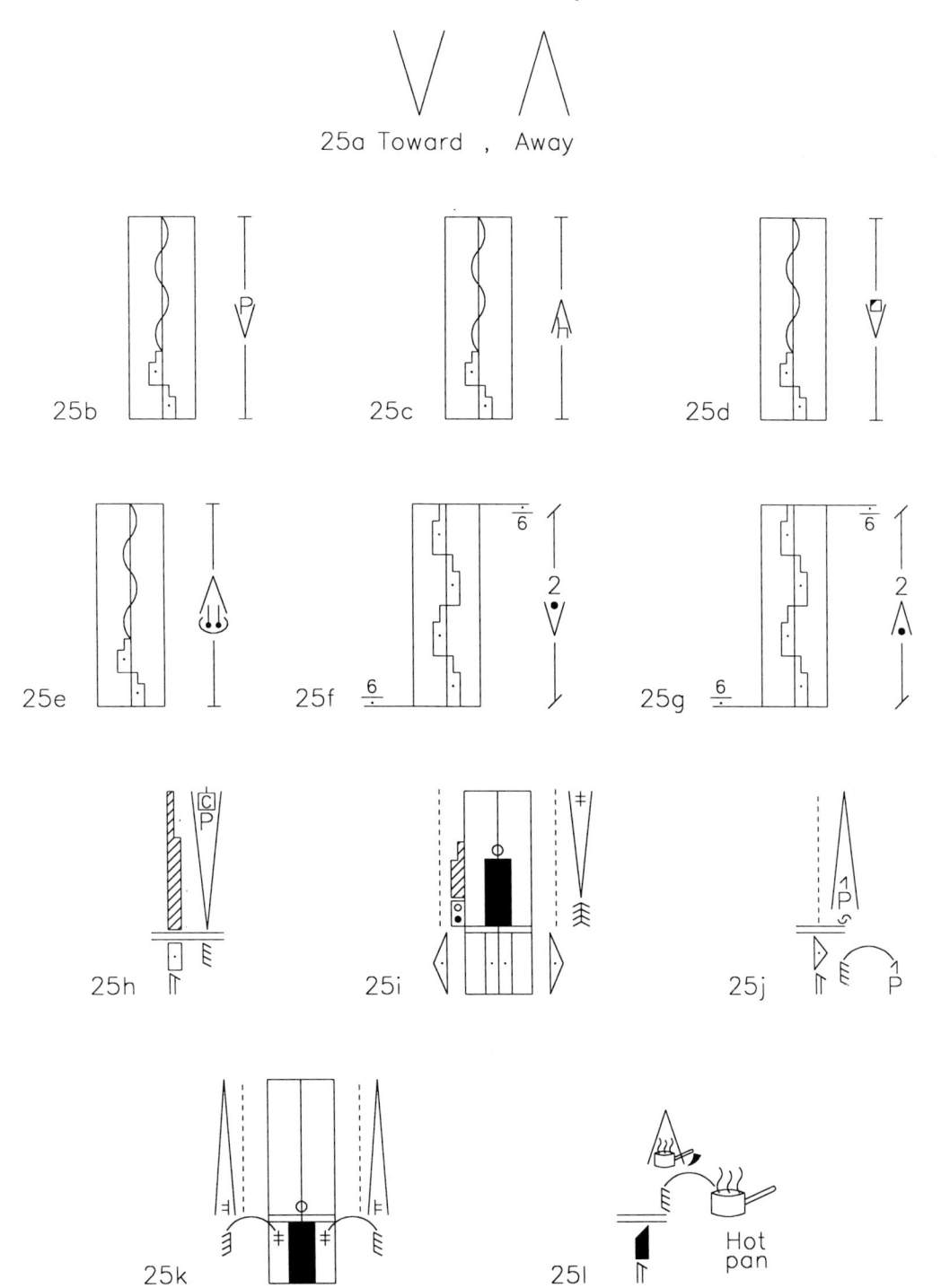

25a Toward , Away

25.4. **Toward, Away from a Directional Point.** In contrast to a gesture arriving at an established directional point around the body, the movement may be one of moving toward that point. Ex. **25m** states that the right arm moves toward place high, but does not arrive. The form of motion of **25m** is not to be confused with **25n** or **25o** which state the direction of progression. As illustrated in **25p**, the path of the motion of **25m** will, of course, depend on where the arm starts. In **25q** the location of the starting point makes this action more defined. What is not indicated is the distance of the motion, but this may not be important, some freedom is undoubtedly desired.

25.5. Because the limb does not have the quality of arriving at a clear destination, the viewer cannot know what the intention was. The performer may initially intend to arrive at that point but for some reason does not complete the movement. The idea is made more obvious to the viewer by the performer looking into the appropriate direction, as given in **25r**. A similar example is **25s** in which the arm moves toward the side middle point, the sense of an 'unfinished' gesture is made more apparent by the head looking to that side.

25.6. Motion away from a defined point is shown in **25t**; the arm was up, it moves away from that point, in what direction is not stated. A gestural statement may have been made; it is over, so the arm moves away. In **25u**, a similar example, when the arm moves away from side middle, the face looks into that direction, perhaps seeing the reason for the withdrawal.

25.7. **Toward, Away from the Body.** A general statement for a gesture toward the body may be needed. The sign of **25v**[42] represents the body-as-a-whole, all parts moving as an entity. In **25w** the arm approaches the body; in **25x** it moves away. A more specific statement can be made, as in **25y** in which the arm approaches the chest, or **25z** which states that the right hand approaches the right hip.

25.8. **Away as Cancellation.** The away sign is also used as a cancellation sign to indicate that the previous indication (or resulting state) is no longer to be in effect. In **25aa**, which starts in a low knee bend, the level of the center of weight is no longer to be in effect, the level of the steps will be their standard level. For this example neither a back to normal sign nor a place high sign is appropriate for the center of weight. For this usage the away sign is drawn within the width of a column. A good example is **25ab** in which the sideward tilt of the chest disappears when the whole torso bends forward high. The chest does not go back to normal, yet its previous state needs to be cancelled. The head is looking sideward in **25ac**, it then 'goes away' from this state, but not with any destination indicated, which is clearly stated in **25ad** or **25ae**.

Advanced Labanotation 89

Toward, Away from a Directional Point

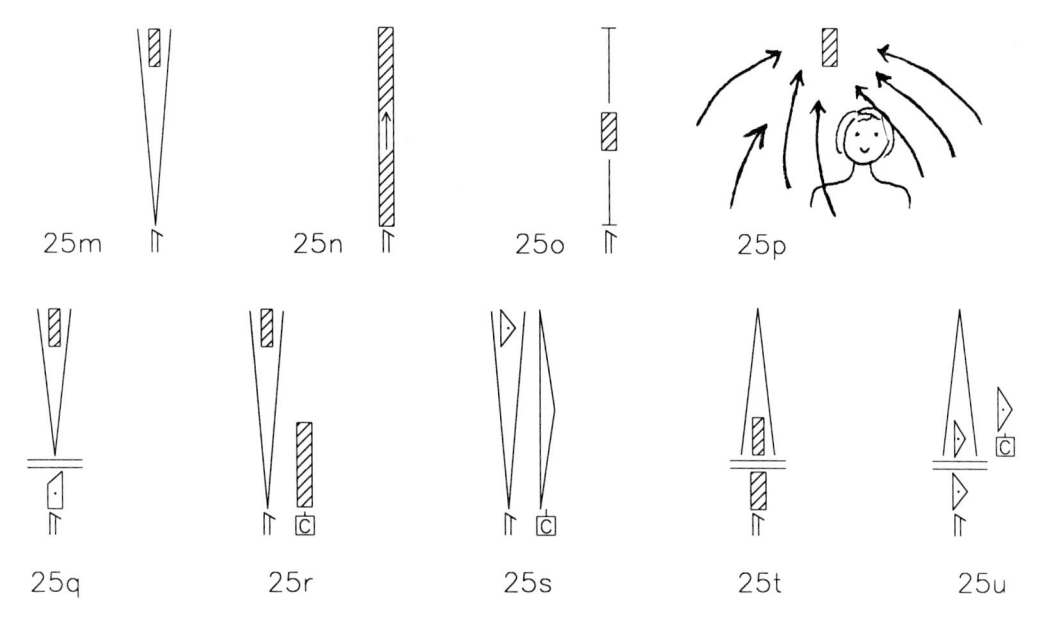

25m   25n   25o   25p

25q   25r   25s   25t   25u

Toward, Away from the Body

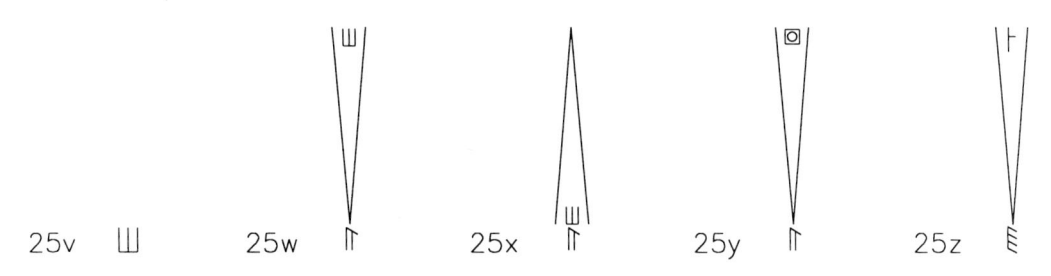

25v   25w   25x   25y   25z

Away as Cancellation

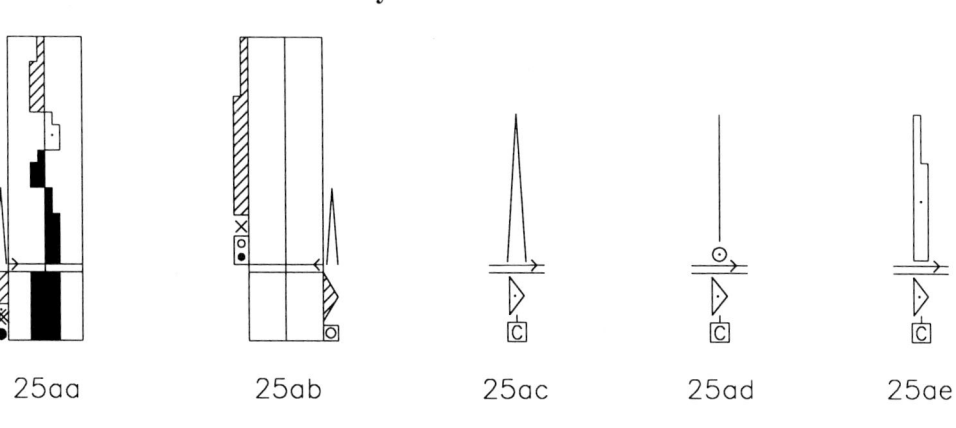

25aa   25ab   25ac   25ad   25ae

25.9. **Destinational Statement.** As is known, every gesture described with a direction symbol is a destination, illustrated in **25af** in which the arm moves forward, pauses and then moves up. A destinational statement of a path of the body-as-a-whole or of a limb can be made using the 'resultant bow'. In **25ag** the aim of the path, the result, is for the performer to end in the downstage right corner of the stage. In **25ah** the arm moves forward high with the destination of the hand touching the cheek of a person identified as P. Ex. **25ai** indicates that the flexion of the arm is for the purpose of the hand to touch the right side of the waist.

25.10. Ex. **25aj** contains a destinational statement both for direction and degree of leg contraction. In contrast, this end result is only approached in **25ak**, the gesture does not reach the 3 degree state of flexion nor the forward low direction. The performer has this instruction in mind, the viewer is only aware of an unfinished movement, a movement without a definite sense of arrival. Note the difference between this elongated 'V' indicating 'toward', and the short 'v' (placed within one square when using graph paper in a Labanotation score) which indicates a sequential, successive movement, **25al**.

25.11. **Contraction and Extension - Destination.** Ex. **25am** describes the arm contracting one degree, while maintaining the side middle direction. It is equal to **25an**, where the side middle direction is restated.[43] In **25ao** the arm moves to a 'neither flexed nor stretched' destination from a three-degree contracted side middle situation. The same destinational movement of **25ao** can be expressed as **25ap**.[44]

25.12. **Motion Toward a Defined State of Flexion or Extension.** Whereas the examples of **25am-25ap** show arrival at a defined destination, we are also concerned with the concept, the intention, of moving toward or away from a defined state of flexion or of extension. As mentioned before, **25aq** indicates arrival at the destination of being contracted one degree. In **25ar** the motion is *toward* that state, the performer has a goal in mind but does not reach it.[45] Similarly the goal of being contracted four degrees is not reached in **25as**. Nor in **25at** is the goal of one degree of extension reached.

Advanced Labanotation 91

Destinational Statement

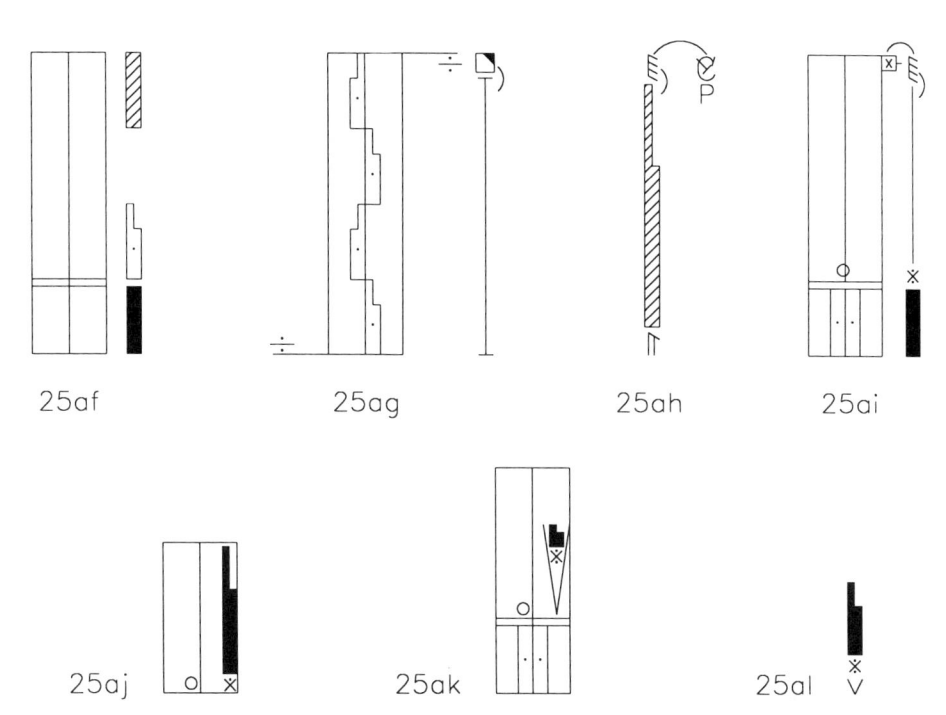

25af 25ag 25ah 25ai

25aj 25ak 25al

Contraction and Extension - Destination

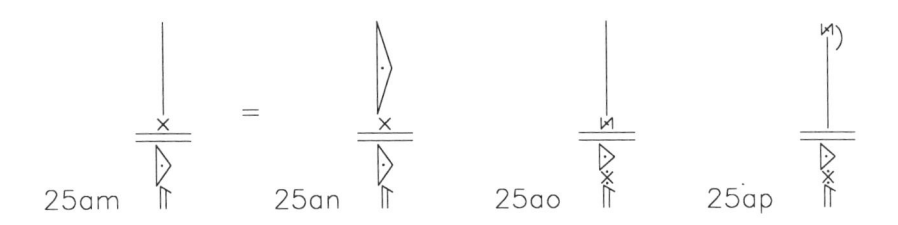

25am 25an 25ao 25ap

Motion Toward a Defined State of Flexion or Extension

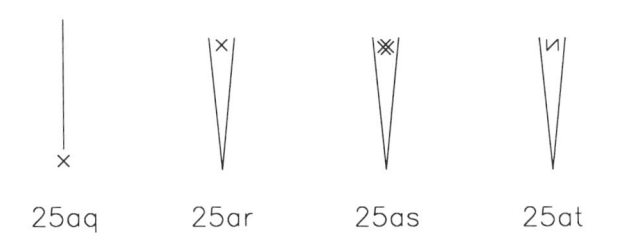

25aq 25ar 25as 25at

25.13. **Motion Away from a Defined State of Flexion or Extension.** One can also have the intention of moving away from a previous state. In **25au** the right arm starts four degrees contracted, and then moves away from that state. The degree of this motion away is not known. The nature of the movement will, of course, be one of *extending*, but the performer is not focussing on that aspect of the movement. Note that the unqualified 'away' sign of **25av** serves as a cancellation, hence the need to repeat the state from which movement is away. The motion away from the extended state in **25aw** will require the motion of *flexing*; the chosen description of the movement does not draw the performer's attention to this fact, awareness is on motion away from the previous state. In the case of **25ax**, the arm starts contracted one degree and then moves away from this state of contraction. Such motion could be either one of extending, or of contracting to a greater degree, the performance is left open, only departure from the previous state is stipulated.

25.14. In **25ay** moving away from the extended state has been given the destination of being folded three degrees. Note that folding actions can be indicated as well as degrees of contracting. From the very folded state at the start of **25az**, the right arm moves away from this state. The motion is, in fact, one of unfolding, **25ba**. These examples illustrate the possibilities of committing to paper the intent, awareness or focus of movement of this kind.

25.15. **Contracting and Extending - Motion Toward.** Ex. **25bb** shows a contraction sign with the degree of contraction left open. In place of the dots for specific degrees, the vertical ad lib. sign is drawn.[46] Thus in **25bc** the *motion of contracting* (no degree, no destination) is indicated.[47] It may happen that artistically what is important in a slow movement is the sensation/awareness of the *motion of contracting* with no destination, no end result in mind. If, however, for such a slow movement featuring the sensation/awareness of *contracting*, arrival at a specific state is also required, the two indications can be combined, as in **25bd**. In this example, from a side middle placement, a sustained motion of *contracting* takes place, and the arrival state of five degrees of contraction is also given. Ex. **25be** is the sign for the *motion of extending*; thus **25bf** shows the motion of *extending* coming from a five degree contracted state; in this example no arrival state is given, thus no specific end result is important.

Advanced Labanotation

Motion Away from a Defined State of Flexion or Extension

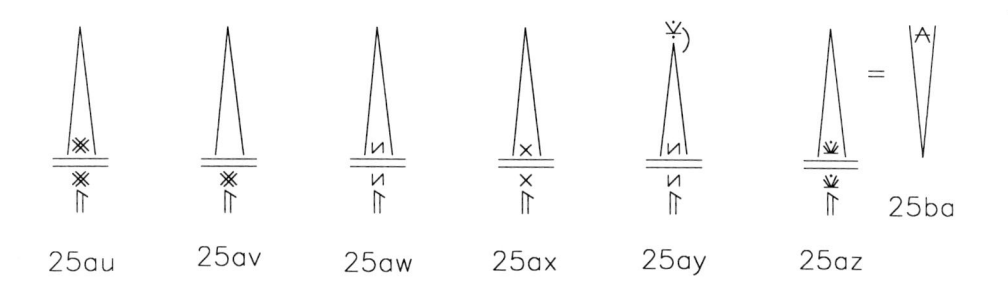

25au   25av   25aw   25ax   25ay   25az   25ba

Contracting and Extending - Motion Toward

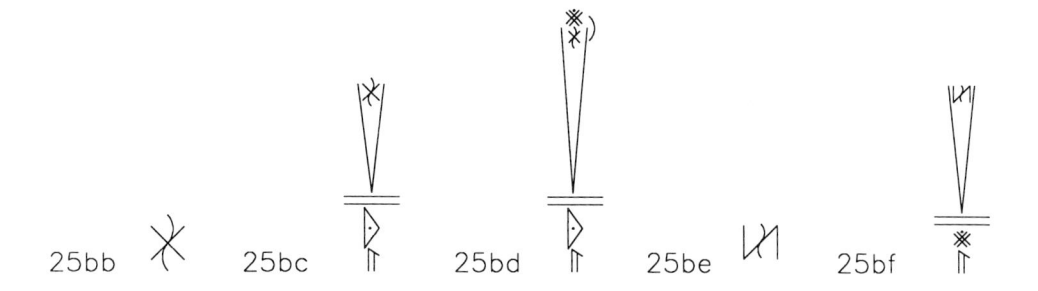

25bb   25bc   25bd   25be   25bf

VII   PATH SIGNS FOR GESTURES[48]

Rather than describing movements of the arms, legs, torso and head in terms of directions, they can also be described using path signs, such as horizontal paths, sagittal (somersault) paths, lateral (cartwheel) paths and diagonal circular paths lying in between. Indeed, many movement instructions use the word 'circle': "Make a full circle of the head.", "March in place, circle arms.", "Swing the lariat (lasso),[49] circling the arm overhead.", and so on.

A path sign placed outside the staff means a displacement of the body-as-a-whole. When placed within a gesture column, path signs are understood to refer to the path made by the extremity of the part of the body in question.

In Sections 26-33 focus will be on circles of the right arm. Circles of the head and torso will be dealt with in Section 34 and those of the hands and knees in Section 35.

26 Straight Path

26.1. Straight paths for gestures can be indicated by the straight path sign combined with a direction symbol. Ex. **26a** indicates a straight path forward horizontal from wherever the arm started, i.e. the extremity of the right arm, the hand (finger tips) describes a path moving forward horizontally. The starting and ending locations are not shown, only the path of the movement, the motion is given.

26.2. Placement of the direction symbol at the end of the path sign, as in **26b**, indicates a destination. Here the arm moves from wherever it was to the specific destination of forward middle, the hand making a straight path through space. In this example the starting position is also not stated.

26.3. A fuller investigation of the concept and use of a straight path gesture may be helpful. In **26c** the starting point for the arm and the destination result in the motion of a straight path as well as a destination. By adding a straight path sign, as in **26d**, the line of the movement should be stressed.

26.4. The destination is given in **26e**, but no starting point, thus the path cannot be known. It may be that in a particular piece of choreography it does not matter. The form of the path, straight, is stated in **26f**, but where it comes from to reach that destination is not known. With statement of the starting point in **26g** the movement to be performed is clear. This could also have been written as **26h**. Other placements of this straight path to a stated destination

Advanced Labanotation 95

may occur, as in **26i** and **26j**. To perform the path of these four examples the arm will have to bend slightly; this is understood and not written.

26.5. The action of **26k** is comparable to **26l**, except that for the latter a destination is given. Exs. **26m** and **26n** give a similar forward horizontal motion in a different setting. These and the next examples start with a flexed arm since this is a more functional state in which to begin such straight paths.

26.6. In the case of **26k** no distance is indicated for this motion. Approximate distance can be shown in the path sign; in **26o** a very short distance is stated; in **26p** a long distance should be covered. Because they are placed within a path sign, these distance signs do not refer to flexion or extension of the limb.

Path Signs for Gestures - Straight Path

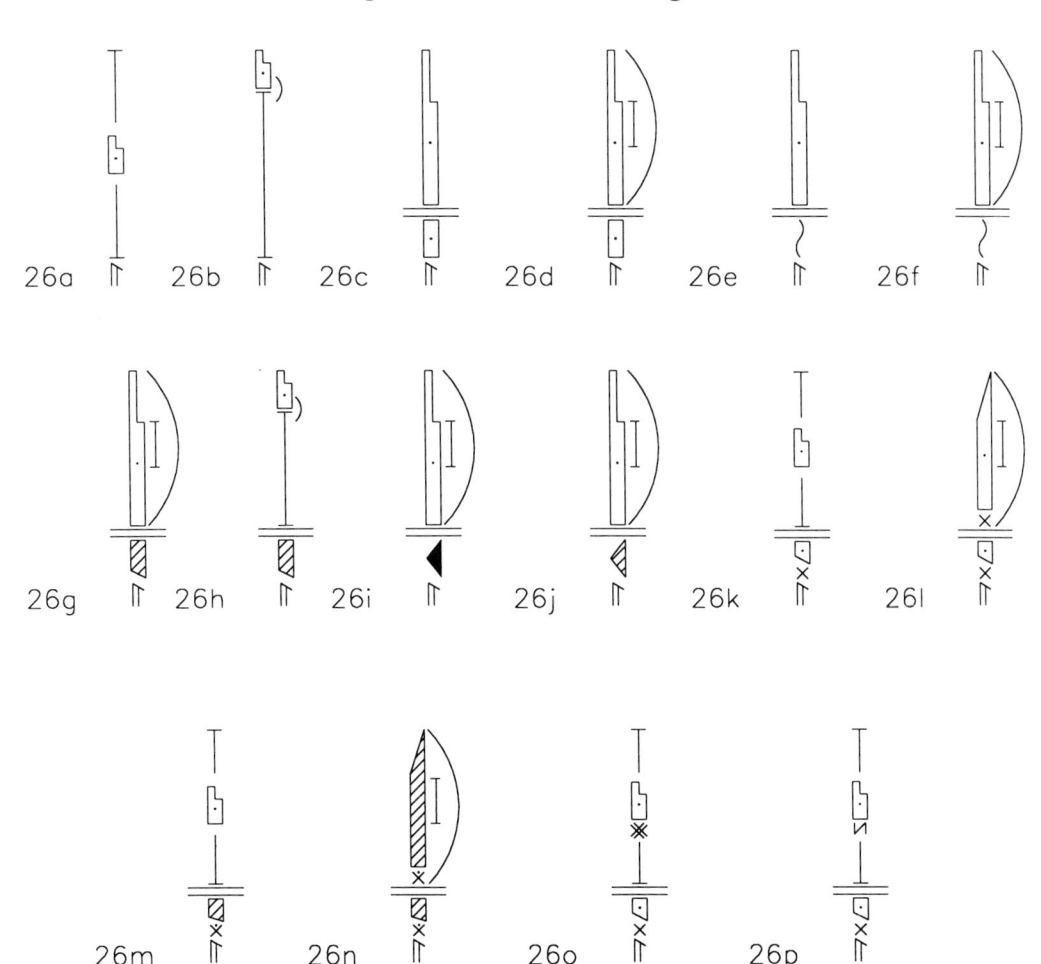

27 Analysis of Circular Paths for Gestures

27.1. Circles of the limb may be *planal* or *conical*. For a limb to describe a planal circle, the limb as a whole and the path it follows lie at right angles to the axis of the circle. When describing a conical circle, the angle between the limb and the axis will be less than 90°; the limb will trace the shape of a cone.

27.2. **Planal Circles.** There are three main forms of planal circles, each of which encompasses two of the three dimensions in the body. Each circle has two directions of motion.

27.3. The horizontal circle of **27a** lies on the plane which encompasses the lateral (side-side) and sagittal (forward-backward) dimensions.

27.4 Exs. **27b** and **27c** show the two main forms of planal circles which incorporate the vertical dimension. In **27b** the arm circles on the lateral plane, passing through the vertical and lateral dimensions around a sagittal axis; thus a cartwheel path is performed. The sagittal circle of **27c** passes through the sagittal and vertical dimensions, circling around a lateral axis; a somersault path. Because of the structure of the body, for the whole arm to achieve this circle, the upper torso will need to be included during the backward part of the circle.

27.5. Between the lateral (cartwheel) and sagittal (somersault) circles lie the diagonal circles. Related to this is a range of possible intermediate circles following vertical planes which lie between the simple lateral and sagittal circles. These may be compared to the vertical segments of an orange, **27d**.

27.6. Planal circles can be performed by the lower arm through rotation in the upper arm. Ex. **27e** illustrates a lateral circle for the left lower arm (a cartwheel path).

27.7. **Conical Circles.** A conical circle described by a limb produces a planal circle at the extremity. The planal circle described lies farther from the body than the planal circle to which it relates. As the angle between the limb and the cone axis decreases, the cone becomes increasingly narrower and the plane described by the extremity moves farther away from the body. Ex. **27f** illustrates a lateral (cartwheel) circle performed in front of the body, the dotted line indicating the shape of the cone made by the arm-as-a-whole; **27g** shows a sagittal (somersault path) circle performed with the arm out to the side. Ex. **27h**

Advanced Labanotation 97

shows a horizontal circle, performed overhead. These placements illustrate cones in the dimensional directions; they can, of course, occur in a range of intermediate locations.

Planal Circles

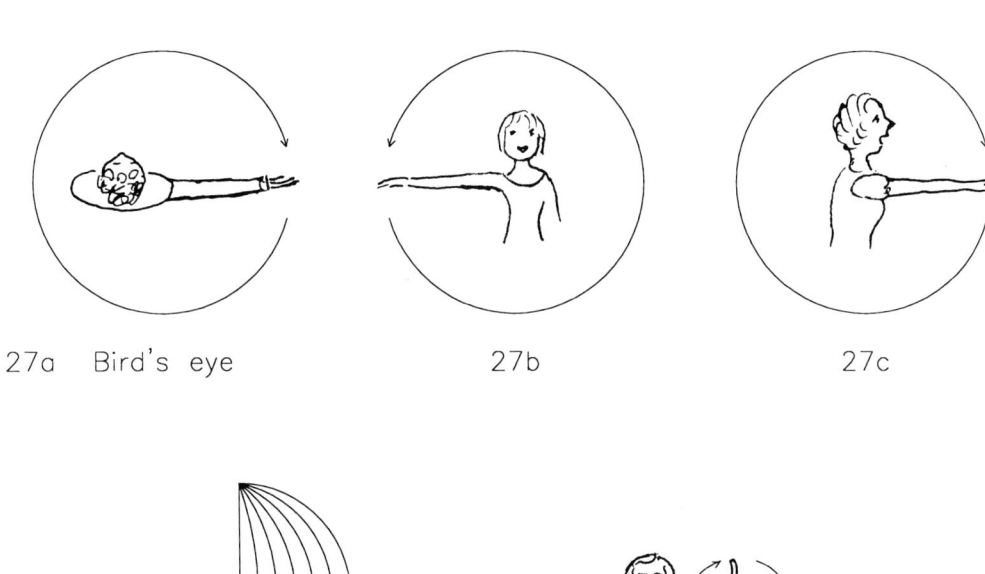

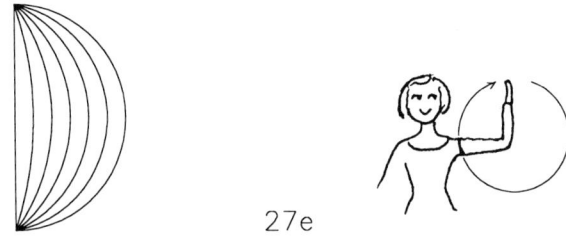

27a   Bird's eye   27b   27c

27d   27e

Conical Circles

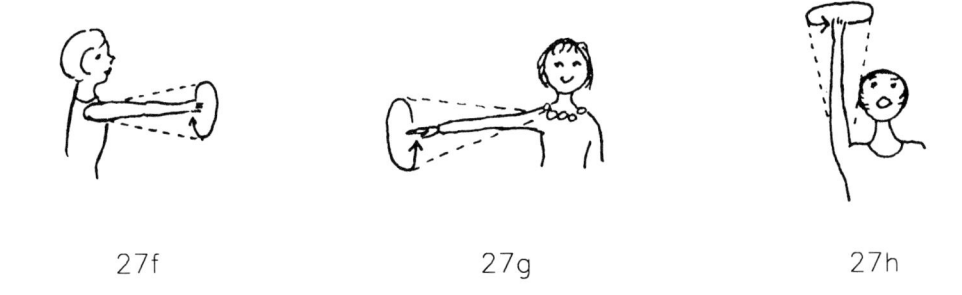

27f   27g   27h

28 Indication of Circular Path for Gestures

28.1. **Horizontal Circular Paths.** Horizontal circular paths are indicated by the signs of **28a** (counterclockwise) and **28b** (clockwise). These signs have an understood vertical axis, whether performed as planal or conical movement.

28.2. Horizontal planal movement will result from a middle level starting point. Ex. **28c** illustrates a planal version of **28a** using direction symbols. Note that the upper body needs to be involved to move the arm into the backward direction and maintain the horizontal line of the path. This movement could also be written as in **28d**, a full counterclockwise circular path starting from right side middle. Here, the notation immediately conveys the message that a circular path is to be performed. While the four direction symbols of **28c** produce a circle, visually **28d** makes an immediate statement.

28.3. Horizontal conical movement will result from starting points at other levels. Ex. **28e** illustrates a conical version of **28b**. The same movement is given in **28f**, described as a full clockwise circular path.

28.4. **Somersault Paths.** The sagittal, wheel-like circle can move forward, **28g**, or backward, **28h**. A planal forward somersault path is spelled out in **28i**, while **28j** spells out a conical backward somersault path. Again, these direction symbols can be replaced by the path signs to give an immediate message as to the kind of path the arm is to follow. Exs. **28k** and **28l** indicate the circles of **28i** and **28j** respectively.

28.5. **Cartwheel Paths.** Lateral (vertical) circles are illustrated in **28m** (to the left) and **28n** (to the right). Ex. **28o** illustrates a planal version of the cartwheel to the left, while in **28p** the extremity follows a cartwheel path to the right. This is expressed with path signs in **28q** and **28r** respectively. Note the abbreviated form of the cartwheel path signs, **28s** and **28t** for **28m** and **28n**, which some people find easier to read than the full sign.

28.6. The circular paths lying on the diagonals pose a choice of description and will be dealt with in Section 30.

Advanced Labanotation

Horizontal Circular Paths

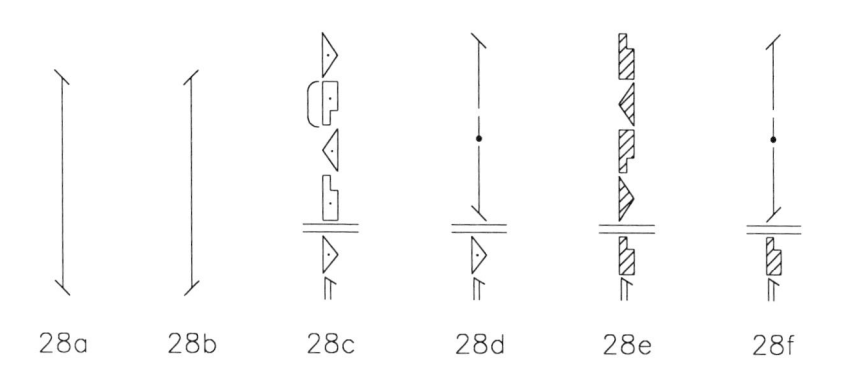

28a 28b 28c 28d 28e 28f

Somersault Paths

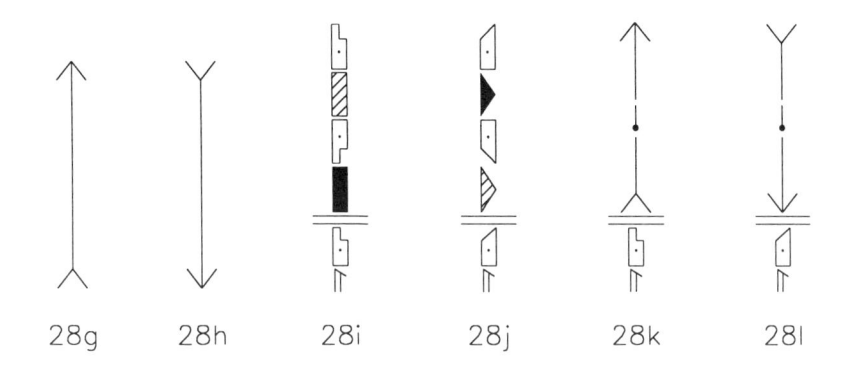

28g 28h 28i 28j 28k 28l

Cartwheel Paths

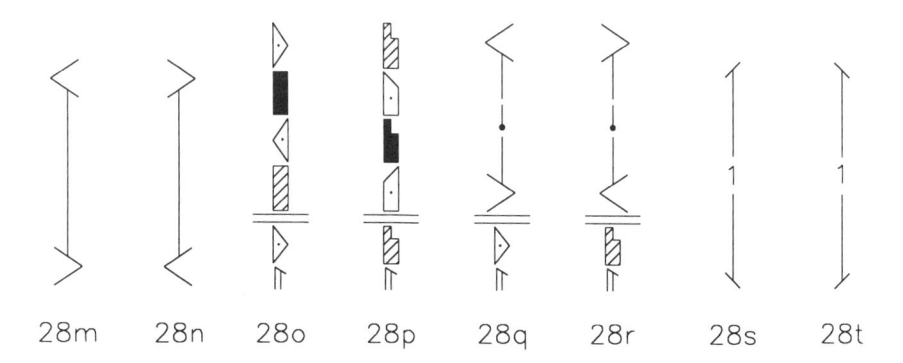

28m 28n 28o 28p 28q 28r 28s 28t

29 Elongated Circular Paths for Gestures

29.1. Circular paths may not always be true circles. Ex. **29a** illustrates a wide, laterally elongated circle, written with Design Drawing; in **29b** it is stretched vertically. Exs. **29c** and **29d** show the same for a figure-eight.

29.2. Such modifications of a shape, such as a circle or figure-eight, can be expressed in movement terms by use of the signs for spreading and closing laterally, **29e**; sagittally, **29f**; diagonally, **29g** or **29h**; and vertically, **29i**, the vertical dimension being stated by combining white and black circles with the spreading sign.[50]

29.3. Thus, in **29j** the cartwheel path is spread laterally, producing **29k**. In **29l** it spreads vertically, with **29m** illustrating the result. The latter could also be considered the result of a lateral contraction, **29n**, causing the circle to spread into the vertical dimension.

29.4. The circle can also be elongated along a right side high-left side low axis, as shown in **29o**, illustrated in **29p**.

29.5. The same device can be applied to sagittal (somersault) circular paths. In **29q** the circling stretches in the forward-backward dimension; in **29r** it stretches vertically, which can also be indicated by a sagittal contraction, **29s**. Illustrations for these would be the same as **29k** and **29m** respectively, but seen from side view.

29.6. For horizontal circles spreading may be lateral, **29t** (illustrated in **29u**), or sagittal, **29v** (illustrated in **29w**). These illustrations are seen from above, bird's eye view.

29.7. Amount of modification can be indicated to some degree. Ex. **29x** (illustrated from bird's eye view in **29y**) states exaggerated sagittal spreading for a horizontal path.

29.8. In writing such circular paths, decisions need to be made as to which description is the most appropriate and practical for the need in hand.

Advanced Labanotation 101

Elongated Circular Paths for Gestures

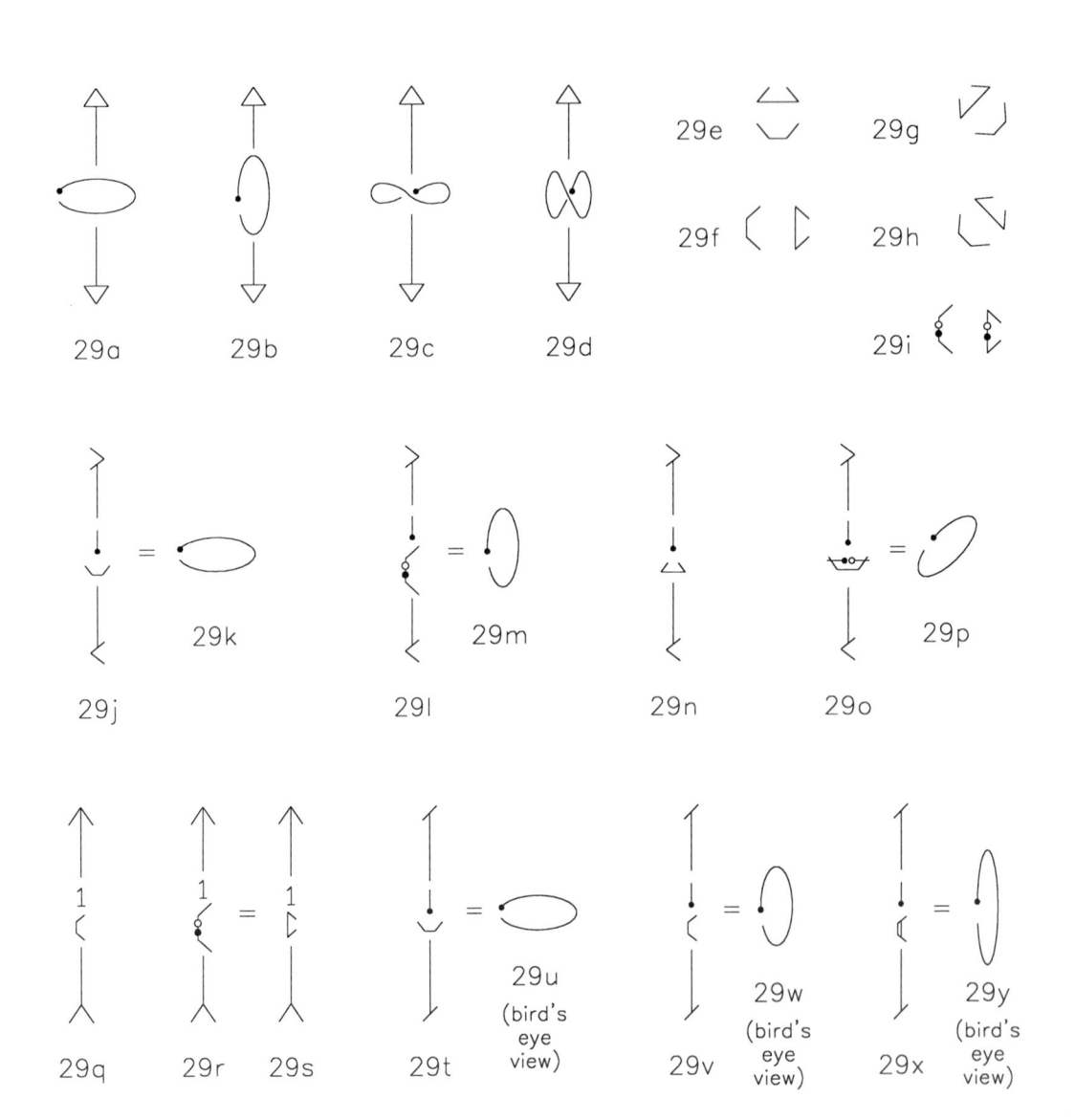

29a 29b 29c 29d

29e 29f 29g 29h 29i

29j 29k 29l 29m 29n 29o 29p

29q 29r 29s 29t (bird's eye view) 29u (bird's eye view) 29v 29w (bird's eye view) 29x 29y (bird's eye view)

30 Diagonal Circles, Tilted Circles for Gestures

30.1. A circle which does not have one of the three main dimensions as its axis, can be described by stating the specific axis used.[51] Ex. **30a** illustrates the understood lateral axis for the forward and backward sagittal paths, indicated with horizontal pins (tacks). Similarly **30b** shows the understood sagittal axis for lateral circular paths.

30.2. **Diagonal Circles.** Diagonal circles lie between the sagittal and lateral circles and thus the axes for such diagonal circles are a combination of the axes for the sagittal and lateral paths. The diagonal directional pattern of **30c** produces a circular path which lies between a somersault and a cartwheel path, the axis therefore being a combination of **30a** and **30b**. This axis can be stated with the two pins of **30d**. Thus, **30e** describes the movement of **30c** as a forward somersault circle around the stated axis. The same circling may be seen or experienced as a cartwheel to the right around this same axis, **30f**.[52] The simplified cartwheel sign is shown in **30g**.

30.3. **Tilted Circles.** The horizontal circle of **30h** may be tilted to produce **30i**. The understood axis for the horizontal path of **30h** is, of course, the vertical up/down, as indicated in parentheses in **30j**. The axis for the tilted circle of **30i** is shown in **30k**, i.e. a forward high/backward low axis. Note that the axis is stated first, then the amount of circling. This same circular path could also be viewed as a tilted cartwheel, **30l**, shown with the simplified sign in **30m**.

30.4. Similarly, the circle written out in **30n** can be seen as a somersault path which has been tilted to left side high/right side low, and thus circling around the axis of **30o**. Equally it could be experienced as a tilted circular path, raised on the left, lowered on the right, the axis being the same, **30p**.

Advanced Labanotation 103

Diagonal Circles

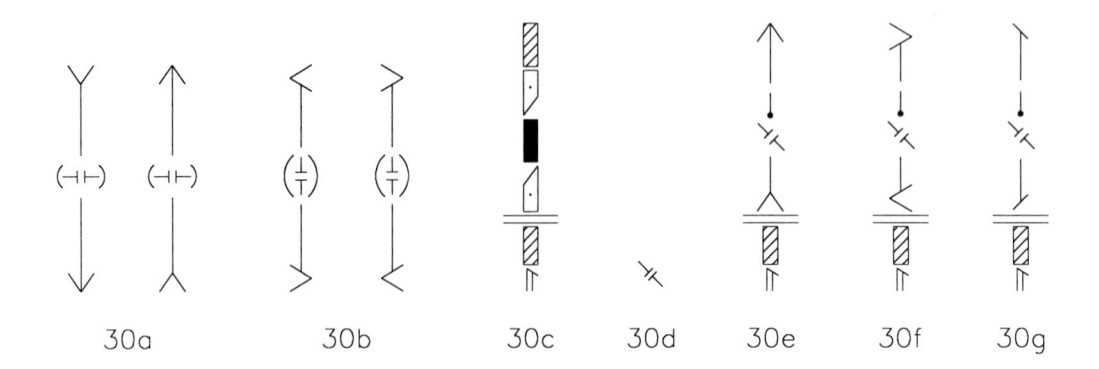

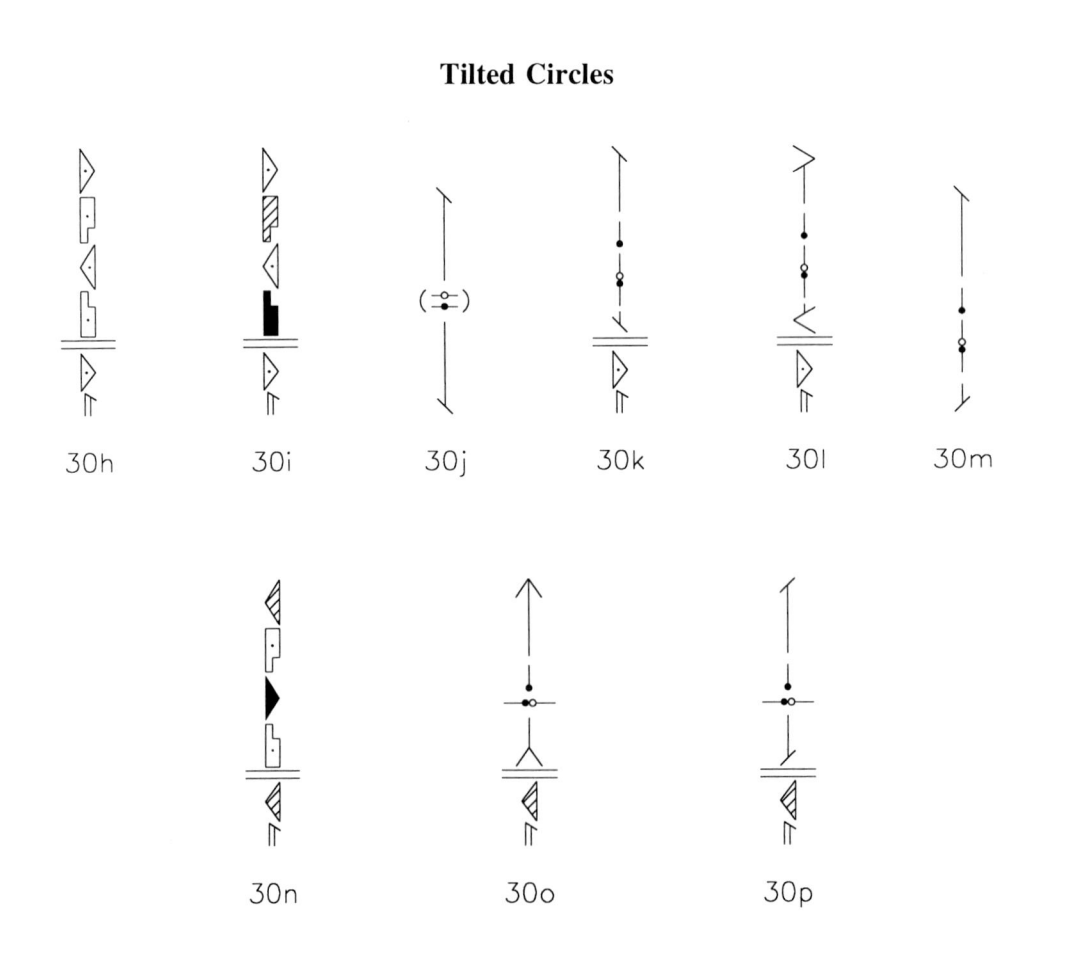

30a 30b 30c 30d 30e 30f 30g

Tilted Circles

30h 30i 30j 30k 30l 30m

30n 30o 30p

31 Location and Size of Circle for Gestures

31.1. Size and location of a planal circle indicated by a path sign is usually clear. Ex. **31a** states a starting location and full cartwheel to the right; it will result in a planal circle, the arm automatically passing through the opposite diametral side right point. For the conical movement of **31b** the circle will pass through the diametral point of diagonal right forward middle.

31.2. The diametral point can be stated by writing a small direction symbol attached to the outer edge of a half-circle curve.[53] This indication is placed in the path sign. Ex. **31c** confirms that the circle of **31b** passes through the right forward middle point, illustrated in **31d**. A modified version of this circle is given in **31e**, in which forward middle is the diametral (halfway) point; this modified circle is slightly off the lateral plane, the previous sagittal axis being slightly displaced toward diagonal left forward-right backward, as illustrated in **31f**. With forward high being the diametral (halfway) point in **31g**, yet another size and location of the circle takes place. This version, illustrated in **31h**, begins to take on the character of a sagittal circle. If left forward low is the diametral point, the resulting small circle could more closely be described as that of a forward somersault, **31i**. The advantage of indicating the diametral point is that the size as well as the placement of the circle is known.

31.3. As indicated in **30e** and **30k**, double pins may be used to indicate the axis when this is more practical for the movement description, rather than statement of the diametral point. In **31j**, the axis provides a differently placed circle from **31b**, the circle being more sagittal. Because the axis is slanted in **31k** (forward high-backward low), the resulting circle will slant backward high to forward low. It should be noted that the sign for a lateral circle is still being used for these modified circles, the diametral point or indication of the axis producing the more three-dimensional placement.[54]

31.4. As can be seen, instances occur where it becomes somewhat arbitrary to determine whether a cartwheel, somersault, or horizontal circular path sign should be used; they become somewhat interchangeable. In fact, with the additional information about axis and diametral point, the basic circular path signs of **31l** can be used. For example, the cartwheel of **31g** could be written as a somersault path, **31m**. (See also 33.2.)

Advanced Labanotation

Location and Size of Circle for Gestures

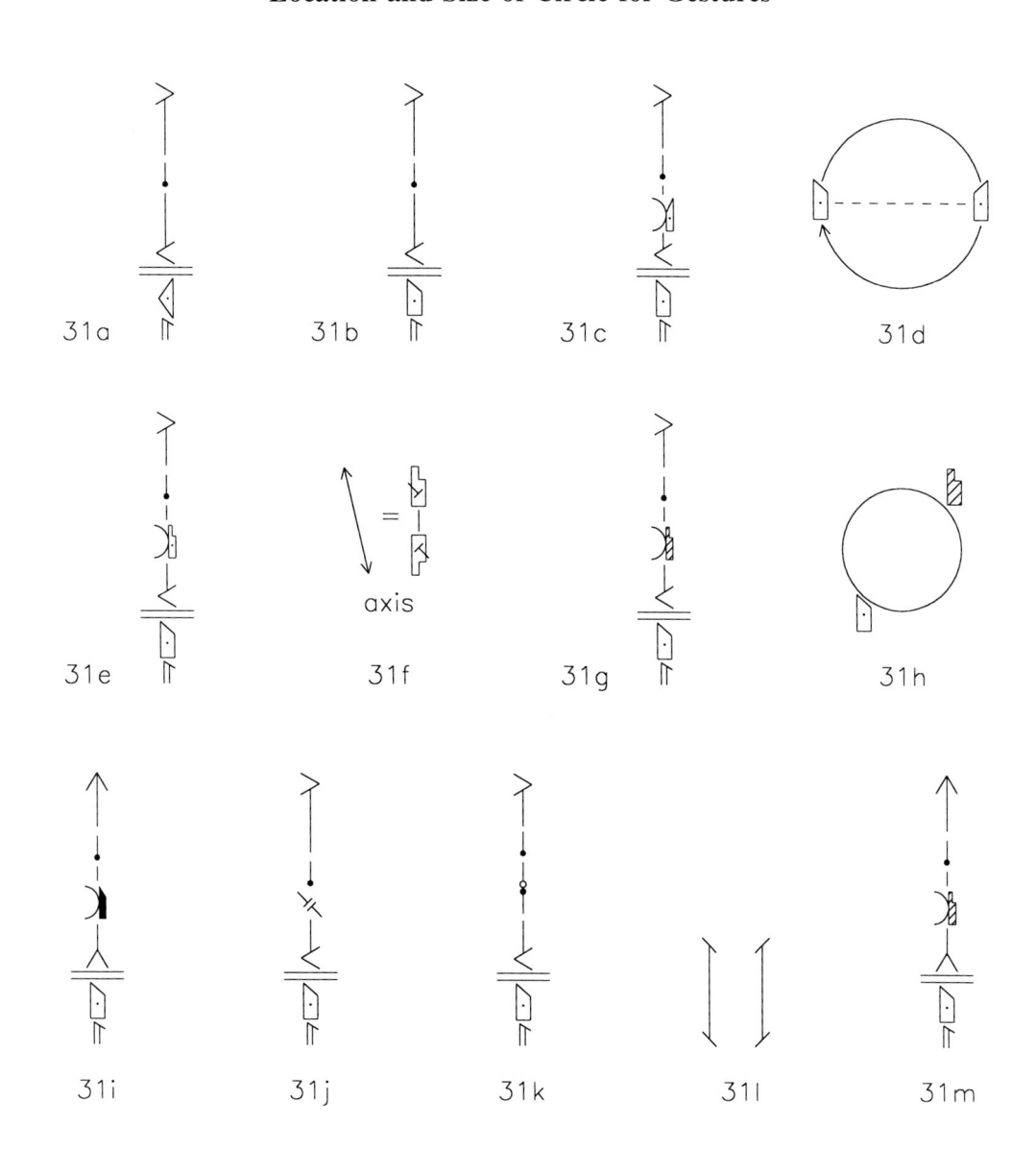

31a 31b 31c 31d

31e 31f 31g 31h

axis

31i 31j 31k 31l 31m

32 Circles Achieved Through Flexion of the Limb; Spirals

32.1. **Circles Achieved Through Flexion of the Limb.** So far we have dealt with circles of the limb-as-a-whole, no specific flexion or extension of the limb being indicated or expected during the circling. Such circles could also be performed with a flexed (bent) limb, the degree of flexion being kept constant. The more flexed the limb, the smaller the circle that will be described by the extremity. Ex. **32a** shows a cartwheel path to the right performed with a contracted arm, the degree of contraction being retained.

32.2. To be considered are circles in which flexion and extension are used to create the circle. Ex. **32b** shows a horizontal, clockwise circle which starts with the arm forward low. From this starting position, with the torso upright, only a small horizontal circle can be achieved in front of the body; with the torso forward, as in **32c**, a larger circle is possible, the arm producing a conical shape. For the circle to be in front of an upright torso it would have to be much smaller and, for the extremity (the hand) to describe a true horizontal circle, the arm must bend. Ex. **32d**, written with direction symbols together with flexion and extension signs, describes a probable performance of **32b**.

32.3. Ex. **32e** shows a lateral circle to the right, starting with the arm forward middle and three degrees contracted. The action might be one of polishing a mirror on the wall in front of you. It is difficult to describe the movement of **32e** through direction symbols. In **32f** the diametral direction and deviations have been written to give the circular idea for an interpretation of **32e**; this, however, lacks the immediate message, the intention to describe a circle. In addition, the axis of the 'circle' has shifted slightly to the right. In **32e** there is no retention for the flexed state, thus some leeway may occur.

32.4. There is also the question of where on the lateral circle the movement begins: rising first, as in **32g**? Moving to the right first, **32h**? Moving down first, **32i**? And so on. Each of these possibilities still uses the same lateral circle. To define which should be used, the diametral point needs to be stated, as in **32j**. This statement will also give an indication of the size of the circle.

Circles Achieved Through Flexion of the Limb

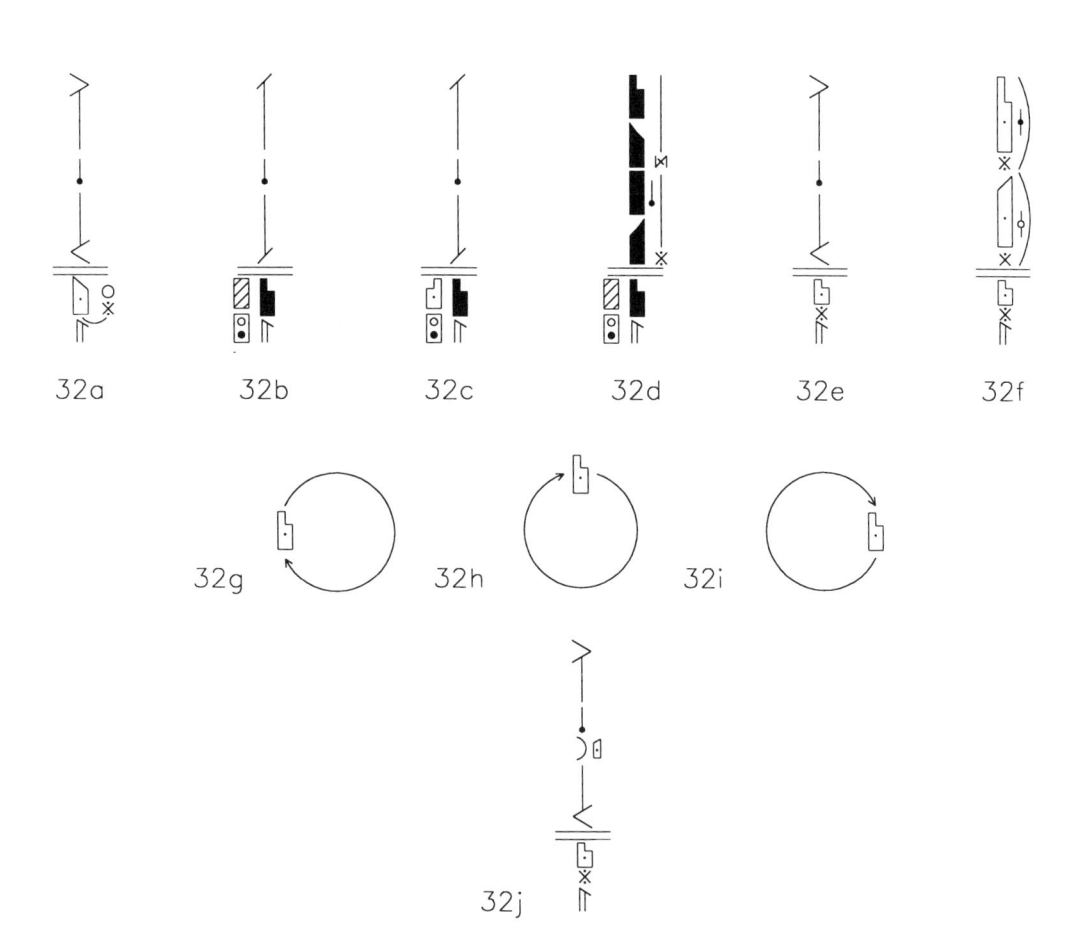

32a 32b 32c 32d 32e 32f

32g 32h 32i

32j

32.5. Spiral Paths. Spiral paths may be planal or conical and are produced through flexion and/or extension of the limb.

32.6. A planal circle can decrease in size thus making a spiral design which lies on the same plane. In **32k**, the arm gradually flexes while performing three cartwheel paths. This pattern, illustrated in **32l**, could also be written with Design Drawing, **32m** (for design drawing see the Advanced Labanotation issue *Shape, Design, Trace Patterns*).

32.7. A reverse pattern, moving from smaller to larger in a sagittal path, is shown in **32n**. Here the arm, starting flexed, gradually extends during three somersault paths. This pattern, illustrated in **32o**, is written through Design Drawing in **32p**, the design being drawn as though on the wall at your right. This same pattern may also be written as if on the wall to your left, **32q**. Note that in this case the Design Drawing has to be reversed.

32.8. **Helical Paths.** A helix[55] is performed through maintaining the size of a repeatedly performed circle while the limb travels in space, **32r**, illustrated in **32s**. In this example no indication is given regarding size of circle. If no change of size, increase or decrease, is added, the size remains the same. However, if the need arises to indicate that the circle size must remain constant, this can be indicated by placing within a diamond the symbol for spatially neither long nor short (the composite sign) as in **32n**, thus indicating the spatial aspect to be neither larger nor smaller, i.e. no change of spatial size. Ex. **32t** gives a statement of size, the indication for spatially small being placed in an addition bracket. Ex. **32u** shows the same helix written as Design Drawing, the number four indicating four circles. That the size of the circling remains the same does not need to be indicated here. When needed, statement of size can be indicated by stating the diametral direction for the circle.

32.9. **Three-dimensional Spiral**. A helix which expands or contracts becomes a three-dimensional spiral. Ex. **32v** shows a spiral which advances forward and also enlarges, the arm ending forward high. This is illustrated in **32w**. The sign for 'increase in size' (grow spatially larger) is added. The same spiral can be written with Design Drawing, **32x**.

Advanced Labanotation

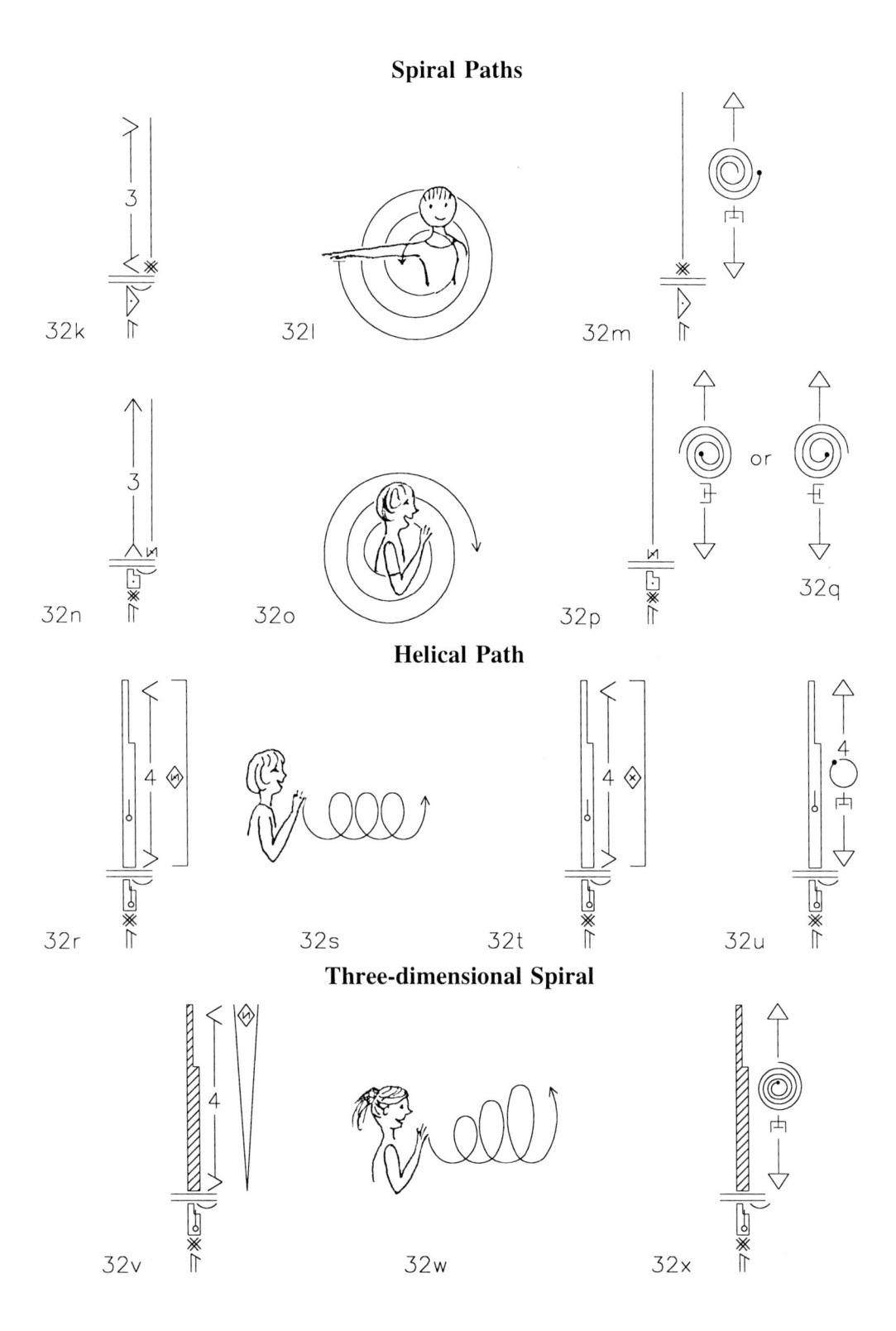

Spiral Paths

32k 32l 32m

32n 32o 32p 32q

Helical Path

32r 32s 32t 32u

Three-dimensional Spiral

32v 32w 32x

33 Indication of 'Surface' for a Gestural Circle

33.1.   As already explored in **32k** and **32n**, circular paths may often be experienced as occurring on a surface in a way comparable to awareness of a surface in Design Drawing.[56] The kinds of paths now being explored will involve unemphasized flexion and extension of the limb. For the three main forms of planal circles there is an understood surface for each. For the horizontal circles of **33a** it may be a surface parallel with the floor, it could also be the ceiling, although this choice is rarer, **33b**. For sagittal circles, **33c**, it is the wall at the right or left, **33d**, the choice depends on context. Cartwheel paths, **33e**, usually occur on the flat wall surface in front, **33f**. In theory, they could be imagined to occur on the wall behind, but this is awkward and not practical.

33.2.   The figure of **33g** shows a person drawing a circle on a horizontal table. In the notation of this, **33h**, the surface sign given here should not be needed, it should be understood. When the table surface is tilted 45° as in a slanted desk, **33i**, the surface is now forward low, **33j**. A further 45° tilt, as in **33k**, and it is comparable to writing on a blackboard or on the wall in front of you, the surface being directly in front, **33l**. At this angle, the circle has, in fact, become a cartwheel, but the horizontal circular path sign can still be used at any angle as long as the surface (or other indication of placement) is stated.

33.3.   Intermediate degrees of slant are shown by combining two pins. The more gentle slant of **33m** is shown with the pins of **33n**. The steeper slant of **33o** is indicated with the pins of **33p**. This tilting of a surface from vertical toward horizontal can also occur for sagittal circles.

33.4.   A vertical surface may also be tilted upward, as illustrated in **33q**. Here it may be envisaged as a slanting ceiling, indicated by **33r**. A further tilt and it becomes the ceiling, **33s**, indicated by **33t**.

33.5.   Vertical surfaces also exist in the diagonal directions, as illustrated in the drawing of **33u**. The vertical surface of 'a' in this drawing is shown as **33v**; that of 'b' as **33w**. These diagonal surfaces may also slant toward the ceiling or toward the floor, as in **33x** and **33y**. Describing circular patterns on these surfaces may be written as Design Drawing patterns, **33z**, drawn on the surface of **33i** or as circular paths, **33aa**, depending on intent.

Advanced Labanotation 111

Indication of 'Surface' for a Gestural Circle

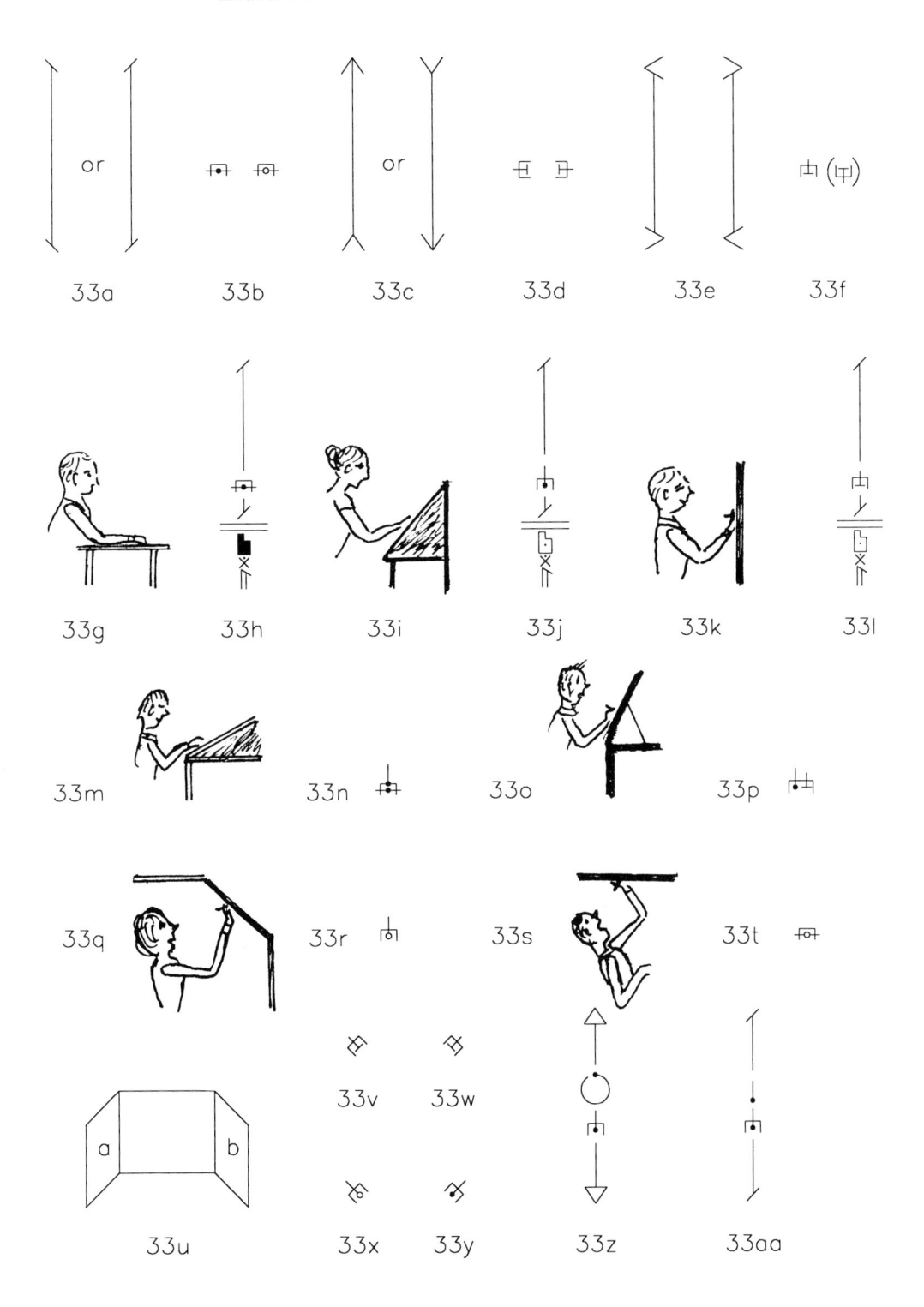

33a   33b   33c   33d   33e   33f

33g   33h   33i   33j   33k   33l

33m   33n   33o   33p

33q   33r   33s   33t

33u   33v   33w   33z   33aa
      33x   33y

34 Circular Paths for Head, Torso and Pelvis

34.1. Circling for the head and torso, for which the extremity of the head describes the path, are usually horizontal paths. Partial sagittal and lateral paths can also be described, often they are made possible through tilting and flexing parts of the spine in the appropriate direction. These will be explained later.

34.2. Ex. **34a** shows a clockwise circular path for the head, starting with the head inclined forward. The head must, of course, be off the vertical for such a horizontal path to occur. Performance of this circular path may vary. A number rather than a pin is used in **34a**, because there is no **complete** change of front during the full circle. There is often the tendency to include rotation in the direction of the circling, thus augmenting the sense of the size of the path. The simple indication of **34a** does not specify use of or elimination of rotation.

34.3. Circling the head without rotating, that is, keeping the nose aligned to the same room direction, may require practice. For the head to circle without any turning, as it does in the directional description of **34b**, a space hold is added, **34c**. This usage of the space hold is derived from the indication of walking a circular path without change of front, **34d**. Rotation of the head in the direction of the circling is given in **34e**.

34.4. In **34f**, an example from Shawn's Fundamental Exercises,[57] the movement is written with direction symbols with repeats indicating the number of circles. The overall pattern is stated more simply in **34g**.

34.5. Wheeling of the torso in **34h** causes a change of Front for the torso, indicated by the black pins. Such wheeling could also be described as rotations around the vertical axis, as in **34i**. Because the turn signs leave little room for the key, it is placed alongside in a bracket.[58]

34.6. Ex. **34j** is a torso exercise in which change of Front of the torso is not included. The circular path is drawn by the extremity, the head. To remain horizontal, much flexibility is needed in the hip joints and spine, particularly in the backward direction. In **34k** this circle is spelled out with direction symbols.

34.7. The pelvic circling of **34l** does not include a rotatary action, i.e. there is no change of front. The pelvis must displace to start a horizontal circle; here the displacement is a shift forward. In **34m**, from a backward shift, the pelvis

Advanced Labanotation

circles sagittally around a lateral axis outside the pelvis. During this circle the pelvis should remain vertical; sagittal pelvic rotation should not occur here, the movement is produced through leg flexion (not notated here).

Circular Paths for Head, Torso and Pelvis

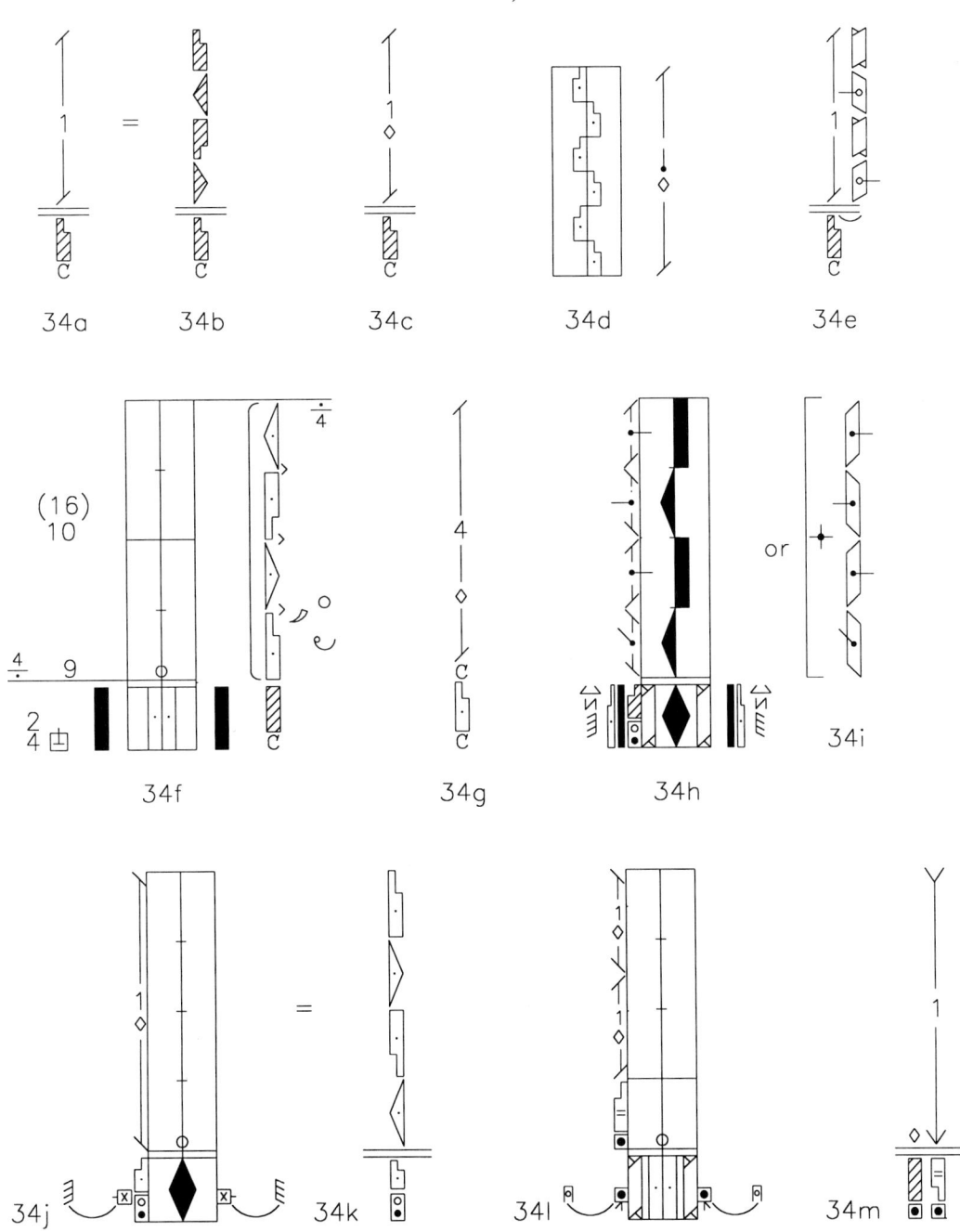

34a 34b 34c 34d 34e

34f 34g 34h 34i

34j 34k 34l 34m

35 Circular Paths for Hands, Knees

35.1. Hand circles occur in many dances and in many cultures.[59] They may be ornamental, pantomimic, or to handle an object.[60] Depending on where the arm is spatially, hand circling may be appropriately described as sagittal paths, lateral paths or horizontal paths. When the arm is moving spatially, it is more practical to use a description based on the build of the wrist, i.e. using the Individual Body Part Cross of Axes. For this clockwise or counterclockwise circling, as analysed when the arm is down, suffices, **35a**. Note that in this example a starting point for the hand is given.

35.2. Ex. **35b** shows the arm in a forward location, the same physical action then follows, the interpretation of the horizontal path sign being made clear through use of the Individual Body Part Key. Without this key the analysis would be of a cartwheel, as in **35c**. A similar movement occurs in **35d** with the arm out to the side. Here, without the key a backward somersault path would need to be written. In neither of these is a starting location for the circling shown.

35.3. In **35e** the backward fold of the wrist indicates where the circle should start. Hand circling while the arm moves is shown in **35f**, the hand movement continues to be physically the same.

35.4. Stirring with the index finger, **35g**, is facilitated by passive reaction in the hand.

35.5. The right knee circles in **35h**. The ball of the foot stays on the ground and the leg reacts passively during the circling which ends with a kick into a lunge. If the circling is to be large, as in **35i**, a greater degree of passive facilitation of the leg will be needed; this is not spelled out here but would be understood. The size of the circling can also be shown as in **35j**.

Advanced Labanotation

Circular Paths for Hands, Knees

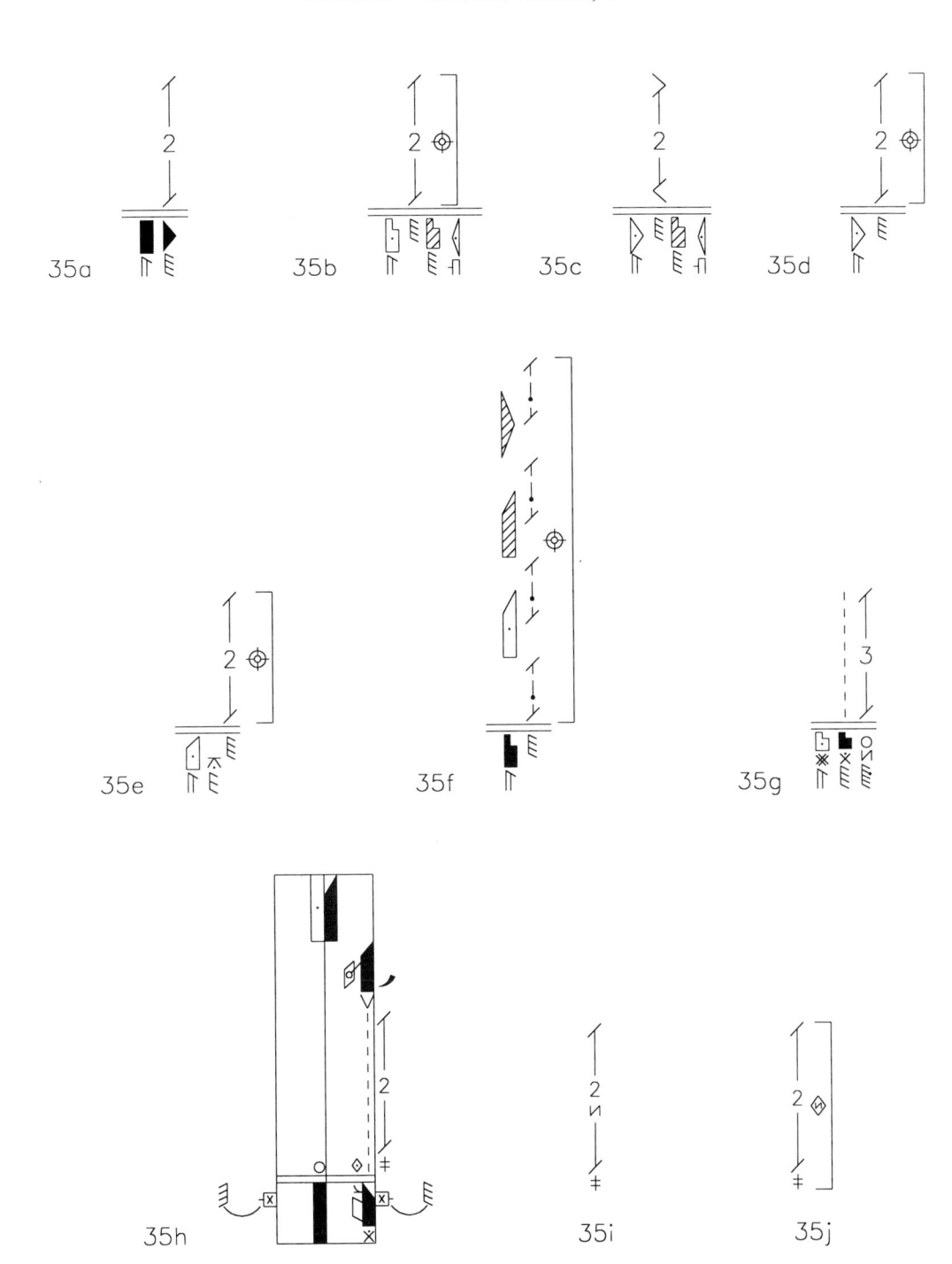

35a 35b 35c 35d

35e 35f 35g

35h 35i 35j

36 Performance Details for Paths for Limbs

36.1. This section deals with certain details in performing paths for gestures which have not yet been explored in this book.

36.2. **Spatial Placement of a Conical Circle.** From its starting position in **36a**, the arm cannot perform a backward sagittal circle as it is located at the axis of that circle. No problem is encounted in **36b** as the arm starts in a situation above the required axis, thus the circle of **36c**, seen from the performer's point of view, will take place. A smaller cone of the same kind will be performed in **36d**, the arm starting just slightly above side middle. Moving away from the axis can be indicated as being linked to the start of the circle. In **36e** a small downward displacement leads into the circular path. This is illustrated in **36f**. The amount of displacement gives an indication of size of the circle.

36.3. In a similar way the starting point can be shown for circular patterns which are not cones. In **36g** the arm is forward low, contracted two degrees. A horizontal circle is to be performed by the extremity, how is this circle to start? Ex. **36h** shows with the black dot four possible starting points (as seen from above). Here the device of **36e** is needed to give the appropriate start. A slight forward movement gives the starting direction in **36i**; this will produce the lower left circle shown in **36h**. A slight displacement to the right would produce the lower left circle of **36h**; a slight movement backward would produce the upper right circle, and a slight displacement to the left would result in the lower right circle. All these circles will be quite small.

36.4. **Spatial Retention for Direction of Gestural Path.** The intention of **36j** is for the arm to continue its lateral path despite the twist of the torso. To achieve this path space holds (white or black) need to be used in the direction symbols once the torso turn begins. A simpler description to achieve the desired arm circle is **36k**. Here the path of the circle is shown to have a spatial retention.

Advanced Labanotation

Spatial Placement of a Conical Circle

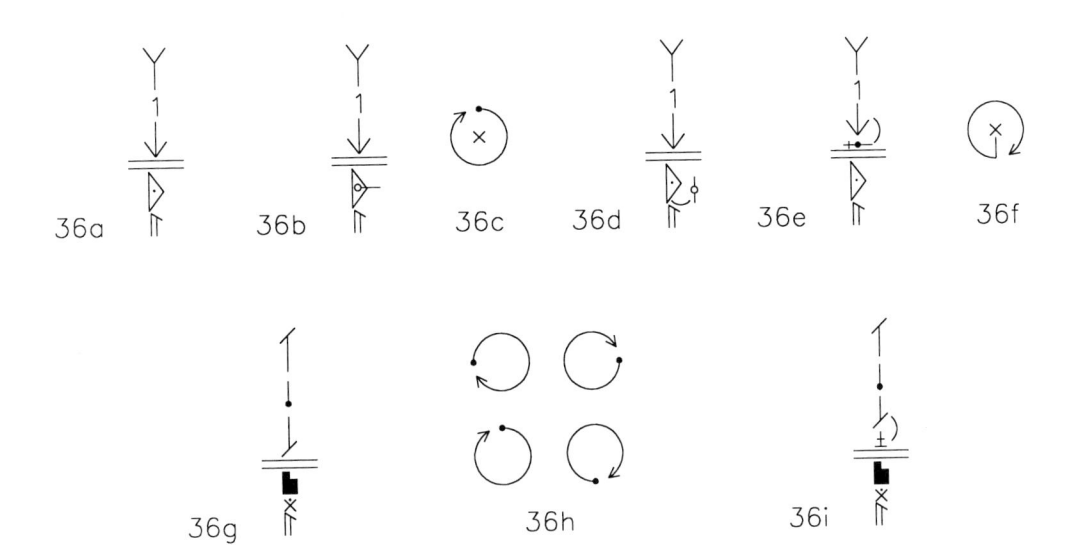

36a 36b 36c 36d 36e 36f

36g 36h 36i

Spatial Retention for Direction of Gestural Path

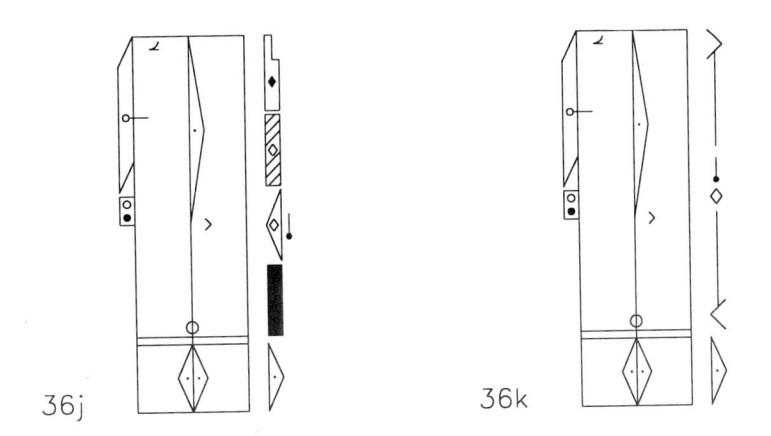

36j 36k

36.5. The same idea, but in an increasingly more complex setting is seen in comparing the next examples. In **36l** the right arm makes two lateral circles while walking in a circle. Because the arm pattern remains related to the Standard system of reference, this same can be written with direction symbols, as in **36m**. Revolving on a straight path to the side in **36n** is accompanied by two lateral circles which remain on the same spatial plane. If written with direction symbols the arm gesture would be described as in **36o**. Determining the constantly changing directions is not easy, thus one welcomes the simpler description of **36n**. Here, as with all steps revolving on a straight path, only the first step is physically to the side, the rest of the steps adjust their physical direction to adhere to the straight path while turning. The question may arise as to whether the arm crosses in front or behind the body. If important this would need to be stated.

36.6. Use of the Constant Cross Key for both the direction of the steps and also the circular arm movement is shown in **36p**. While the physical step directions keep changing, the sideward progression is constant, thus the symbols clearly indicate the direction of travel. This appears similar in result to **36n** because both start facing front. Should the performer start facing stage left, as in **36q**, the forward direction for the right arm at the start and for the forward steps, will be toward the audience, producing the same physical sequence, both for the steps and for the arm gesture as in **36p**. The steps will move toward the front of the stage, but start sideward right in relation to the performer.

Advanced Labanotation

Spatial Retention for Direction of Gestural Path (continued)

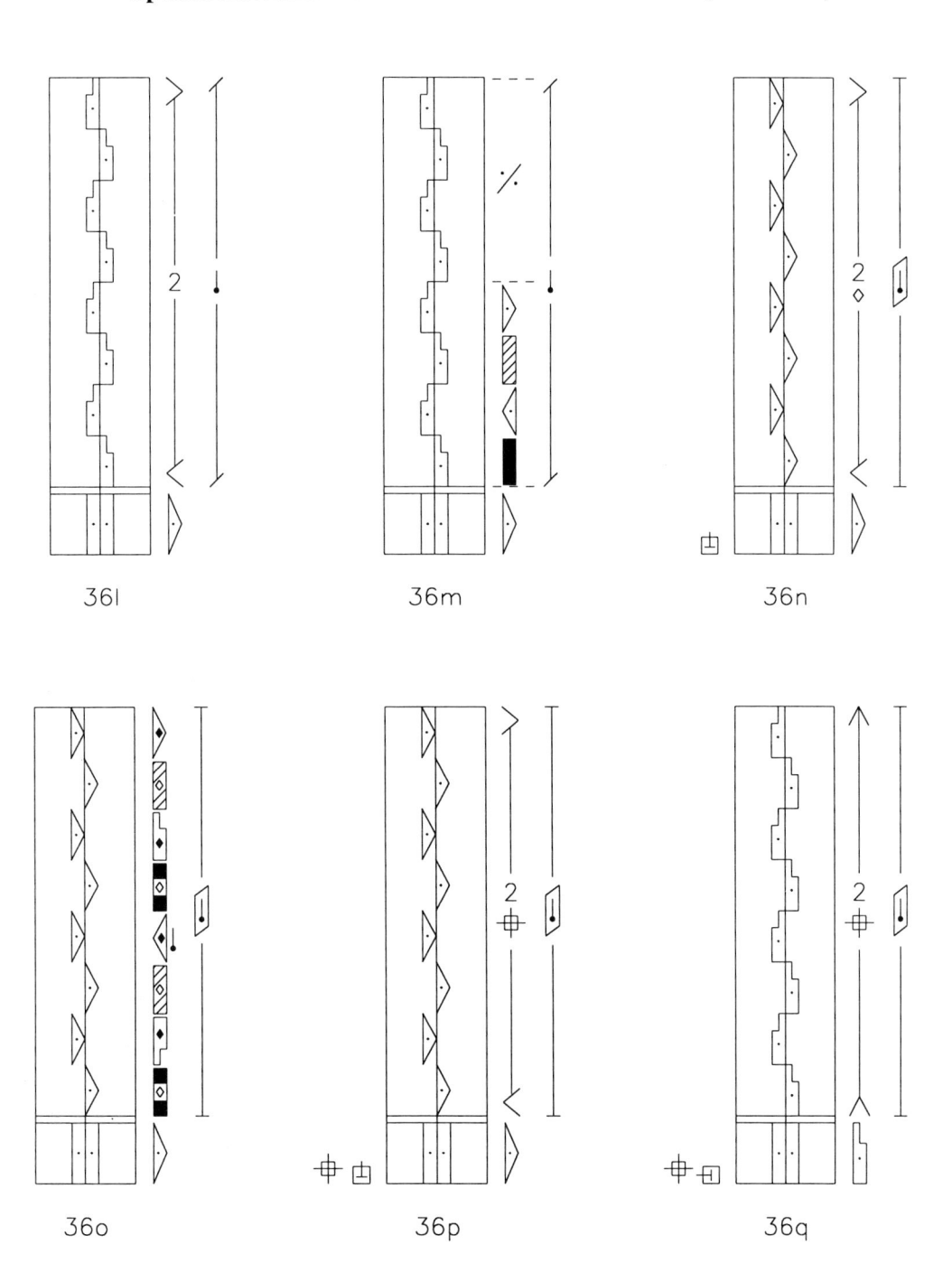

36l 36m 36n

36o 36p 36q

Spatial Variations

36.7. **Timing of Gestural Circles.** The advantage of using direction symbols to describe gestural circles is that changes in timing can easily be seen. In **36r** the timing indicates a swing which begins rapidly and then increasingly slows down. The reverse is true for **36s**, the start is slower and the gesture gains speed, ending with an accent as it arrives at its destination. As can be seen, this advantage is lost when path signs are used, **36t**; one assumes an even distribution.

36.8. Speed and changes in speed can be shown by using the Time Sign[61] for speed, **36u**. The arm circle of **36v** is shown to decrease in speed, the indication being put in an addition bracket alongside the movement. An increase in speed is shown in **36w**.

36.9. The lower part of the basic sign for speed can be used by itself to indicate a decrease in speed, here applied to the triple backward arm circle of **36x**. In contrast, the speed is increased in **36y**. These smaller signs have the advantage of being able to be placed within a direction symbol. In **36z** the arm gesture slows down as it rises.

Advanced Labanotation

Timing of Gestural Circles

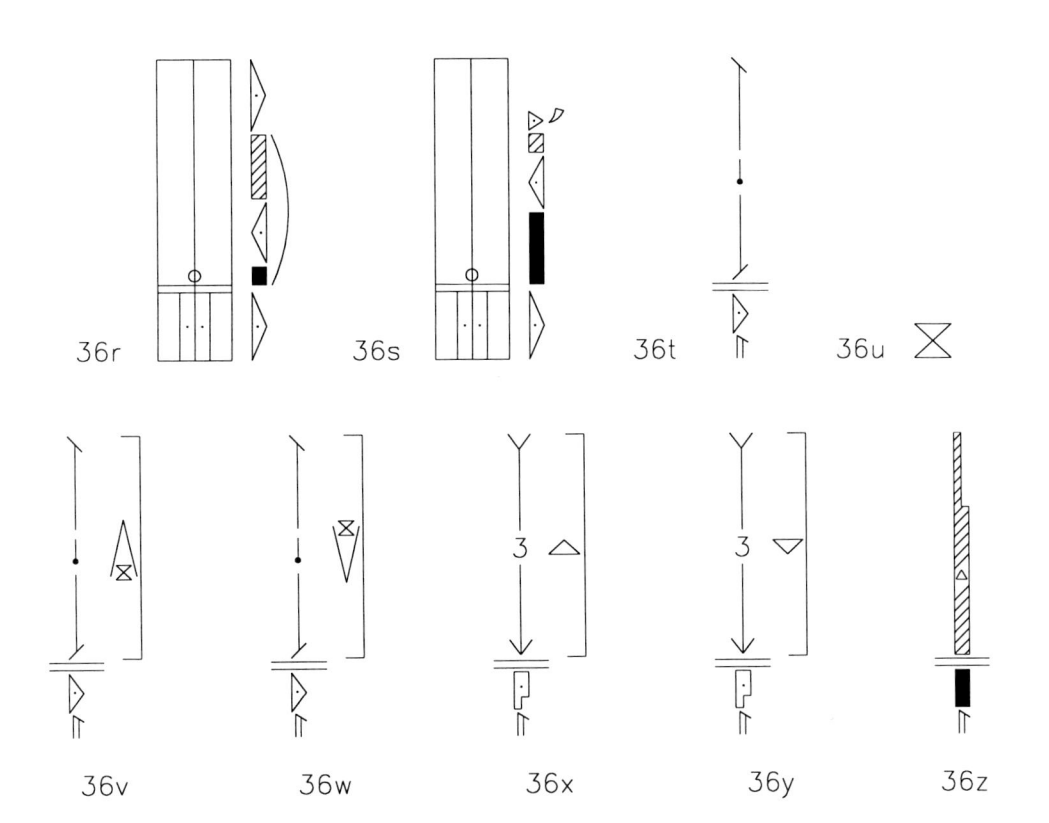

36r   36s   36t   36u

36v   36w   36x   36y   36z

VIII   DISTANCE

37 Length of Steps

37.1. **Natural Step-length.** Although a standard step-length has been established for notation purposes, in general practice step-length will vary according to the build of the individual, each middle level step being the length of the person's normal pace. This variance is not being dealt with here. Distance is also affected by the direction and level of the steps. Steps in low level as in **37a** tend naturally to be larger than steps in middle level, **37b**. Steps in high level, **37c**, are naturally shorter, the reach of each leg being diminished in that level. Steps in the backward direction, as in **37d**, tend to be smaller than forward steps. The crossed steps in **37e** are normally shorter than the open ones; crossing behind usually means an even shorter step, **37f**. Indication of the size of these different directional steps is usually not needed.

37.2. The rotational state of the legs affects distance. Parallel feet, **37g**, facilitate a longer forward stride, the length of the previously supporting foot adding to the distance. With a comfortable turn out, **37h**, this advantage is slightly diminished, and, with outward leg rotation, **37i**, even more so.

37.3. **Standard Step-length.** Standard step-length is determined as follows. With the longitudinal axes of the feet in line, as in **37j**, the distance is judged from the heel of the back foot to the heel of the front foot. The feet are considered to be one standard step-length apart when the heels are two foot-lengths apart *on the line of the path of the step*. From this relationship the feet can turn out, keeping the heels in place, **37k**, the resulting position is still one standard step-length apart (heel to heel). Ex. **37l** shows the same step-length, ie. heel to heel, for a sideward step with outward leg rotation. Here, with both feet in line to the right, as illustrated in **37m**, (i.e. the left foot much turned inward) the distance between the heels can be seen to be the same.

37.4. Statement of a standard length can be made; in **37n** the crossed step and the backward step are to be neither long nor short, i.e. the standard step-length. The key of **37o** states that each step is short, the exception being the first step in the second measure. Without the key, each step would be a natural length, except for the one which is indicated as being exactly of standard step length. In **37p**, the standard length sign placed in a bracket together with the sign of **37q** for a step, a transference of weight on the feet,[62] indicates that all the steps within the bracket are to be of standard size, even the crossed steps.

Advanced Labanotation

Natural Step-length

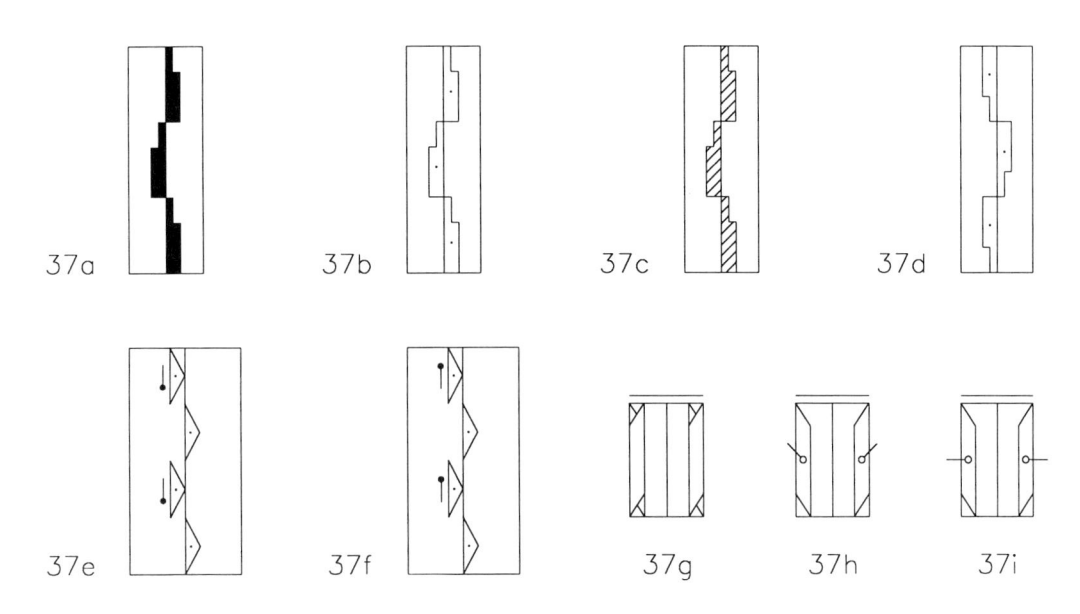

37a 37b 37c 37d

37e 37f 37g 37h 37i

Standard Step-length

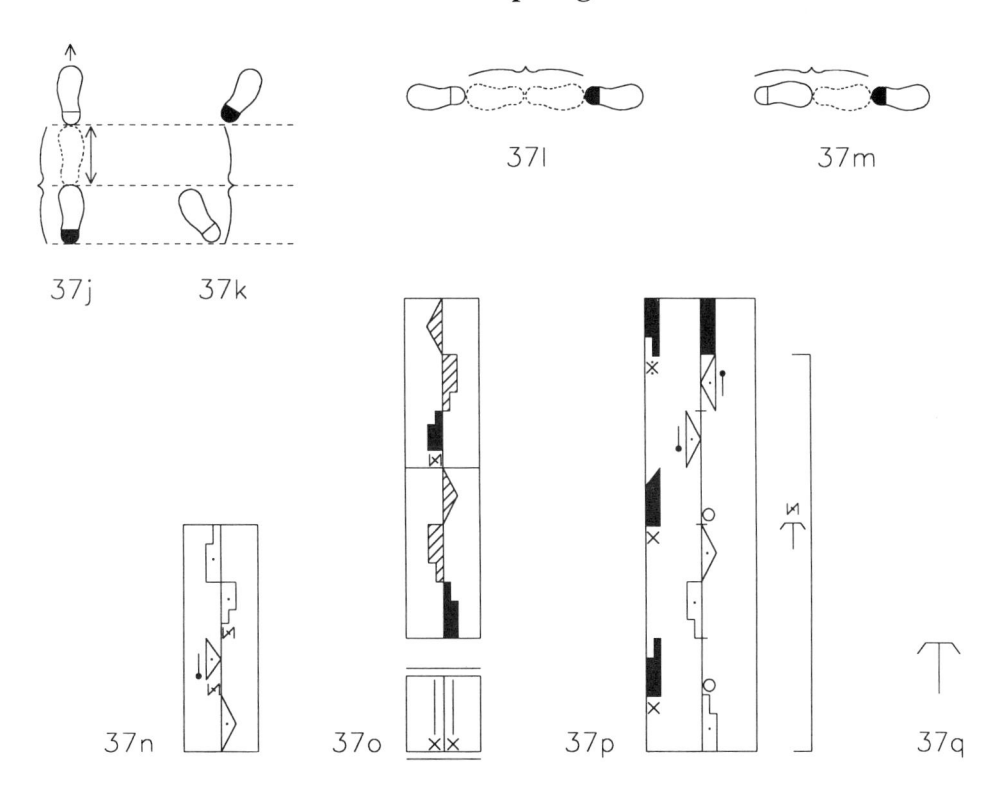

37j 37k 37l 37m

37n 37o 37p 37q

124   *Spatial Variations*

37.5. **Modifying Step-length - General Scale.** Step-length can be modified using measurement signs. The double X (very short, very narrow) sign indicates a very small step, **37r**; the single X sign indicates a small (short, narrow) step, **37s**. A natural (normal) sized step, **37t**, is indicated by an unmodified direction sign (shown as 'Dir' in the chart). Ex. **37u** states a long step and **37v** an extra long step. Stepping out wider and wider with the right foot is indicated in **37w**, using the general scale. These general descriptions of step-length, though not precise, are satisfactory for most needs. The intermediate degrees of shortening or lengthening the steps are often not needed.

37.6. **Modifying Step-length - Specific Scale.** When a more precise indication of step-length is needed the measurement signs are modified to indicate exact distances. Ex. **37x** shows the comparison between the general scale and the specific six scale; the sign for 'neither long nor short' indicates the standard length. In the 6/6 scale each degree of shortening indicates a reduction of 1/6 of the standard step length. In **37y** the performer's steps become increasingly smaller. The sixth degree of narrowing is not used as it is identical with the direction place.[63] The 8/8 scale[64] is seldom used for step-lengths.

Note that when dots are added to the measurements signs it is immediately clear that the specific scale is being used. To indicate use of the specific scale when only the basic narrow and wide signs are used, a statement that the single X represents a shortening of 1/6 must be made, as indicated in **37z**. If nothing is indicated, the general scale is automatically understood to be in effect. In **37aa** the wide signs are to be interpreted as if in the specific scale.

37.7. Ex. **37ab** shows the right foot stepping farther and farther away, ending in a split. Use of the dots provides the message that the specific scale is being used. The diagram of **37ac** below gives the specific scale for widening steps compared with the general scale. Note the indication below of the equivalent step-lengths. Each degree of extension indicates an increase of 1/4 step-length until two step-lengths are reached. From here on, experience has indicated that there is less need to be so specific, hence between the double and triple wide signs, each degree indicates 1/3 increase and the final (triple with dot) degree produces a 'split' (stride), that is, the greatest possible widening, usually 3 1/2 step-lengths.[65]

The general scale:	⋈			⋈		⋈			⋈	
The specific scale:	⋈	⋈	⋈	⋈	⋈	⋈	⋈	⋈	⋈	
Step length:	1	1¼	1½	1¾	2	2⅓	2⅔	3		

37ac

Advanced Labanotation

Modifying Step-length - General Scale

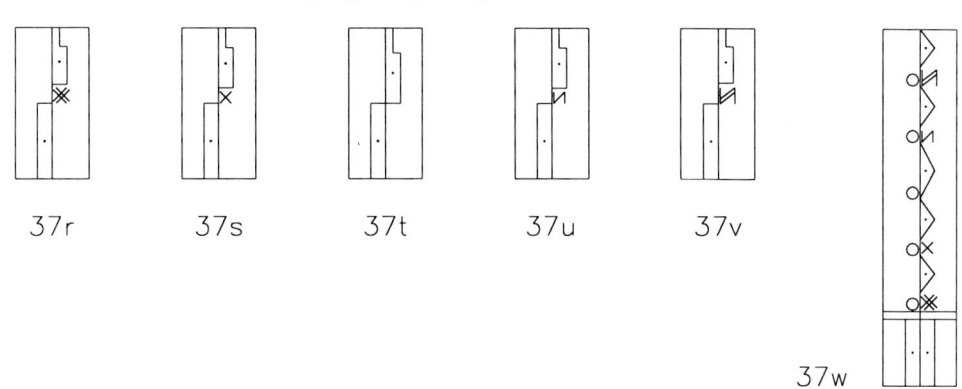

37r   37s   37t   37u   37v

37w

Modifying Step-length - Specific Scale

37x The general scale: | Dir | × | ※ | ▫ |

The specific six degree scale. | Dir | × | × | × | ※ | ※ | ※ or ▫ |

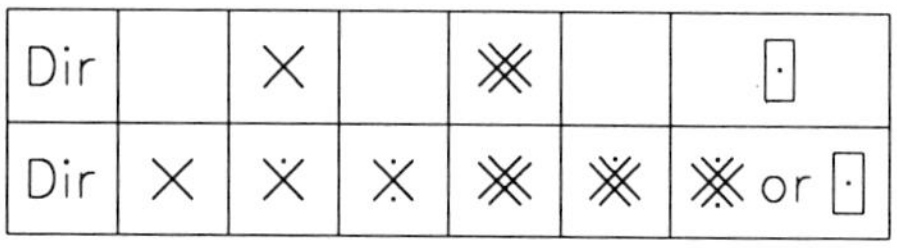

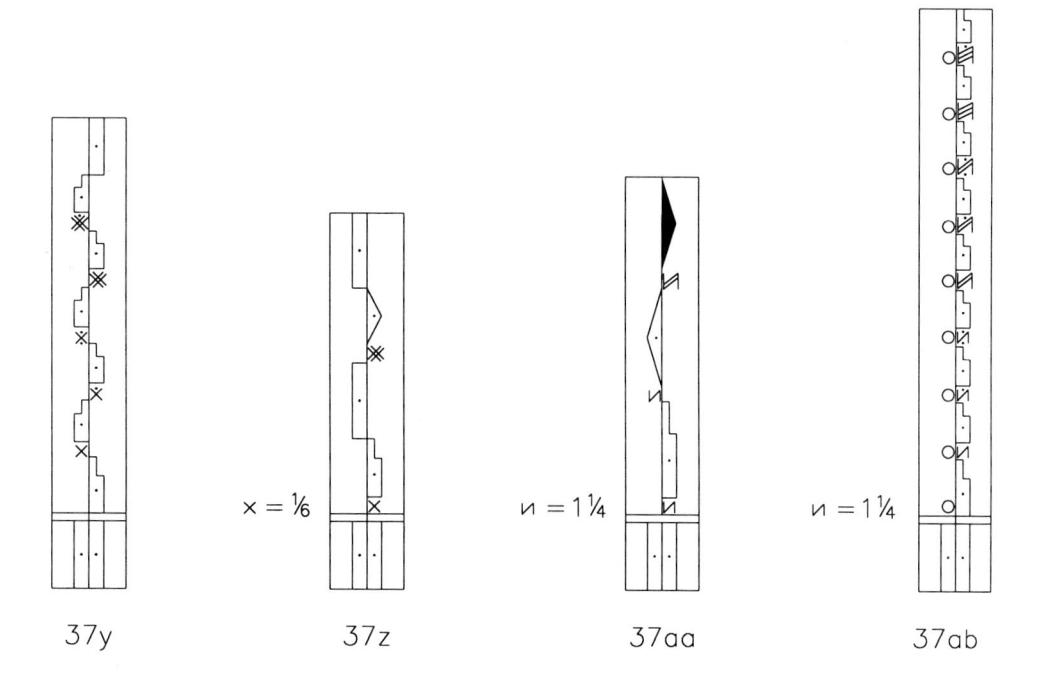

37y   37z   x = ⅙   37aa   ɲ = 1¼   37ab   ɲ = 1¼

126   *Spatial Variations*

37.8. **Length of Steps - Modifying Distance.** Modification of step-lengths can also be indicated within a straight path sign, as in **37ad**. Here the question arises as to whether the overall path is to be much smaller than normal, or if each step is to be of double narrow size. Ex. **37ae** states that each step should be very small, the double circle indicating 'each one'.

37.9. This indication of distance for a path is also applied to circular paths. A very small circle is to be performed with 12 steps, **37af**. In **37ag** the same circle is to be performed with 16 steps, but only the steps on the right foot are to be very small. Note the sign for a step on the right foot. Usually the indication for size of step is placed before the step symbol in the support column, but in the case of very fast steps there may not be room.

37.10. **Increase or Decrease of Distance.** In **37ah** each of the eight steps is to become increasingly longer. (See Section 25 for the toward, increase sign.) The performer must gauge how to spread this increase in distance over the designated number of steps. No eventual size of step is indicated here.

37.11. The size of the steps are shown to be getting smaller in **37ai**. Exactly how small is stated for the last of the 12 steps which is to be very small. An increase or decrease in the size of step can be shown also for a circular path, as in **37aj**, in which the steps are becoming longer. Performing this requires some measuring out, a full circle must be achieved. Since the shape of the circle should not be affected, less circling will need to be accomplished with the first steps and more toward the end, illustrated in **37ak**.

37.12. The 'increasingly small' indication of **37al** may need to have its meaning specified. For **37am** it is not clear to what the sign refers, no link to the steps or the path is given; the ending degree of bend for the last step suggests it refers to bending the legs. To avoid doubt, **37an** clearly states that it is the legs to which the increasing smallness (flexion) relates. Note that for the action of *flexing* (no stated degree), the vertical ad lib. sign is used to indicate 'degree is open'. This usage illustrates the difference between statements of distance for supports (steps) and flexion for leg gestures. A definite degree of leg flexion to be achieved during a series of steps can be shown by the indication of **37ao**.

37.13. Statement that the X sign refers to size, i.e. to space, distance, is shown in **37ap**. In **37aq** the increase in size of steps is stated in an addition bracket in which the sign for 'steps', is used together with the sign for increasing spatial length. A path sign cannot be used for this example as neither a straight nor a circling path occurs.

Length of Steps - Modifying Distance

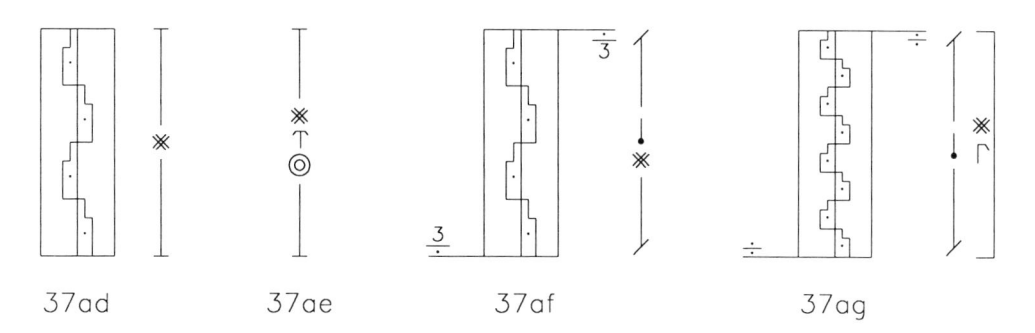

37ad　　37ae　　37af　　37ag

Increase or Decrease of Distance

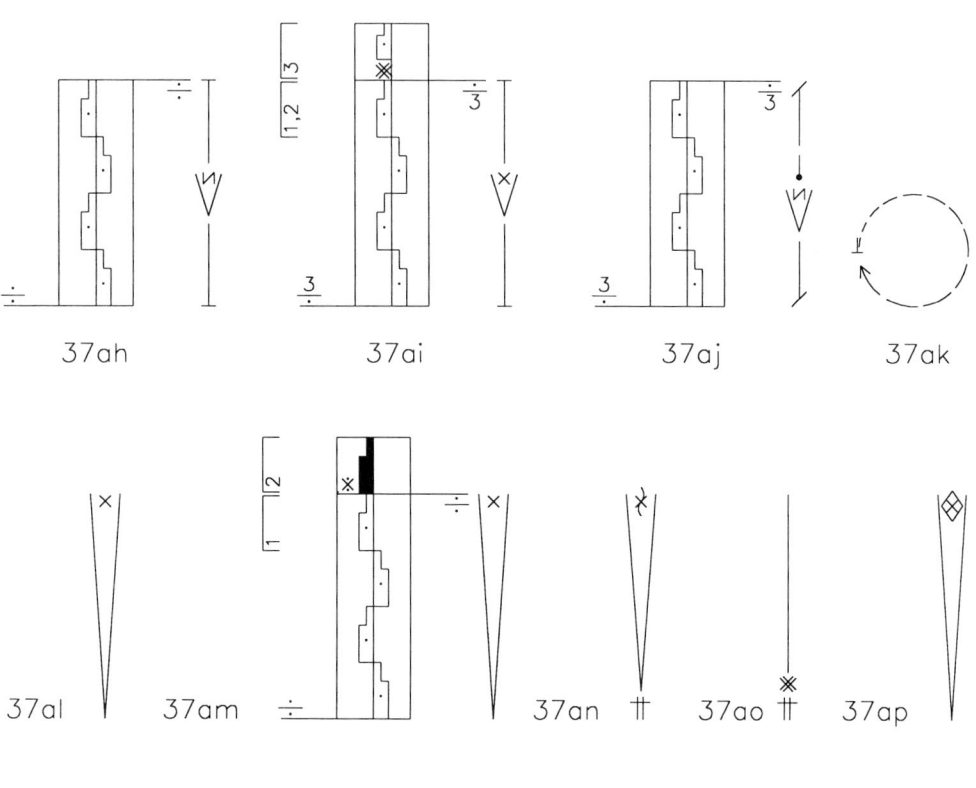

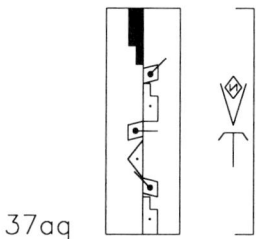

37ah　　37ai　　37aj　　37ak

37al　　37am　　37an　　37ao　　37ap

37aq

38 Distance, Aim of Path

38.1. **Distance in Terms of Units.** Distance to be traveled can also be specified in terms of step-lengths by placing the appropriate number in a box.[66] In **38a** the equivalent of 2 step-lengths is traveled in the forward direction while jumping in 2nd position. Ex. **38b** shows that a distance of 3 step-lengths is covered, here the direction sign is omitted, the overall direction is obvious from the step directions. When step-length is not a factor to be considered, the distance traveled can be left open as in **38c** in which the ad lib. sign provides freedom in the distance traveled, it is left open to the individual performer. Here the openess is specifically stated; the ordinary path sign also allows freedom in distance.

38.2. Distance between performers can be stated in terms of step-lengths as in **38d**, where B is 3 step-lengths in front of the performer. The step-length stated here is understood to be that of the performer unless otherwise specified. Such specification can be indicated where needed, at the beginning of the score or in the glossary. In **38e**, for example, the number in a box refers to the amount in terms of meters; **38f** states that each number in the box indicates two foot-lengths.

38.3. **Relative Location for Aim of Path.** The aim of a path, the ending location, can be indicated in relative terms. This destination can be described as distance from an established point. In the first three examples here, focus is on moving away from a partner (P). In **38g** no indication is given as to how far away from the partner the path ends. In **38h** the path away leads to a location far from P; in **38i** it is very far from P. One will interpret this description subjectively, how much distance is far or very far is not specified.

38.4. The resulting location of a path can also be described in terms of distance from an area, rather than a point. The sign for area is a square, **38j**. Ex. **38k** indicates a spatial area, a sign which is useful when people are working in a large space, each having his/her own established area.[67] Ex. **38l** designates the area where P is. Thus **38m** shows a path ending near the area where P is, wherever that might be.

Advanced Labanotation

Distance in Terms of Units

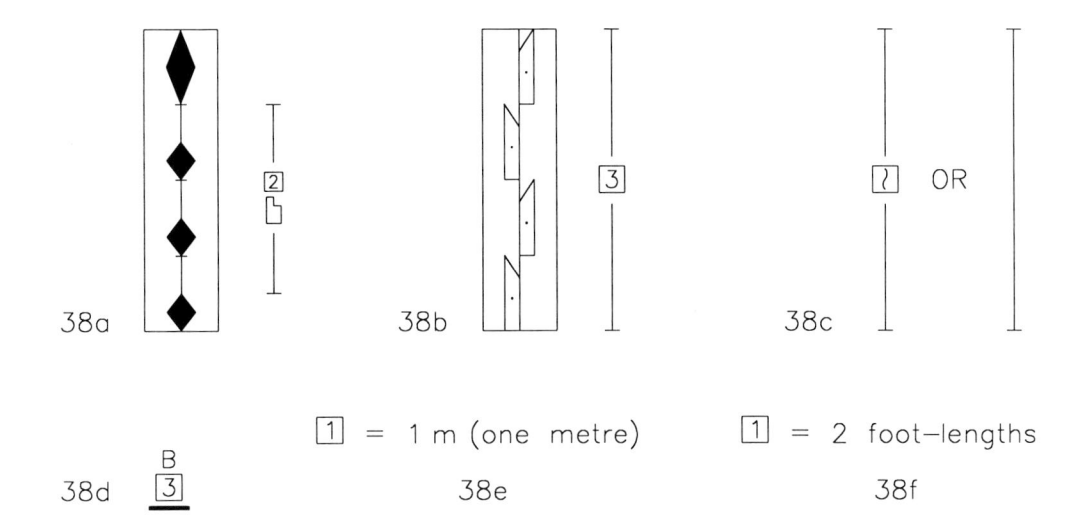

38a 38b 38c

38d 38e 1 = 1 m (one metre) 38f 1 = 2 foot-lengths

Relative Location for Aim of Path

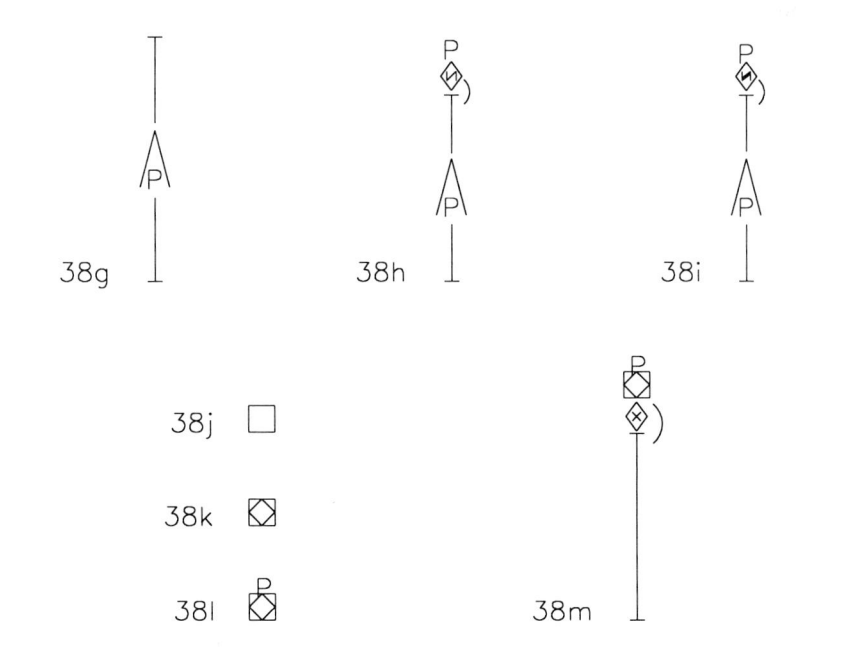

38g 38h 38i

38j
38k
38l 38m

39 Distance for Leg Gestures

39.1. **Distance for Touching Leg Gestures.** When standing with a straight touching leg gesture, the distance between the feet will usually depend on the level of the support. In **39a**, for example, when in a low level support, the distance between the feet is greater than with the middle level support of **39b**; distance in **39c** is even smaller because of the high level support.

39.2. When a straight gesturing leg touches the floor, and no hip inclusion or displacement occurs, only one distance from the support is possible. A bent leg allows more leeway, modification of the degree of knee bend may occur.

39.3. There is no distance between the bent touching leg gesture in place and the supporting foot in **39d**. The level of the support dictates the degree of knee bend. In **39e** the gesture is shown to be slightly to the right, under the right hip. The pin is tied to the direction symbol, **39f**, to clarify that the pin is a modification of the main direction and not a relationship pin. A further distance to the right is indicated in **39g**, a third-way toward the side low direction. In **39h** the sideward low gesture is one third of the way toward place low. (For intermediate directions see Part I.) Beyond this point the gesture is described as a right sideward low direction, **39i**.

39.4. Modifications of **39i** are indicated as the distance from the main support, indicated by placing a measurement sign in the support column. This usage relates to the idea of distance of a step. In **39j** how far away the foot is placed to take the step (the distance) is shown in the support column. Because in **39k** this same statement of distance applies to the placement of the toe in a gesture, the right foot being very close to left foot, the diamond is added to make clear that distance is being described, not limb flexion. In **39l** the toe is less close, but closer than normal to the support. In **39m** the toe is further away than normal and in **39n** as far away as possible while keeping the gesturing leg bent.[68] When the support is in low level, as in **39o, 39p, 39q** and **39r**, there is a greater range in distance between the placement of the right toe and the left support.

39.5. In the sequence of **39s**, as the degree of bend of the supporting leg increases, the right foot touches further to the right, ending with a low support and a wide distance for the touch. Note the differences between the following examples, the degree of bend for the leg gesture is the same in each pair, but the distance of contact slightly modifies this degree. In **39t** the foot is near the supporting leg, touching with the heel slightly off the floor; in **39u** the touch is far from the supporting leg. In **39v** and **39w** the gesturing leg is bent two degrees, touching first near and then far from the supporting leg.

Distance for Touching Leg Gestures

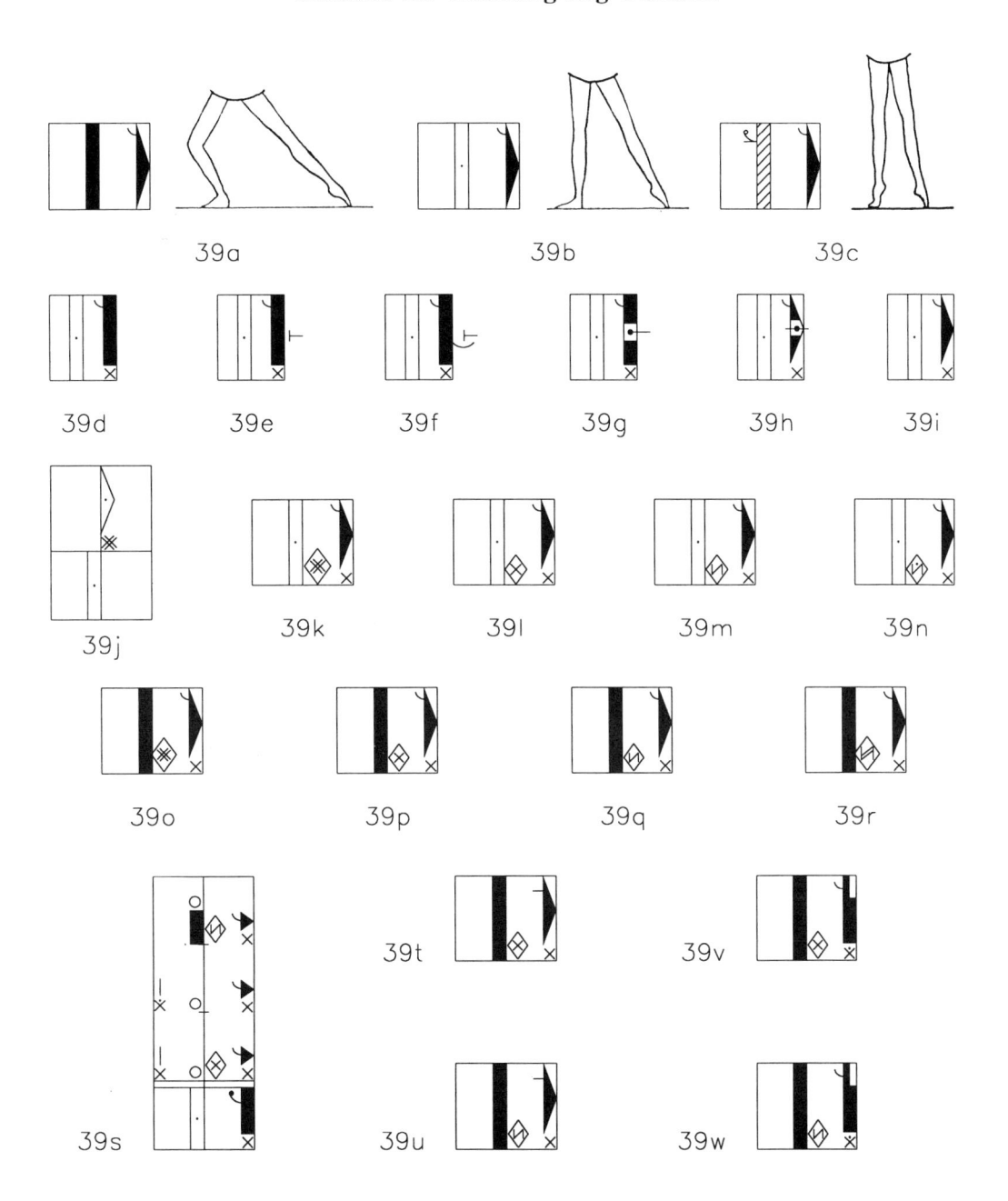

39.6. **Distance for Leg Gestures Off the Floor.** When a leg gesture is off the floor, distance from the floor may need to be stated. The following examples feature the right leg gesturing forward low. An expected difference occurs depending on the level of the support. Because of the high support, in **39x** the foot is obviously farther from the floor than in **39y**. For leg gestures the distance *between the foot and the floor* can be indicated in the same way that distance is shown *between the foot and the support* for touching leg gestures. Ex. **39z** shows the right leg at the standard 45° angle, with the foot pointed, illustrated in **39aa**.

39.7. With a flexed ankle, **39ab**, the extremity of the leg in the same forward low gesture will be farther from the floor, **39ac**. Note that for the leg direction, the line of the leg to the heel is the factor to consider, shown in these two examples with a dotted line. However, if the observer is aware of the extremity of the leg and its nearness to the floor, this is what will be recorded. In **39ad** the foot is shown to be nearer the floor, more or less the same as the intermediate direction of **39ae**. In **39af** the distance is even smaller, approximately the level of **39ag**. The three levels of **39aa**, **39ae** and **39ag** are identified as a), b), and c) in the illustration of **39ah**, a) being the standard forward low. These are relative statements. There is an advantage in writing the general leg direction and then adding the distance from the floor, as in **39ad** and **39af**, rather than indicating an intermediate direction symbol.

39.8. Ex. **39ai** describes a brushing leg gesture in which the foot ends only slightly off the floor. This is very similar to **39aj** in which the foot is shown to release just off the floor - as a rule the distance of one inch (2.5 cm).

In the jump of **39ak**, illustrated in **39al**, the legs hardly rise from the floor; **39am** indicates that the feet should be far from the floor, resulting in a high jump, **39an**, with the legs still at the side low 45° angle.

Advanced Labanotation

Distance for Leg Gestures Off the Floor

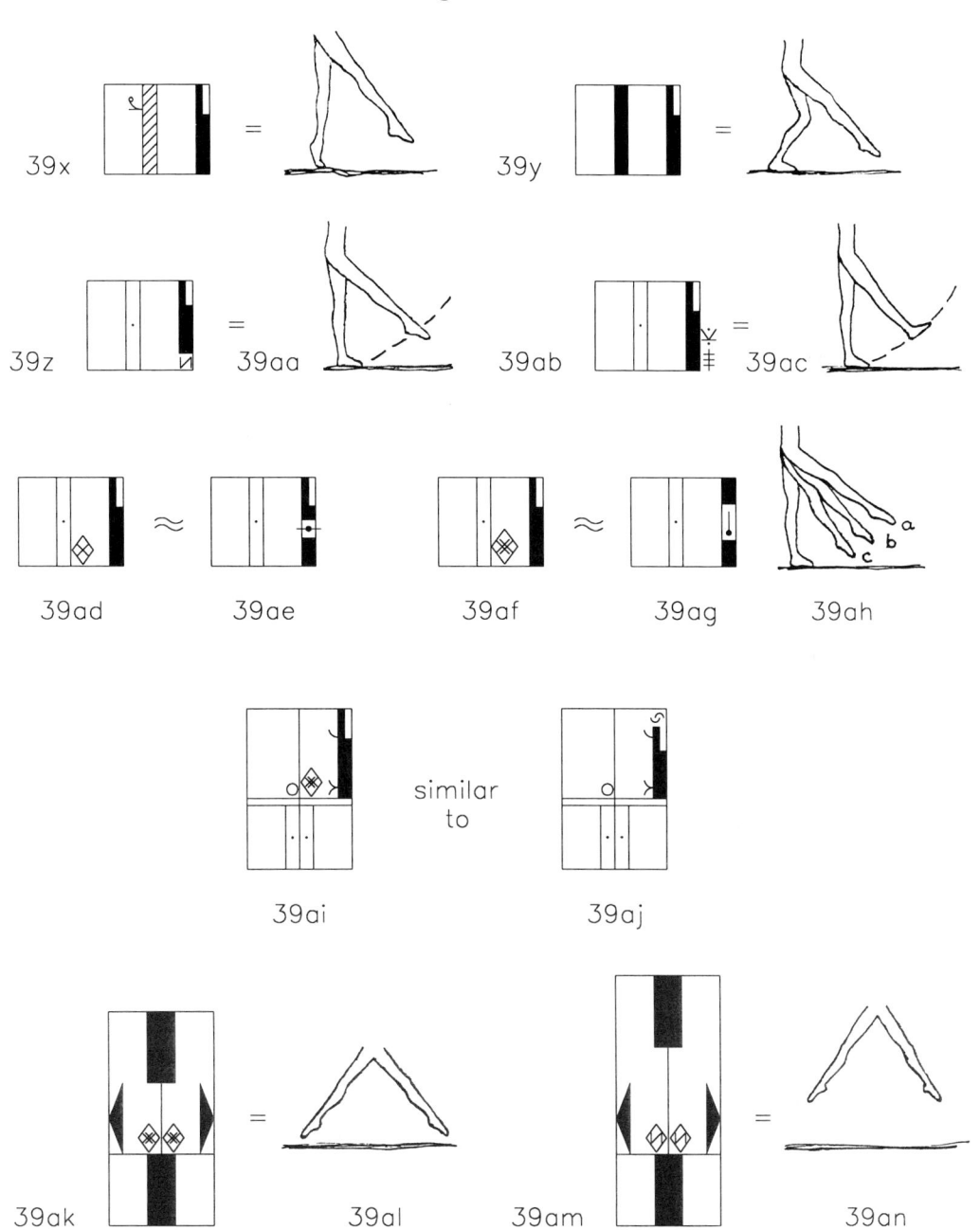

39x 39y

39z 39aa 39ab 39ac

39ad 39ae 39af 39ag 39ah

39ai similar to 39aj

39ak 39al 39am 39an

Spatial Variations

39.9. **Distance of Leg Gestures from the Center Line.** During a jump with the legs apart, the greater or lesser spread of the legs can be indicated with the signs for abduction and adduction.[69] The general degrees of lateral spreading (abduction) are shown in **39ao** and **39ap**. Lateral closing (adduction) are shown in **39aq** and **39ar**. These indications can conveniently be added to the basic statement of leg direction without needing to make use of intermediate direction signs. Ex, **39as**, illustrated in **39at**, shows a standard jump with the legs opened to side low. In **39au** the legs are shown to be wider apart than standard; here an abduction sign is written for each side, one centered lateral spreading sign can conveniently be placed across the staff center line, as in **39av**, illustrated in **39aw**.

39.10. Ex. **39ax** shows the same jump with the legs closer together than standard, less spread. This is indicated with the lateral adduction sign modifying the side low gestures. An adduction sign can be used for each side, or, one centered sign can suffice, as in **39av**. This narrower spread is illustrated in **39ay**. This particular jump can be performed with the legs even closer together, the double adduction sign being used, **39az**, illustrated in **39ba**.

39.11. Sagittal abduction and adduction can also be shown. Sagittal spreading (abduction) signs are show in **39bb**, the greater degree being **39bc**. Sagittal closing (adduction) also has two general degrees, **39bd** for slight, **39be** for the greater degree. Note the use of the right and left signs; placed either side of the center staff line they are more easily read.

39.12. The leap of **39bf**, illustrated in **39bg**, can be performed with the legs more spread, **39bh** and **39bi**, or with the legs closer together, **39bj** and **39bk**. The resulting performance of these indications may vary from person to person, exactness in placement is not easy to achieve, rather the idea of these spatial differences is stated in a simple way.

Distance of Leg Gestures from the Center Line

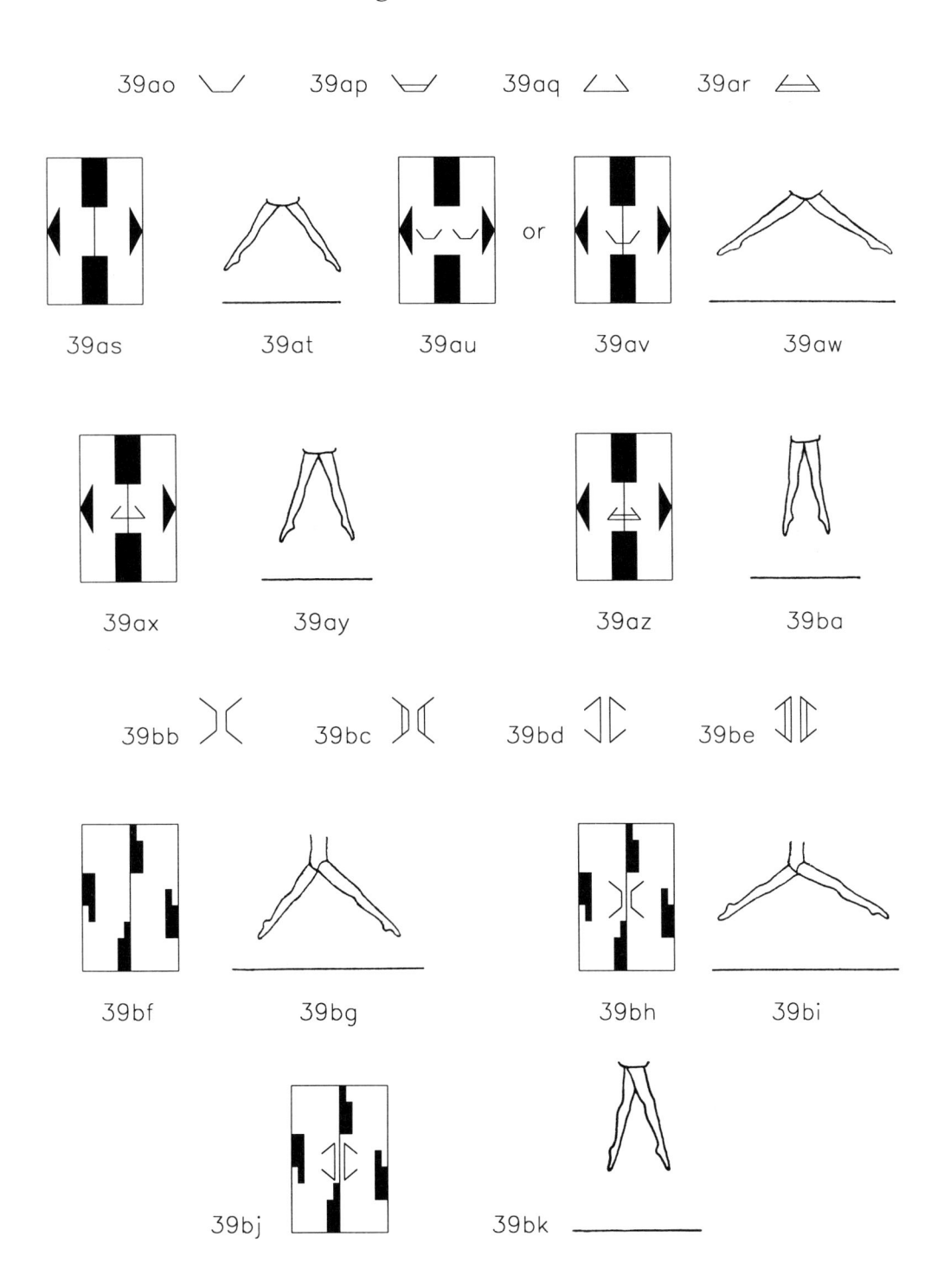

39ao   39ap   39aq   39ar

39as   39at   39au   39av   39aw

39ax   39ay   39az   39ba

39bb   39bc   39bd   39be

39bf   39bg   39bh   39bi

39bj   39bk

40 Sign for Distance

40.1. While Knust established a number in a box to indicate distance, its meaning is only evident when the specific unit of measurement is added, as in **38e** and **38f**. At the 1973 ICKL Conference, the need was put forward for a sign for distance, the basic meaning of which is more self evident. The sign of **40a** was suggested by Edna Geer. A similar indication used in draughtmanship and in carpentry is **40b**; this sign can also be drawn vertically. Statement of distance can be centered in the sign, as in **40c**, **40d**. If the distance sign needs to be drawn rather small, the distance statement can be placed just above it to make reading easier, **40e**.

40.2. The distance sign is particularly applicable to gestures for which other details are not specified. When using DBP (Direction from Body Part, for which see <u>Advanced Labanotation</u> *Floorwork, Basic Acrobatics*) for gestures in a structured description, the distance of the extremity of the limb to the reference point is known from the degree of flexion or extension of the limb. In **40f** the arm is three degrees bent, the hand (the extremity) sideward middle of the right hip.

40.3. In the more open statement of **40g**, the hands address each other, each being sideward horizontal of the other hand. Where this sideward relationship is placed around the body (in front, overhead, to one side, etc.) is not stated. To give an idea of distance between the hands, an indication such as **40h** can be added; here the statement is of far apart. Another placement of hand and foot, **40i**, shows the right hand to be a very small distance above the left foot. Here the application of the distance sign of **40c** is visually appropriate. If there is not room on the staff for placement of such indications, use of the basic sign for relating (a relationship of some kind)[70], **40j**, can be appropriate for showing distance. In **40k** the hands relate in being some distance apart. When there is not room in the staff, such statements can be placed outside. In **40l** the right hand addresses the top of the head at a distance.

40.4. This distance sign can be combined with the box sign. In **40m** the statement is made that the number refers to step-lengths. Ex. **38b**, for example, can be written as **40n**, 3 step-lengths being covered during the four steps. While open statements usually allow freedom in matters of distance, a specific instruction regarding freedom can be given when needed, **40o**.

Advanced Labanotation

Sign for Distance

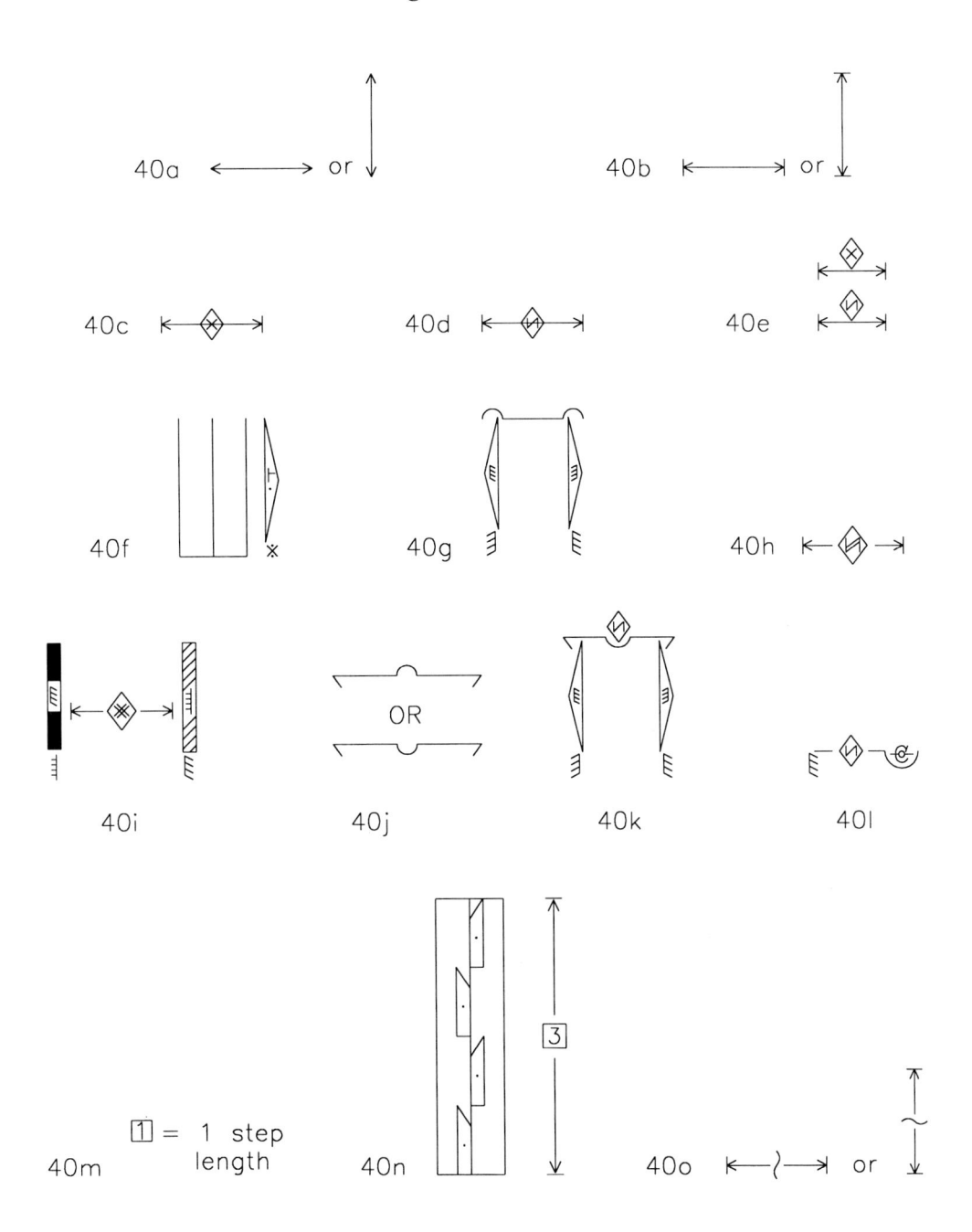

40a 40b 40c 40d 40e

40f 40g 40h

40i 40j 40k 40l

40m ① = 1 step length 40n 40o

IX ORIENTATION

41 Focal Point

41.1. **Orientation in Relation to Focal Point.** The sign for focal point is a black circle, **41a**.[71] Identification of the focal point is given at the start of a score, or at the point in a score where the need arises. Person 'P' (often representing a partner) is indicated as the focal point in **41b**. In **41c** a chair is shown to be the focal point. When performers are in a circular formation or traveling on a circular path, the center of the circle is automatically understood to be the focal point. To indicate relationship to the focal point, the sign is combined with the appropriate meeting line. In **41d** the focal point is in front of the performer; in **41e** it is to the right, in **41f** it is diagonally backward right.[72] These orientation indications are usually placed to the left side of the staff, where the Front Signs (orientation to the room directions) are placed, **41g**. In **41h** the steps occur on a circular path and so the change in orientation is shown as relationship to the center of the circle.

41.2. **Focal Destination for a Turn.** A pivot turn may be designated as ending with a particular relationship to the focal point. To indicate this, the focal point is placed on the appropriate side of the turn sign. Ex. **41i** shows the range of such destinations for turns to the right; the same method applies to turns to the left, **41j**. At the start of **41k** the focal point is to the right of the performer, the turn to the right ends facing the focal point; after the sideward step, the turn ends with the focal point at the performer's left. In the group arrangement of **41l** the eight people in a circle start facing front. The composite turn sign indicates that each should turn either right or left (whichever is the shorter) to end facing the center of the circle.[73] Final focal Front indications are usually added, even when the turn sign incorporates the focal destination.

41.3. The destination of a turn can also be indicated in relation to the established room directions. In **41m** the group of eight people start facing the center of the circle. Each then turns either right or left to face the front of the room, indicated by the middle level tack which relates to the Front Sign. The destination of the left turn in **41n** is stated as stage left. In **41m** and **41n** the new Front sign is stated for readers who glance up the left side of the staff to check orientation.[74]

41.4. With a focal point already established, a turn sign combined with a focal point can be used for a part of the body, thus indicating the final facing position for the front of that part. In **41o** the chest turns (twists) to the right until

Advanced Labanotation

facing the focal point. Ex. **41p** shows the head turning to the right to end with the focal point on its right.[75]

Orientation in Relation to Focal Point

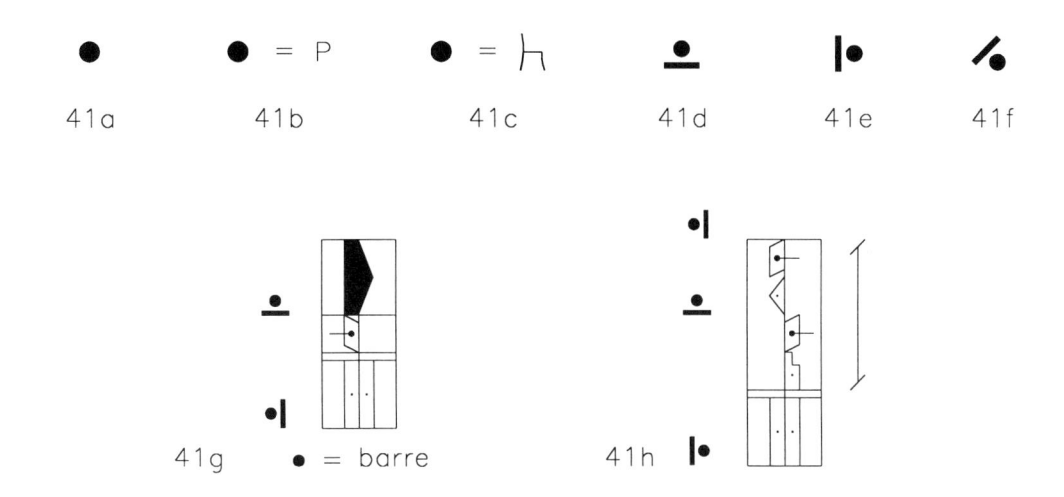

41a 41b ● = P 41c ● = ⌂ 41d 41e 41f

41g ● = barre 41h

Focal Destination for a Turn

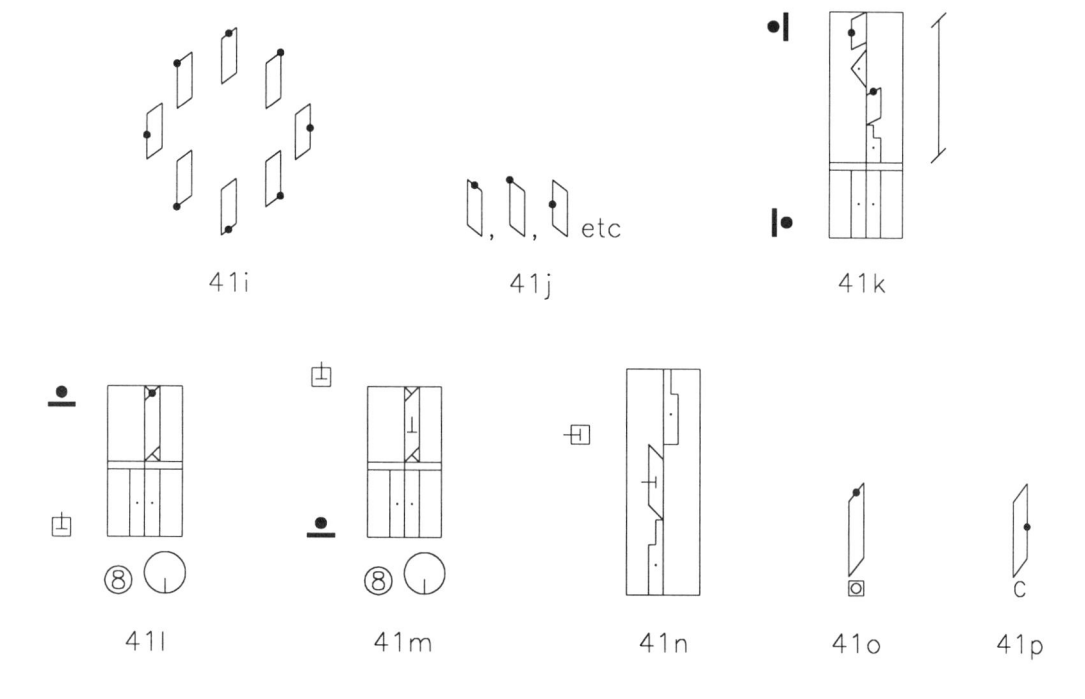

41i 41j 41k

41l 41m 41n 41o 41p

140   *Spatial Variations*

41.5. **Focal Point System of Reference.**[76] One can move toward a focal point, away from it, to the right in relation to it, and so on. Directions can thus be based on a focal point in a way comparable to the Constant Cross of Axes. Instead of the audience or front wall of the room being the forward direction, the direction toward the focal point is forward, thereby establishing backward, sideward, etc. When the performer changes location and/or facing directions, the individual's personal directions will change in relation to the established focal point.

41.6. The key for this system of reference, **41q**, is a Standard Key with a focal point sign attached.[77] When placed outside the staff, all directions relate to the previously stated focal point. All levels for gestures or steps relate as usual to the vertical. For a group, such indications will produce radial or tangental movements, whether the group has a central focal point or the performers are spread across the stage, all relate directional movements to one identified focal point. In **41r**, illustrated in floor plans of **41s** and **41t**, the dancers come together into a smaller circle in the first measure and then radiate out, whirling away from the circle's center point.

41.7. For individual incidental indications, individual direction symbols can be modified by addition of the focal point key. In **41u** it is placed as a pre-sign to the directional movement; in **41v** it is placed alongside in an addition bracket.

41.8. Such incidental indications can also be shown by attaching the focal sign to the end of the direction symbol.[78] Exs. **41w**, **41x** and **41y** all indicate movements toward the focal point, level being judged in the normal way. Exs. **41z**, **41aa** and **41ab** all mean movements away from the focal point, while **41ac**, **41ad** and **41ae** mean to the right side, i.e. the direction which is to the right when facing the focal point.[79]

41.9. In **41af**, K is designated as the focal point. As each performer lunges toward the focal point, the right arm gestures upward toward the focal point, while the left arm gestures away. The arms then draw in as the performers step away from the focal point. This pattern is performed four times changing sides, during which each person makes a full turn to the right. Configuration of performers is shown in **41ag**.

Advanced Labanotation

Focal Point System of Reference

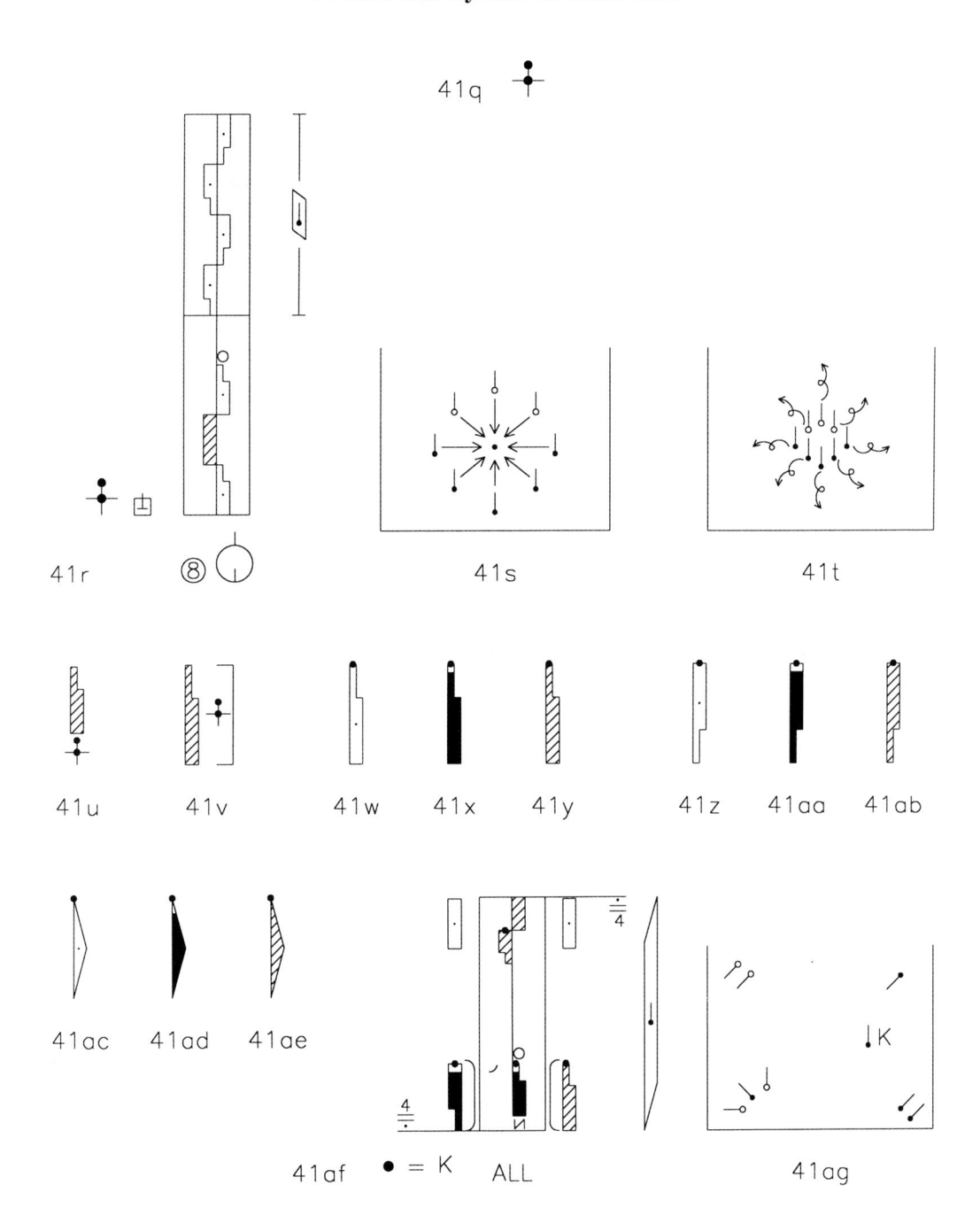

41q

41r ⑧ 41s 41t

41u 41v 41w 41x 41y 41z 41aa 41ab

41ac 41ad 41ae

41af • = K ALL

41ag

42 Line of Dance

42.1. In ballroom dancing the established Line of Dance, also called the General Direction of Progression (GDP), progresses around the room in a counterclockwise direction along the four walls of the room.[80] As they travel counterclockwise, turning and taking their individual step directions from each one's Standard Key, the dancers need to be aware of their facing direction, their Front, in relationship to this line of direction. Ex. **42a** shows how the dancer (solid line) may weave around the general direction of progression (dotted line).

42.2. The sign for the GDP Key is given in **42b**. This key is stated at the start of a score to indicate that facing indications using this key are to be judged according to the Line of Dance.

42.3. The GDP Front Signs, derived from the Key, are black pins within a box.[81] The following examples show where the dancer's Front is in relation to the GDP. In **42c** the dancer faces the GDP; in **42d** his back is to the GDP; in **42e** the dancer's front is turned $1/4$ clockwise from the GDP and therefore the dancer faces the nearest wall. Ex. **42f** states that the dancer is facing to the left, $1/4$ away from the GDP, his/her right side being directed toward the GDP. In **42g** the dancer's front has turned $1/8$ left in relation to the GDP, so that the GDP is at the dancer's right forward direction.

42.4. Ex. **42h** shows a ballroom sequence for a man who starts facing the center of the room. After a sideward and two backward steps, he turns a $1/4$ right to face the GDP. After two more forward steps, a $1/4$ right turn places him facing the nearest wall, i.e. away from center, so that his side-close-side steps travel into the GDP. Following the $3/8$ turn to the left, his forward step crosses the GDP on the left diagonal; similarly, as a result of the subsequent $1/4$ turn to the right, the forward step crosses the GDP on the right diagonal. After two sideward steps he again turns $1/4$ to the left and steps across and back on the left diagonal.

42.5. When the dancer arrives at a corner of the room, the GDP makes $1/4$ turn left and the dancer has to adjust to this new GDP direction. This is indicated as in **42i**, the key for the GDP being followed by a $1/4$ turn sign, The dancer turns $1/4$ to the left, but, because the GDP has also turned left, the new facing direction for the dancer remains forward along the GDP, illustrated in **42j**.[82] In **42k** the GDP turns $1/4$ left at the corner, but here the dancer turns $1/4$ to the right, thus he will end facing backward in relation to the GDP, as in **42l**.

Advanced Labanotation

Line of Dance

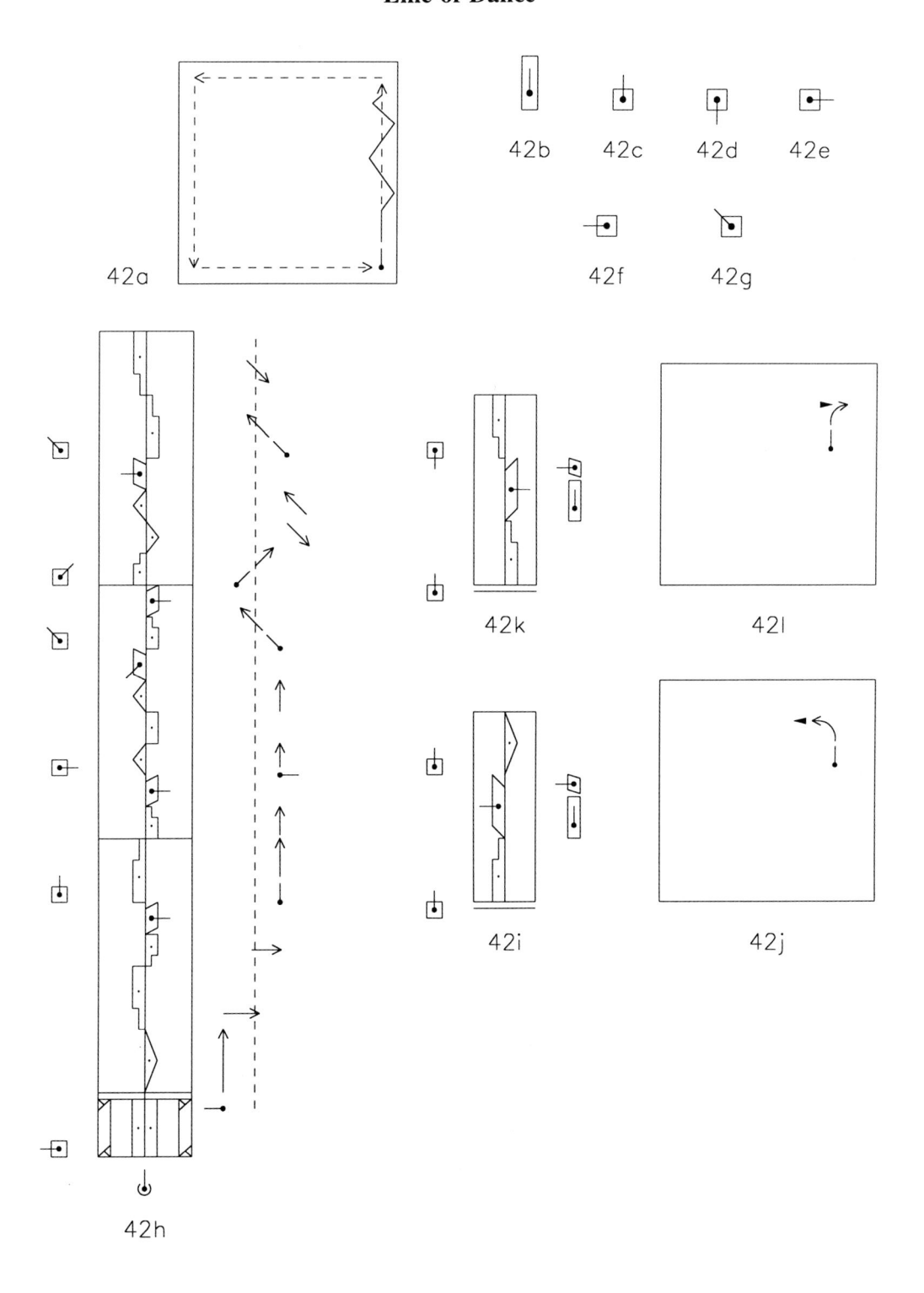

42a

42b   42c   42d   42e

42f   42g

42h

42i

42k

42j

42l

43 Front in Relation to the Path; to the Periphery

43.1. Front in Relation to the Path. In Follow-the-Leader dances such as the Mediaeval Farandole, the path can vary according to the whim of the leader, causing it, for example, to snake in and out, traveling on a straight line, then coiling in to a spiral. The participants usually walk with forward steps but, when holding hands, these may be diagonal and, when interesting variations are included, the individual's relationship to this frequently changing path may need to be stated. Ex. **43a** shows a typical Farandole path.

43.2. The key for Front in Relation to the Direction of the Path is **43b**, the arrow being derived from its use on a floor plan. (See 25.4 for Direction of Progression for gestures.) Front signs for this system of reference are thus: **43c** for facing the line of the path, forward steps will continue the path; **43d** for having one's back to the line of the path, for which backward steps will continue the path; **43e** shows the performer's right side to be toward the line of the path, thus requiring steps to the right to continue the path.

43.3. In the sequence of **43f** any number of people are facing the direction of the path and walking forward. After two steps they turn $1/4$ left, the sideward step on the right foot being in the line of the path. A further turn takes them to stepping backward, following which the half turn brings them back to facing the line of the path and walking forward.

43.4. Turn signs can also be related to the direction of the path: **43g** means turn right until the line of the path is on your left; **43h** states turn left until your back is to the line of the path; **43i** means turn left until the path is on your left, and so on. The amount of turn needed can only be known from where you were previously. In **43j**, illustrated in the floor plans of I and II, the forward progression of a line of people is interrupted by all turning left to face the focal point, the center of the incomplete circle. At that moment all raise their arms. This may lead to an Under the Arches sequence, or, as here, the general path may be continued, all turning right to face the line of the path.

43.5. **Movements related to the Direction of the Path**. The Key of **43k** can be used to indicate that gestures and torso movements as well as the direction of steps relate to the Direction of the Path. The sequence of **43l**, illustrated in **43m**, shows a line of people holding hands and facing different directions in

Advanced Labanotation

relation to the direction of the path; note the ad lib. sign within the starting front sign. All are walking into the direction of the path and swaying the torso into and then away from the line of the path, possibly expressing an inebriated state.

Front in Relation to the Path

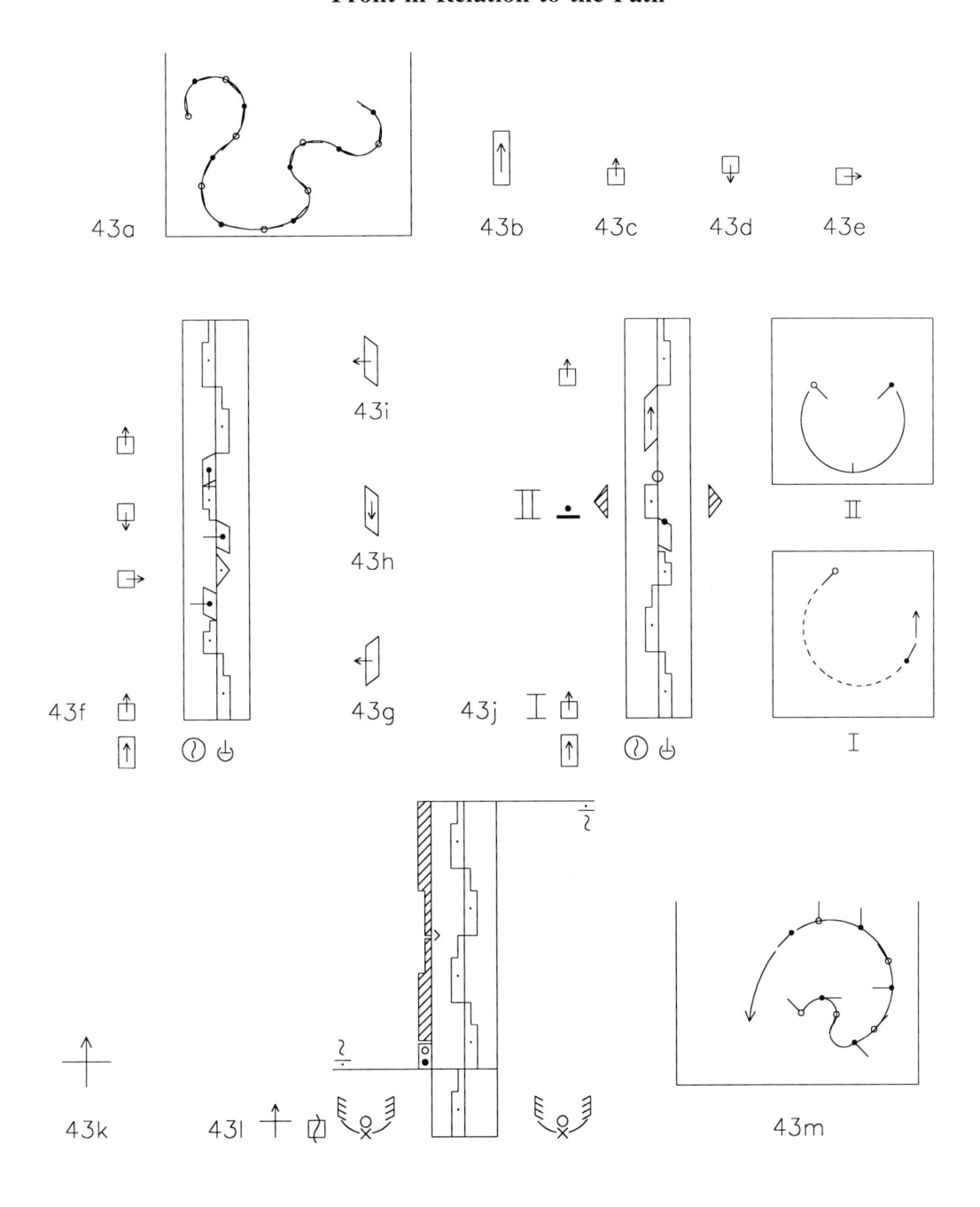

43.6. **Front Oriented to the Periphery.** A different form of orientation, i.e. determining Front, can occur when one is performing in an arena. Such a need occurs in skating and also in circus performance. The statement of **43n** is needed. Here the front orientation is established with a meeting line. The sign for the periphery of the area (the arena) is used. This periphery is shown to be in front of you and the center behind you.[83] Thus, the forward pointing front sign, **43o**, means facing the periphery, **43p** means having one's back to the periphery, i.e. facing the center. The statement of **43q** means that your left side will be to the periphery.

43.7. It will be noted that these are the same front signs as those used in ballroom in relation to the Line of Dance. The statement of **43n** at the start of a score makes clear that this particular usage is required, therefore one is not concerned with the Line of Dance as in ballroom dancing.

43.8. In **43r** which begins with the Peripheral Orientation statement, six female performers are spread around an arena, illustrated in **43s**. The opening position is facing to the left (right side of the body to the periphery). After the $\frac{1}{4}$ turn to the right they are facing out, toward the audience around the ring, **43t**.

43.9. Circular areas or arenas may in addition require an indication of an established point; in a circus this will be the entrance, the break in the ring where the performers enter. For these locations see 44.25.

Front Oriented to the Periphery

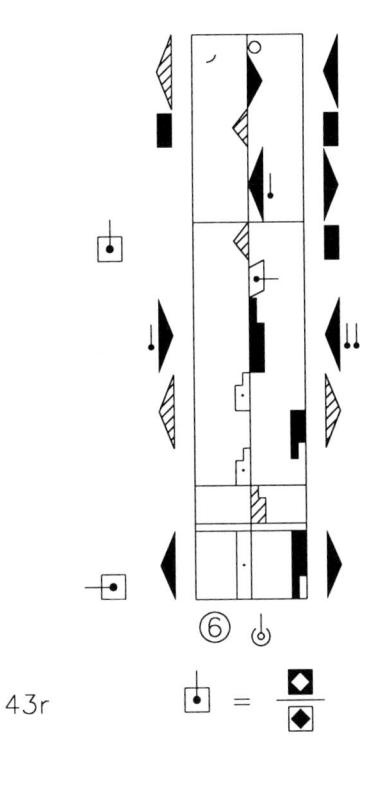

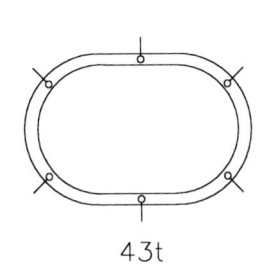

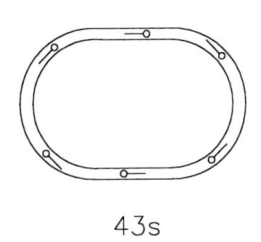

43n 43o 43p 43q

43r

43t

43s

44 Area Signs

44.1. Area signs are an abstract representation of the different areas of the stage or room. These signs range from general statements to specific indications.[84]

44.2. **Basic Signs.** The basic sign for an area is **44a**. The general need is to refer to areas in the room or on stage; for these the stage terms are commonly used. Ex. **44b** shows the left corner of the foreground (downstage left); **44c** indicates the downstage center area; **44d** the downstage right corner area; **44e** the stage left center area; **44f** the center of the stage or room; **44g** the stage right center area; **44h** shows the upstage left corner area; **44i** the upstage center area; and **44j** the upstage right corner area. The diagram of **44k** shows an average sized stage plan, here the area signs are appropriately placed as an illustration. Note that **44c** should not be interpreted as meaning the whole of the front part of the stage, it represents the area of **44l**. To show the whole sweep of the front area, **44m**, the signs of **44n**, condensed to **44o** are used, (see 44.8).

44.3. **Application of the Stage Area Signs.** A general application of location, as is used in Motif Description, may be to indicate where the performer is to start before traveling. In **44p** it is the upstage left corner. The arrival point at the end of traveling can be shown as in **44q** where the destination for circling clockwise is the center of the stage. Motion toward an area can also be indicated; the path in **44r** is to approach (but not arrive in) the center of the stage. An area of the room may be designated as a focal point; in **44s** it is the downstage right corner area. These applications are applicable also to Structured Description in Labanotation.

44.4. Indicating the location on stage is particularly important at the start of a choreographic score. The appropriate statement is placed to the left of the staff, next to the front sign. In **44t** a person is shown to start in the upstage center area, in a low 2nd position, facing back. This location is shown on the floor plan of **44u**.

Advanced Labanotation

Basic Signs

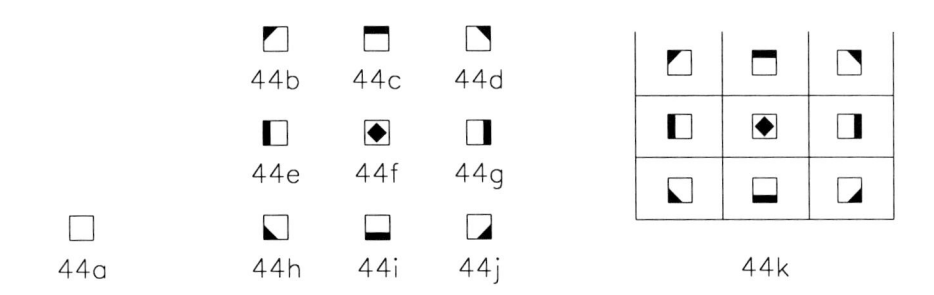

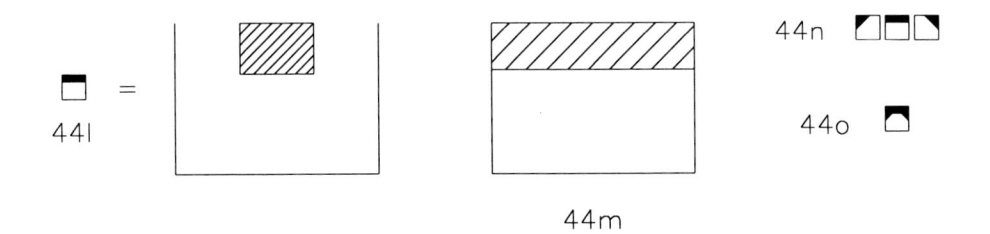

44a 44b 44c 44d 44e 44f 44g 44h 44i 44j 44k

44l 44m 44n 44o

Application of the Stage Area Signs

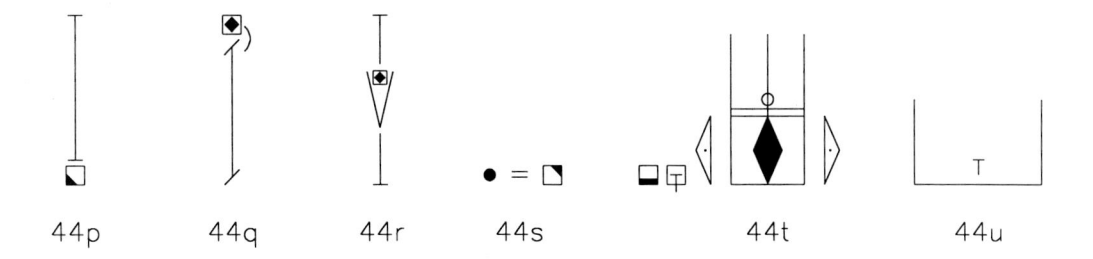

44p 44q 44r 44s 44t 44u

44.5. The woman in **44v** runs from the center stage right area to end center stage. This is illustrated in **44w**. A similar example is **44x** where three women, standing close together, repeat a folk dance step eight times while moving gradually to end center stage, illustrated in **44y**.

44.6. The location of entrances and exits also need to be stated (for indication of wings see 45.1-4). In **44z** the performer takes two preparatory steps before leaping on stage from the upstage left wing. This is illustrated in the floor plan of **44a**. The exit in **44ab** is into the middle wing on stage right, this is illustrated in **44ac**.

A clear floor plan can often make use of stage area signs redundant, however, a reinforcement of the information can be helpful and, in taking in the sense and progression of the movement, the reader's eye may glean information from one place before observing it in another.

Advanced Labanotation 151

Application of Stage Area Signs (continued)

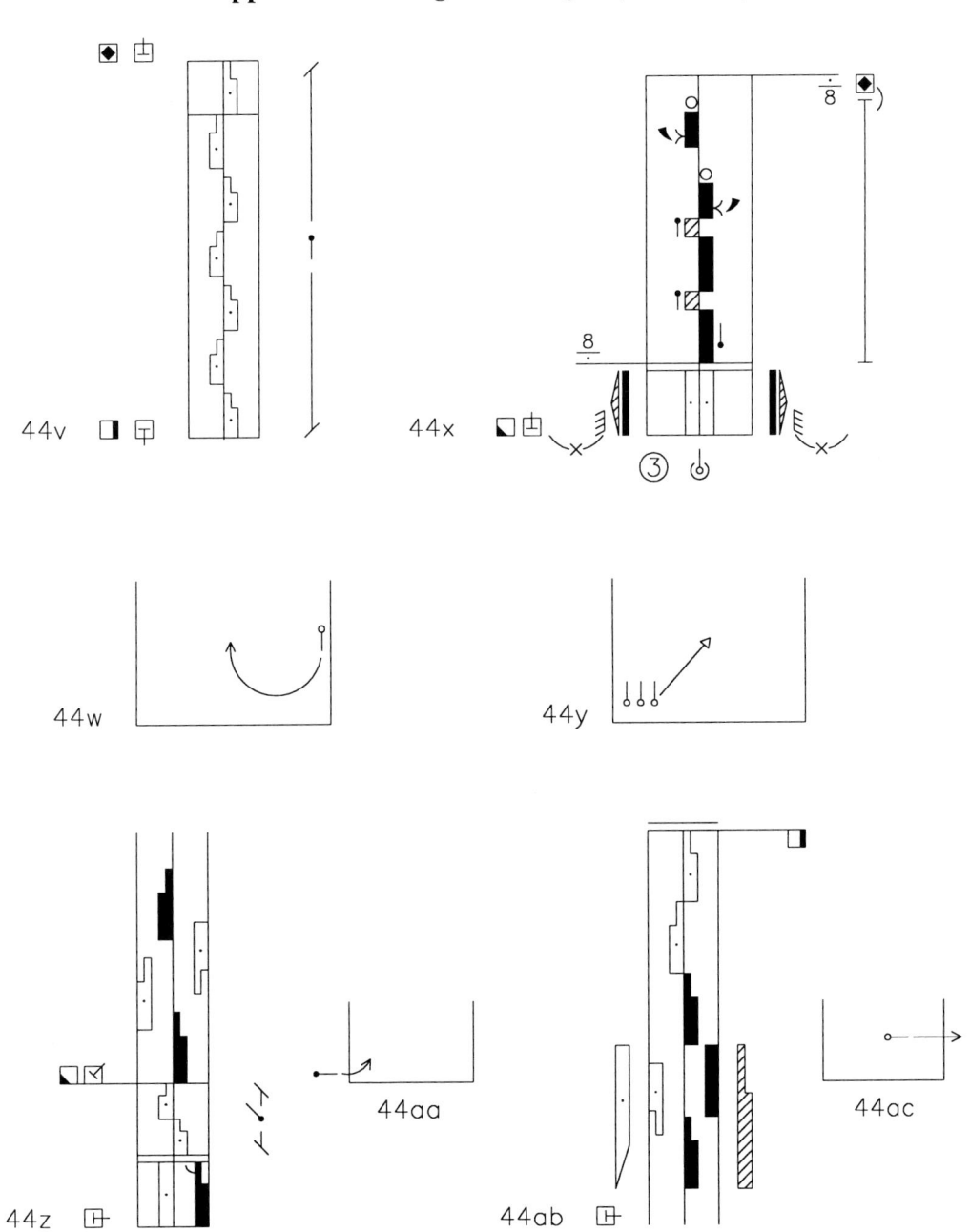

44v

44w

44x

44y

44z

44aa

44ab

44ac

152   *Spatial Variations*

44.7. Ex. **44ad** is an example of a partial entrance on stage; here the person leans and raises his/her arm so that the hand enters the stage and is visible to the audience.[85] A long pole is being brought on stage in **44ae**, the pole emerging first and the performer being seen only after taking three steps.

44.8. **Intermediate Areas**. An area between two stated areas is shown by linking the two area signs. Ex. **44af** indicates an area location between upstage right and center upstage; **44ag** an area between upstage right and the stage right center area. For such statements, the area signs can be placed side to side or one above the other. When drawn within one sign, as in **44ah**, the indication is for both areas. The areas of stage right and the adjacent corner areas is shown in **44ai**.

44.9. **Use of Narrow and Wide Signs.** A narrow sign placed inside an area sign indicates an area closer to the center of the stage or room. Thus **44aj** identifies an area between downstage center and center stage, and **44ak** an area between upstage left and center stage.

44.10. A wide sign inside an area sign indicates an area off-stage, i.e. outside the main performing area. The off-stage area behind the center upstage area, **44al**, is an indication which may be needed before a center upstage entrance is made. A less frequently used sign is **44am** which indicates an area, such as an apron stage, which lies in front of the proscenium arch and may on occasion be used, or it could be used to indicate the pit, if springing into the pit is needed. Ex. **44an** gives an overview of most of the signs discussed so far.

44.11. **Placement of Performers.** The next examples refer to a group of performers and their placement in relation to the stage/peformance area. These general indications have been found useful in recording large group dances, such as movement choirs. Ex. **44ao** indicates that any number of performers are spatially wide, distributed over the whole center of the performance area. In **44ap** they are grouped spatially closer at the center. The sign of **44aq** means around the periphery of the stage; **44ar** shows the area between the periphery and the center. The statement of **44as** means an arrangement in the peripheral ring. Outside the stage, beyond its periphery is shown as **44at**, an indication applicable to a circular arena where performers are waiting off-stage to enter.[86]

Advanced Labanotation

Application of Stage Area Signs (continued)

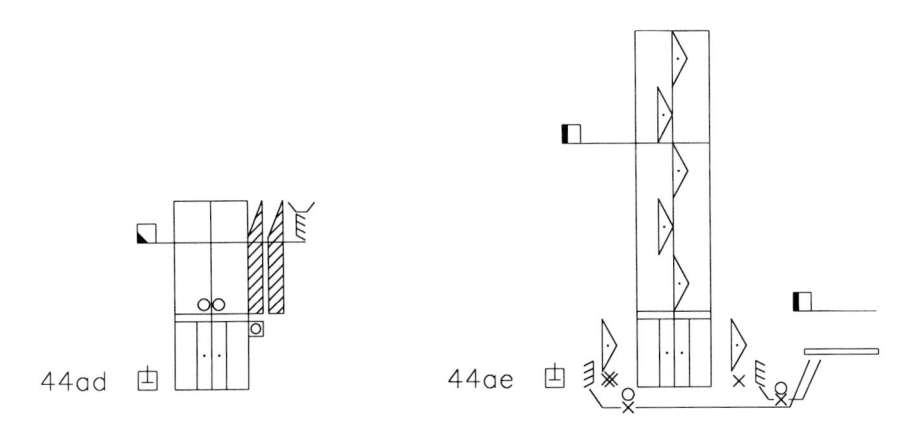

44ad 44ae

Intermediate Areas; Use of Narrow and Wide Signs

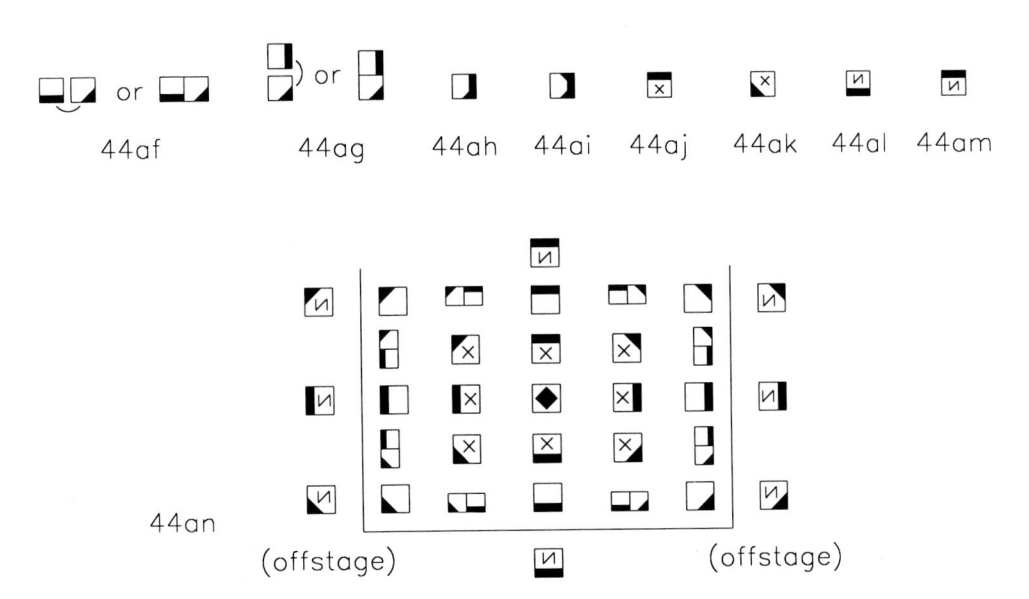

44af   44ag   44ah   44ai   44aj   44ak   44al   44am

44an

(offstage)   (offstage)

Placement of Performers

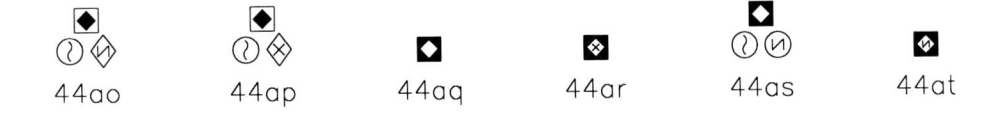

44ao   44ap   44aq   44ar   44as   44at

44.12. **Offstage Actions.** Preparations for entrances may occur off-stage as may the exiting landing from a leap or other movements not seen on stage. Preparations in the wings often include arranging a partner in a lift which has to be in place for the entrance. In **44au** the man needs a good impetus to get into his large entrance leap.

44.13. The performer in **44av** makes a running horizontal dive into the downstage right wing, landing on a mattress, indicated here as 'M'. This leaving the stage could also be written as **44aw**.

Advanced Labanotation

Offstage Actions

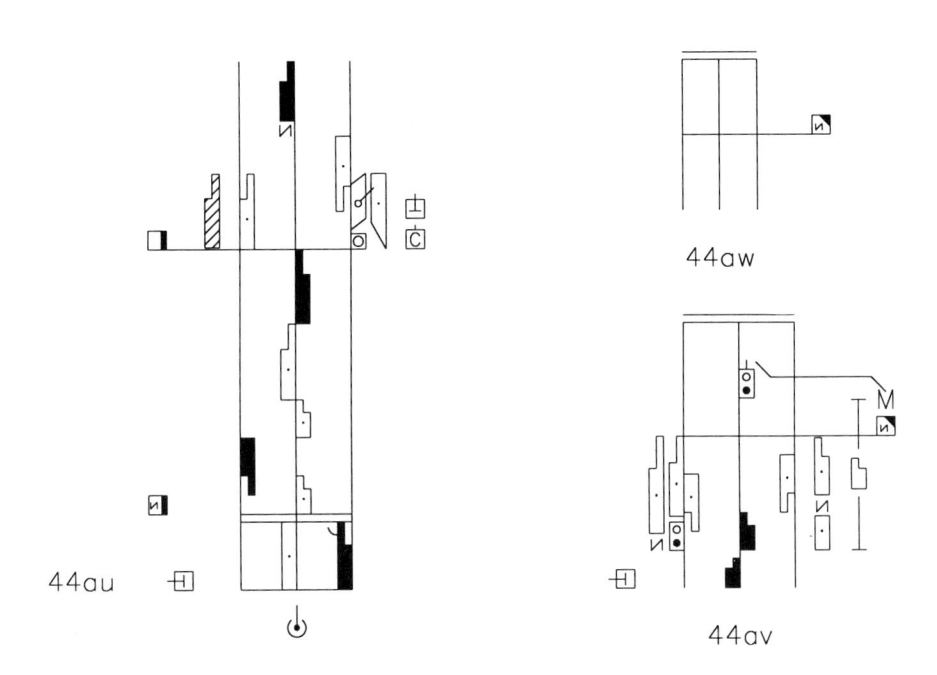

44au

44av

44aw

44.14. **Further Subdivisions Using Strokes.** The following additional subdivisions of the main areas may seldom be required in general practice but serve the purpose when such details are important. Subdivisions of the main areas can be stated by adding small strokes (tick marks) to the squares. The following examples indicate sections of the downstage left area. Ex. **44ax** means the front left corner of the downstage left section; **44ay** means the front part; **44az** the right front section; **44ba** means the left side; and **44bb** means the center section of this area. Exs. **44bc**, **44bd**, **44be** and **44bf** are determined similarly.

The middle of the main center area of the stage is identified as in **44bg**.

44.15. Additional identification of parts of such areas is also possible by combining two detailed indications, as in **44bh** which indicates the front points where the two stated areas meet, or **44bi** which shows the comparable point but closer to the central area on stage.

44.16. The chart of **44bj** shows the subdivisions of the right side area with details of the adjoining areas. Such specificity may be required in particular contexts where a person may need to move between objects placed in that general work area.[87] In **44bk** three people are shown to be located in specific parts of the stage right area. Their location is visually spelled out in **44bl**.

44.17. The chart of **44bm** is a condensation of **44bj** and shows the range (circled here) around that stage area with the contiguous neighboring parts included. This slight enlargement of the stated area may be needed for a performance limited, but not totally confined to that area. This freedom can be expressed as in **44bn** (also see 44.23).

44.18. Details for off-stage areas can be specified. Ex. **44bo** indicates the center of the apron stage area; **44bp** means the front edge of this area, while **44bq** indicates that part nearest to the stage.

Advanced Labanotation

Further Subdivisions Using Strokes

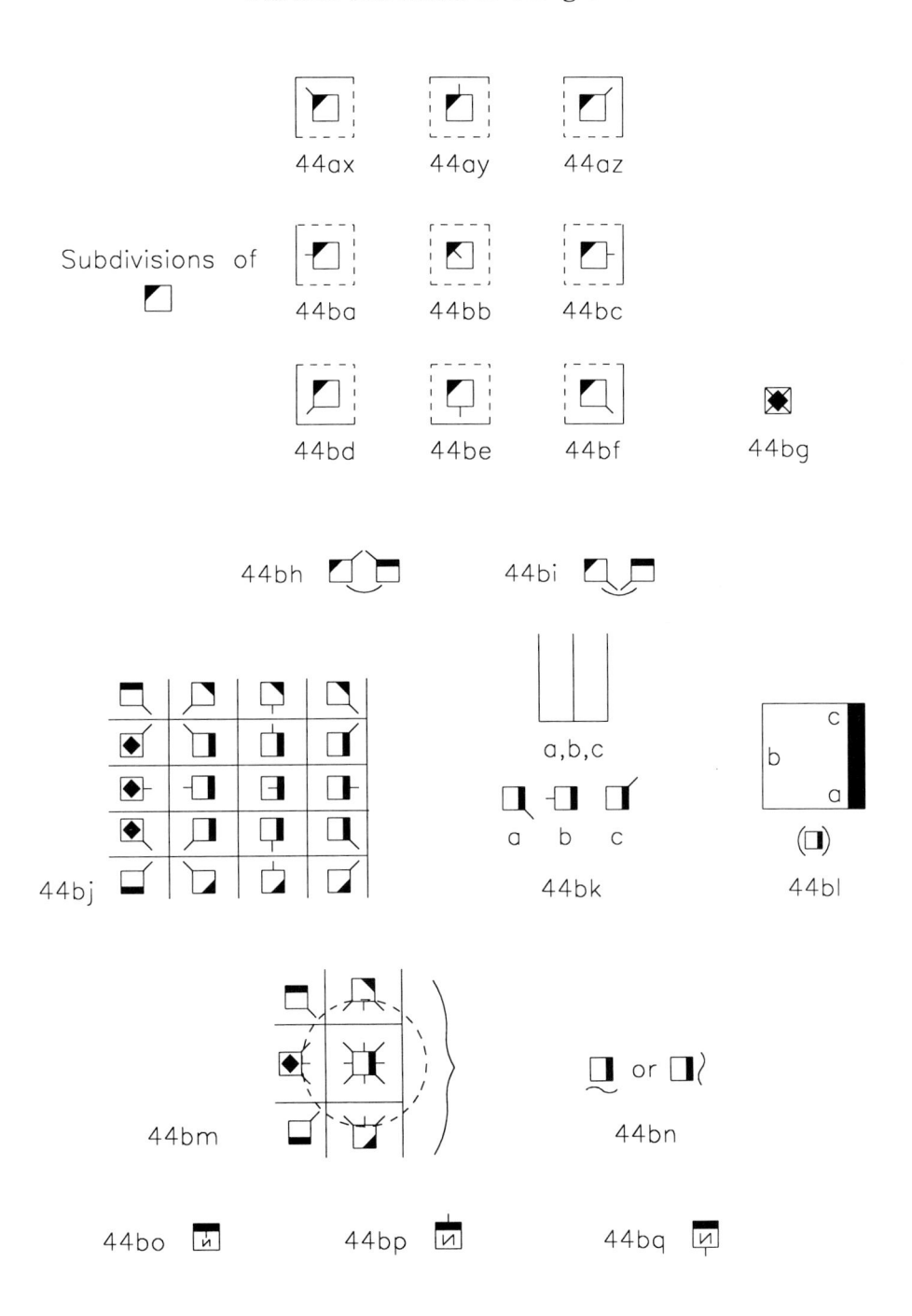

Subdivisions of ◰

44ax 44ay 44az
44ba 44bb 44bc
44bd 44be 44bf 44bg

44bh 44bi

44bj 44bk 44bl

44bm 44bn

44bo 44bp 44bq

44.19. **Unspecified Area.** The sign for 'an area related to space'[88] is useful in certain contexts, for example, when a large group of people, working in a large general space, should divide up into smaller groups, each taking their own area within which to work. Ex. **44br** is the general sign for an unspecified area. By adding tick marks, the nine specific inner areas can be shown, **44bs**, **44bt** being the center.

44.20. In **44bu** the position of working parts of a manufacturing bench are identified.[89] The basic unspecified area sign is valuable to indicate an example such as **44bv**. Here the instruction is to travel on any path to arrive at that place where you were in measure 32. Note use of a number in a diamond to indicate a music measure (bar).

44.21. **Areas Above or Below Stage Level.** Stage scenery may involve different levels, perhaps a platform, or a lower level, a trap door, which would be identified in the glossary. Shading of a small square symbol placed next to an area sign, can indicate the level of a area above or below stage level. Ex. **44bw** states an area above stage level, possibly a platform or raised stage. Ex. **44bx** describes an area beyond downstage center and below the normal stage level, for example, an orchestra pit. In a similar way the location of a trap door can be defined, in **44by** it is between the upstage right corner and the center area. A number in a square may indicate how many step-lengths the area is above or below the normal level. Ex. **44bz**, for example, is an area upstage right raised four step-lengths above the floor.[90]

44.22. **Indications for Floor, Water.** The basic sign for an area, the small square, is also used to indicate the floor (the ground). Within this box is placed a T (from the Latin 'Terra'), **44ca**. This T is often better drawn with a slight slant, as in **44cb**, to distinguish it from a middle level tack, as used in the front sign for facing upstage. The sign of **44cc** means water (from 'aqua'); and **44cd** means specifically the surface of the water.[91]

Advanced Labanotation

Unspecified Area

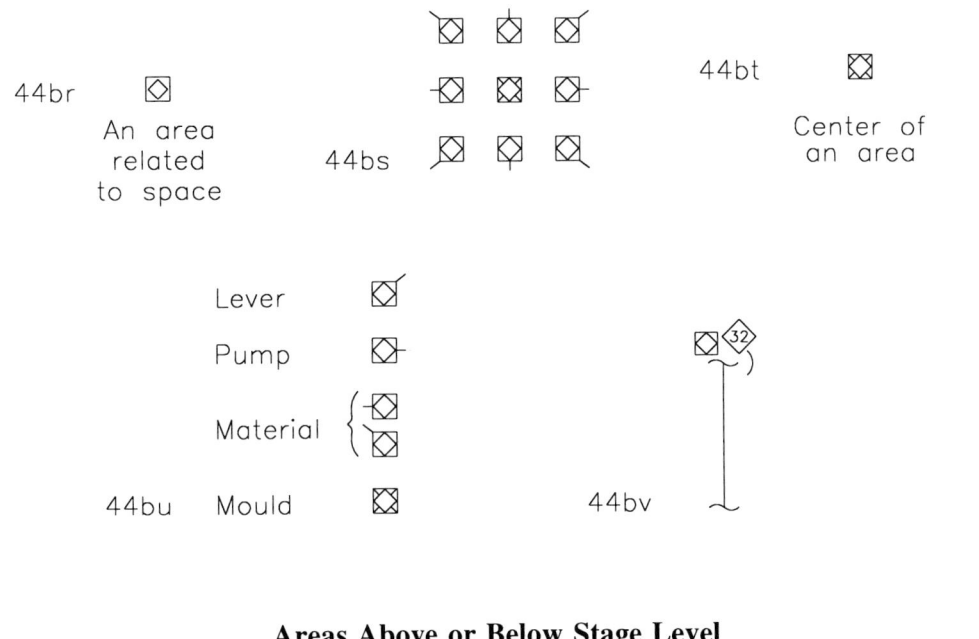

44br   An area related to space

44bs

44bt   Center of an area

44bu   Lever   Pump   Material   Mould

44bv

Areas Above or Below Stage Level

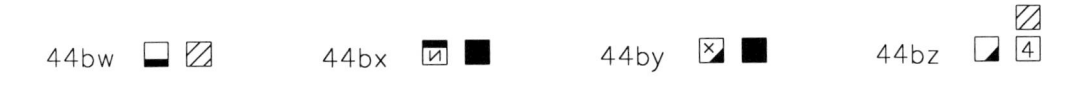

44bw   44bx   44by   44bz

Indications for Floor, Water

44ca   44cb   44cc   44cd

44.23. **Miscellaneous Area Indications.** The need for a free, general statement may require the sign of **44ce** which means anywhere in an area of some kind, usually it refers to a stage area. In contrast **44cf** states approximately at center stage. Similarly, **44cg** means anywhere in the undefined area,[92] The sign for 'any front' in a defined area is **44ch**. More or less facing front (the audience) can be shown as **44ci**.

44.24. The difference between the front area and the forward direction (the audience) on stage is not always clear. In **44cj** the face is looking to the central area at the front of the stage, whereas the in **44ck** the face is looking toward the audience, wherever on stage the performer is standing or where his/her front is directed. (For specific points in the audience see 46.6.)

44.25. Location in a circular arena may need to be shown. Ex. **44cl** shows the eight main areas. The back area, **44cm**, is usually the entrance, with **44cn** being the 'front', the opposite area. The side areas are shown as in **44co**, and the center area as **44cp**. Indication of additional detail can be applied in the same way as with the standard stage area signs, for example, **44cq** means near the front area.

Advanced Labanotation

Miscellaneous Area Indications

44ce

44cf

44cg

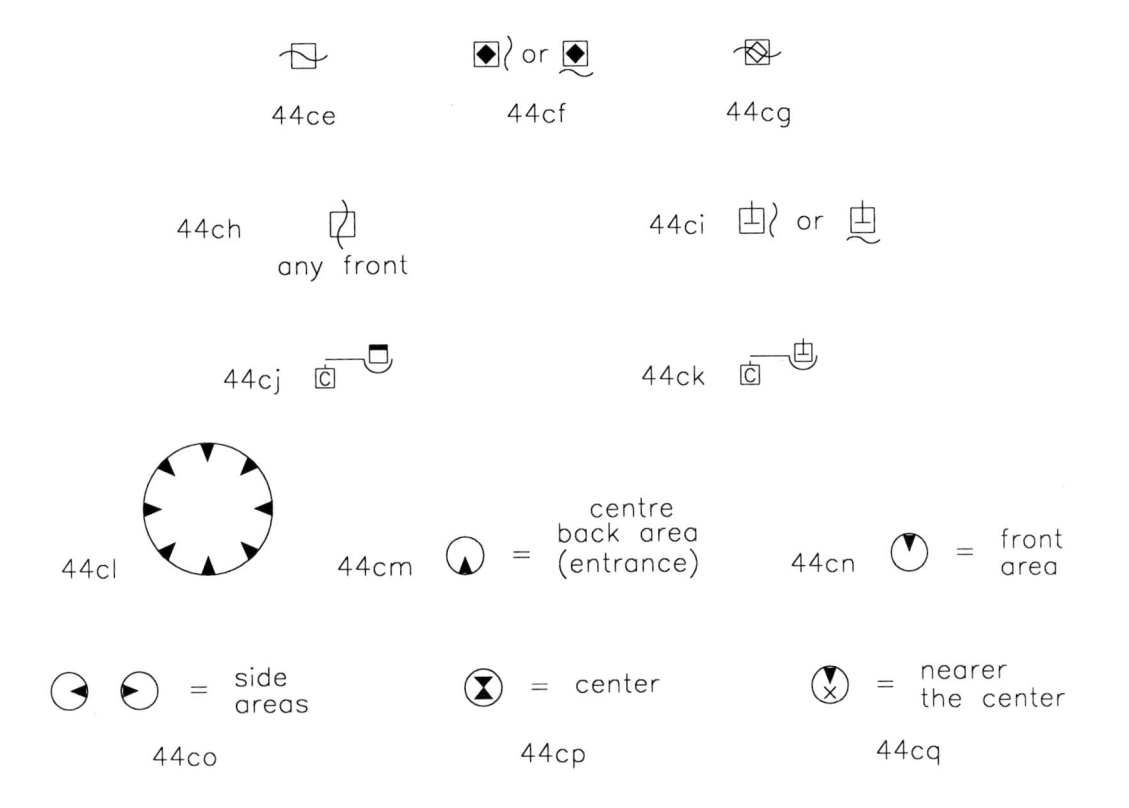

44ch   any front

44ci

44cj

44ck

44cl

44cm ◯ = centre back area (entrance)

44cn ◯ = front area

44co ◯ ◯ = side areas

44cp ◯ = center

44cq ◯ = nearer the center

45 Wings, Lines on Stage

45.1. **Indication of Wings on Stage.** From which wing a performer may enter or into which wing he/she should exit usually needs to be shown. Generally speaking, the signs of **45a** indicate exiting into the front wings, left and right, illustrated in the stage plan of **45b**. Ex. **45c** states exiting into the back wings, left and right, illustrated in **45d** in the floor plan. The simple statements of **45e** are understood to mean the middle wings, left and right, as illustrated in **45f**.

45.2. The intermediate wing downstage of the center left wing is written in **45g**, the two appropriate area signs being tied, this is illustrated in **45h**. In **45i** the performer is exiting in the wing upstage of the center left wing, shown in the floor plan of **45j**.

45.3. While stages vary in the number of wings that are set up, the most is usually five, illustrated in **45k**. By numbering these wings the required exit can readily be shown. Because the corner exits of **45a** and **45c** take care of the front and back exits, only three side exits usually need to be shown.

45.4. Exiting through the second left wing can be written as **45l** by adding the number to the stage left area sign. In **45m** the stage right 4th wing is indicated. These signs are, of course, applicable to both entrances and exits. It should be noted that when the entrance or exit wing is clearly shown on an accompanying floor plan, the simple indication of stage left or stage right will suffice. If a comedy entrance or exit in front of the fore-stage tabs (the proscenium arch exit below the first wing) is required, **45a** can be used, its modified meaning being given in a glossary.

Advanced Labanotation

Indication of Wings on Stage

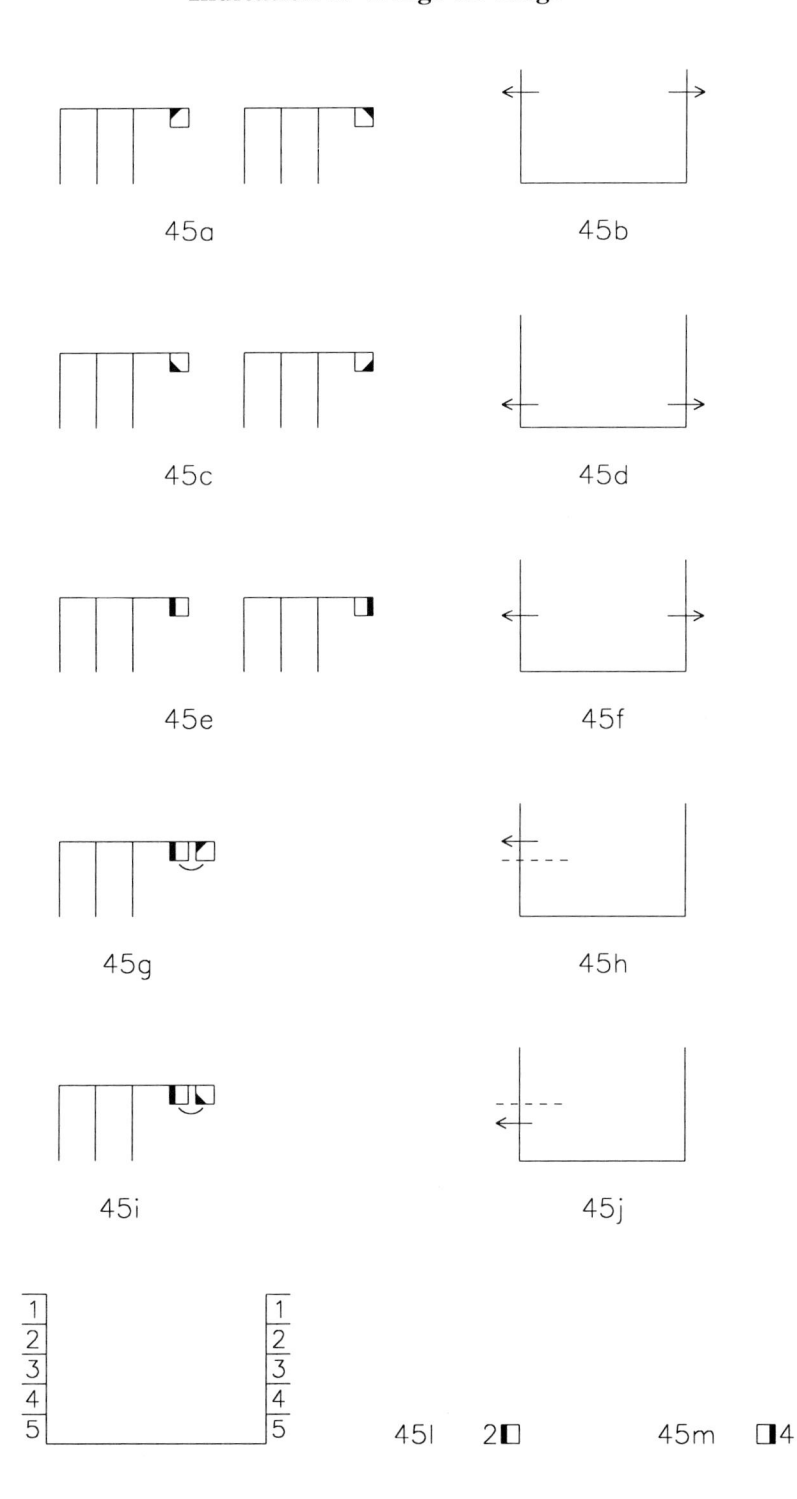

45a

45b

45c

45d

45e

45f

45g

45h

45i

45j

45k

45l 2

45m 4

164   *Spatial Variations*

45.5. **Lines on Stage.** It is often important on stage to show that dancers are standing on the center line which runs from the front of the stage to the back; also frequently used are the quarter line marks and the eighth line marks. The diagram in **45n** illustrates these imaginary lines on stage. Indications for the locations of these lines are often painted at the front of the stage. Ex. **45o** illustrates a floor plan drawing indicating the center and quarter lines, often used in a theatrical score. Ex. **45p** is the symbol for the center line; this can also be written as **45q**.[93] Ex. **45r** is the stage left $^3/_8$ line; **45s** the left $^1/_4$ line; and **45t** the left $^1/_8$ line. A comparable set of signs exist for the stage right divisions, **45u** illustrates the first such division in the stage right area.

45.6. Also important are the center and quarter lines running laterally from stage left to stage right; these are shown as follows: **45v** is the lateral center line; this can also be written as **45w**. Ex. **45x** shows the downstage $^3/_8$ line; **45y** the downstage $^1/_4$ line, and **45z** the downstage $^1/_8$ line. A comparable set of signs exists for the upstage lateral divisions, **45aa** shows the first such division in the upstage area.

45.7. These indications can be combined to show both lateral and sagittal stage placement. Ex. **45ab** shows the performer to be on the center line of the upstage $^1/_4$ line. This could also be written as **45ac**. Placement on the downstage $^1/_4$ line and stage left quarter is stated in **45ad**. The statement for exact center is **45ae**; note the alternate sign for exact center given in **44bb, 44bg**.

45.8. Where small stage plans need to be written, the center line can be indicated as in **45af**. It is important that the basic stage plan shape is clear and that it not be drawn like the original sign for the body-as-a-whole, **45ag**.[94]

Advanced Labanotation

Lines on Stage

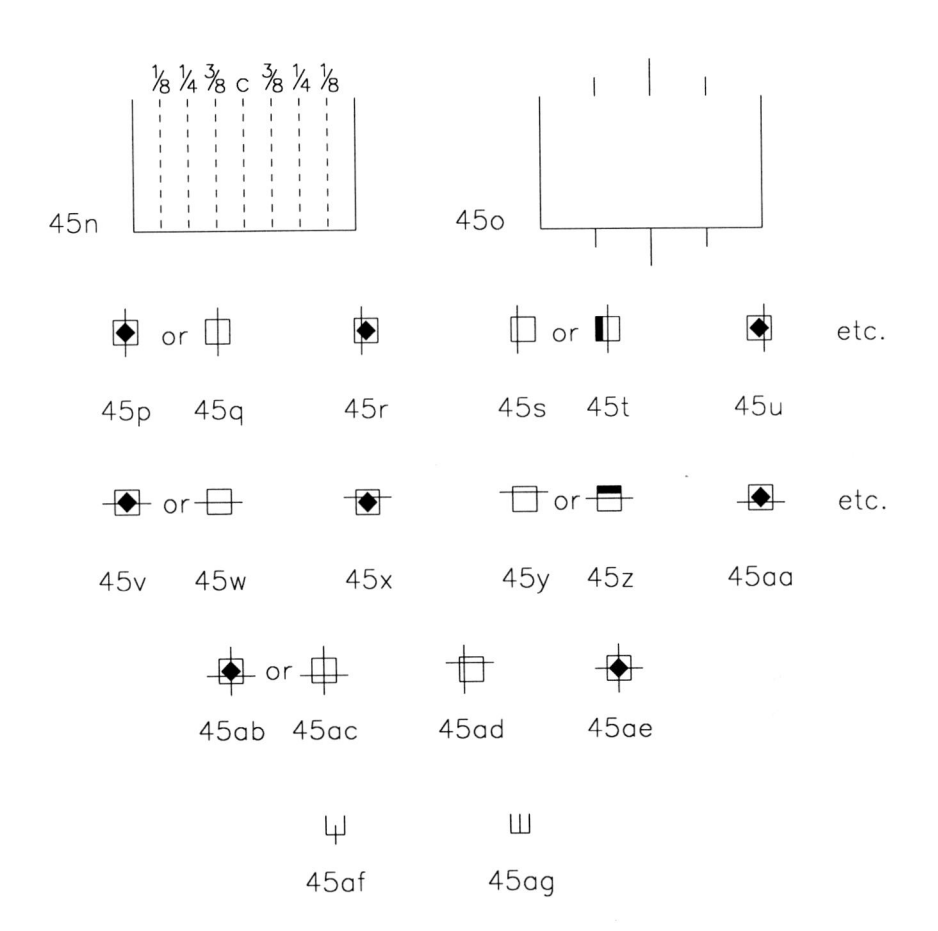

⅛ ¼ ⅜ C ⅜ ¼ ⅛

45n   45o

◆ or ▯   ◆   ▯ or ▮   ◆   etc.

45p 45q   45r   45s 45t   45u

◆ or ▯   ◆   ▯ or ▬   ◆   etc.

45v 45w   45x   45y 45z   45aa

◆ or ⊞   ⊟   ◆

45ab 45ac   45ad   45ae

⊔   ⊔

45af   45ag

45.9. **Specific Stage Diagonals.** A diagonal path on stage may need to be slightly shallower or steeper than the standard 45° angle. The steps in **45ah** should follow a true 45° diagonal line on stage. If the stage is square, the performer, starting center stage, will follow the diagonal line from upstage left to downstage right, as in **45ai**. However, most stages (or rooms) are not square and the progression of **45ah** will not be toward the stage right corner, **45aj**. To make the path shallower, as in **45ak**, either the facing direction or the step direction should be changed. In **45al** the same front is maintained and intermediate step directions are used. In **45am** the front direction is modified to halfway between the diagonal and stage right; with this front ordinary forward steps can be used.

45.10. Often the choreography calls for facing downstage right with the step direction being adjusted unobtrusively by the performer to produce the path of **45ak**. To keep such adjustment simple, the device of alerting the reader to see the floor plan is stated in **45an**. It should be noted that in general usage, when **45ah** is written, the performance of **45ak** is often expected. As a rule the indication on the floor plan takes precedence over the movement description.

45.11. A path on stage may need to follow an unusual diagonal line, or a group of performers may need to be placed on a particular diagonal line, for example, line a) or line b) shown in the floor plan of **45ao**. The appropriate stage area signs can be stated with a line connecting them, **45ap** representing the line a), with **45aq** representing line b), it being understood that here it is the center of the stage right area that is being defined.

45.12. For specialized needs the device of numbering the walls and alphabetizing the corners of the stage can be established at the start of a score to indicate particular lines on stage. In **45ar** the numbering is established in a clockwise direction with the addition of letters for the corners. The line and the direction of travel can, for example, be shown as **45as**, or as **45at** when in the reverse direction.

45.13. When required an even more detailed plan such as **45au** can be established. Here lines a), b) and c) have been indicated on the plan as examples. In the score these can be abbreviated to **45av**. Such devices are not generally needed when careful floor plans accompany the movement description. However, in special circumstances they can prove valuable.[95]

Advanced Labanotation

Specific Stage Diagonals.

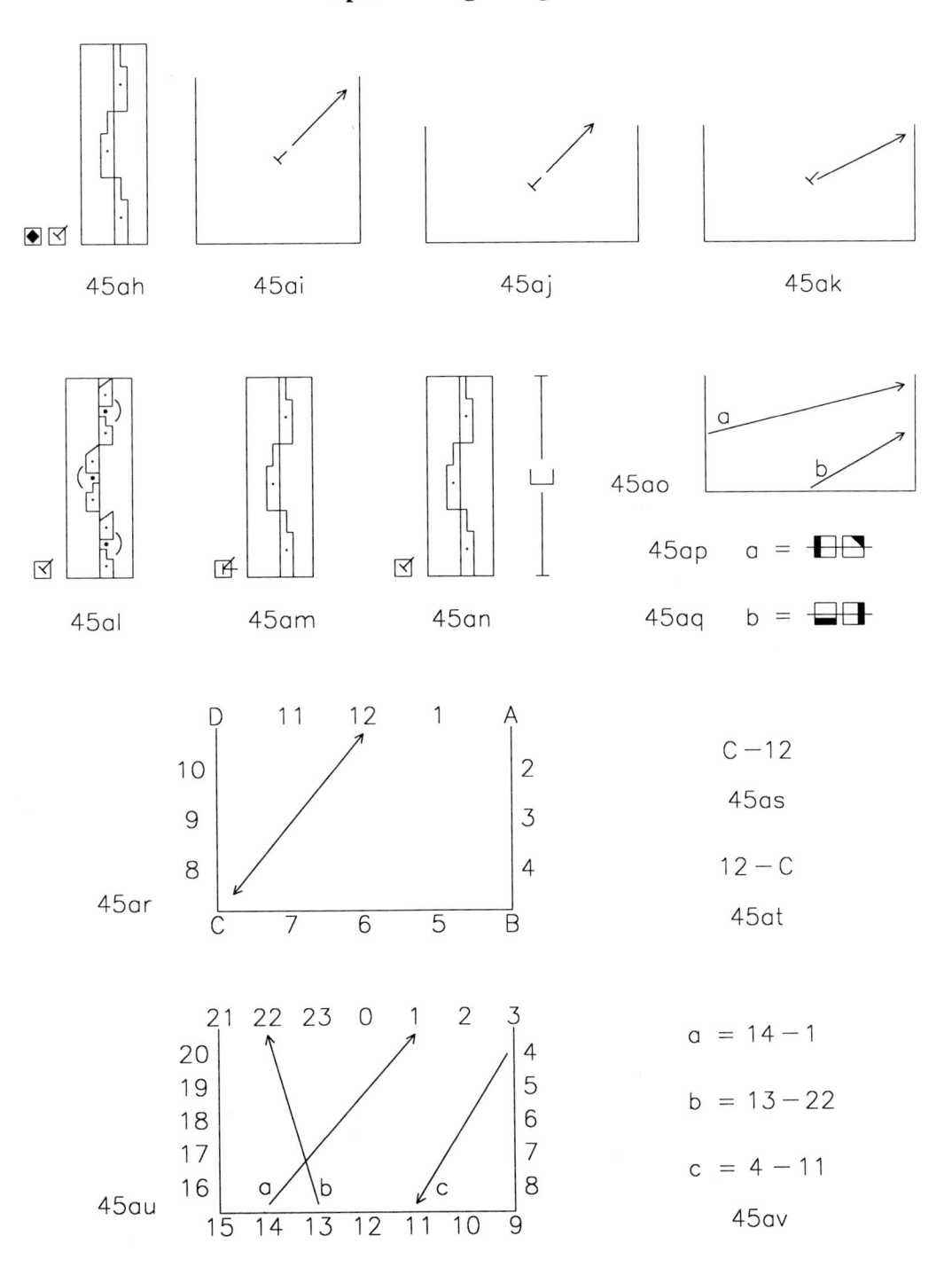

45ah   45ai   45aj   45ak

45al   45am   45an   45ao

45ap   a = ▭▬

45aq   b = ▬▭

45ar

D 11 12 1 A
10   2
 9   3
 8   4
   C 7 6 5 B

C − 12
45as

12 − C
45at

45au

21 22 23 0 1 2 3
20   4
19   5
18   6
17   7
16 a b   c   8
 15 14 13 12 11 10 9

a = 14 − 1

b = 13 − 22

c = 4 − 11

45av

46 Fixed Points in a Defined Space

46.1. The specific points of the physical room or stage can be designated. These are located at the surfaces, edges and corners, and their location is judged from the center of the room, midway between the four walls, the floor and the ceiling. The key for this system of reference is **46a**. Pins (strokes) are added to define the main points, **46b**.

46.2. The level of these fixed points is shown by use of the white pin (high), tack (middle level), or black pin (low level). Ex. **46c** shows the lower left front corner; **46d** the upper left front corner; **46e** the center of the ceiling. Note that, because there is not room to place the pin for 'above' within the basic sign, this need has to be expressed either through use of the two side high pins, as in **46e**, the point between them (place high) being understood. Alternately the above pin can be placed above the key, **46f**. As a rule two pins are used to show intermediate points, as in **46g**.

46.3. By using the Fixed Points Key, as in **46h**, all directions are to be judged from this key. This means all directions for gestures refer to a spot in the room. For example, a right side high symbol would refer to the middle of the right upper edge of the room. The stated direction also applies to supports, but level for supports are to be understood in the usual way. In this example the three performers are standing in different areas of the stage, facing different directions. In the starting position their arms are all directed to the center of the upper edge of the foreground. As all travel toward the right upstage corner, their arms are directed first to the lower upstage right corner, then to the upper point in that same corner. The performers are converging on a common aim. The Fixed Point Key remains in effect until cancelled by another key, usually the Standard Key, as shown here.[96]

46.4. Only the details essential to our purpose are given in **46i**. A group of 16 people, arranged around the edges of three sides of the stage, are all looking at the center of the lower edge of the left center side of the stage. Gradually their gaze rises as they follow an ascending light within the building.[97]

46.5. In **46j** the performer begins facing front, the right arm extended forward high. The motion which follows is one of drawing away from the forward high fixed point.

Advanced Labanotation   169

46.6. **Fixed Points in the Audience.** The front sign in **46k** indicates looking at the audience. In the floor plan of **46l** each performer looks into the forward Constant Direction from where they are standing. Thus the sign means 'audience' only in a general sense. In some plays, particularly comedies, the performer may actually look at specific parts of the audience. In Denmark's Royal Theatre it is the custom to bow first to the royal box. The plan of **46m** includes the main levels of the spectators. An S (for spectators) in a box, **46n**, is combined with a pin to indicate the appropriate part of the audience. The front lower part of the orchestra seating is shown as **46o**; the upper back balcony is **46p**; the Danish royal box is indicated by **46q**. Other parts of the audience are indicated in this manner.

Fixed Points in a Defined Space

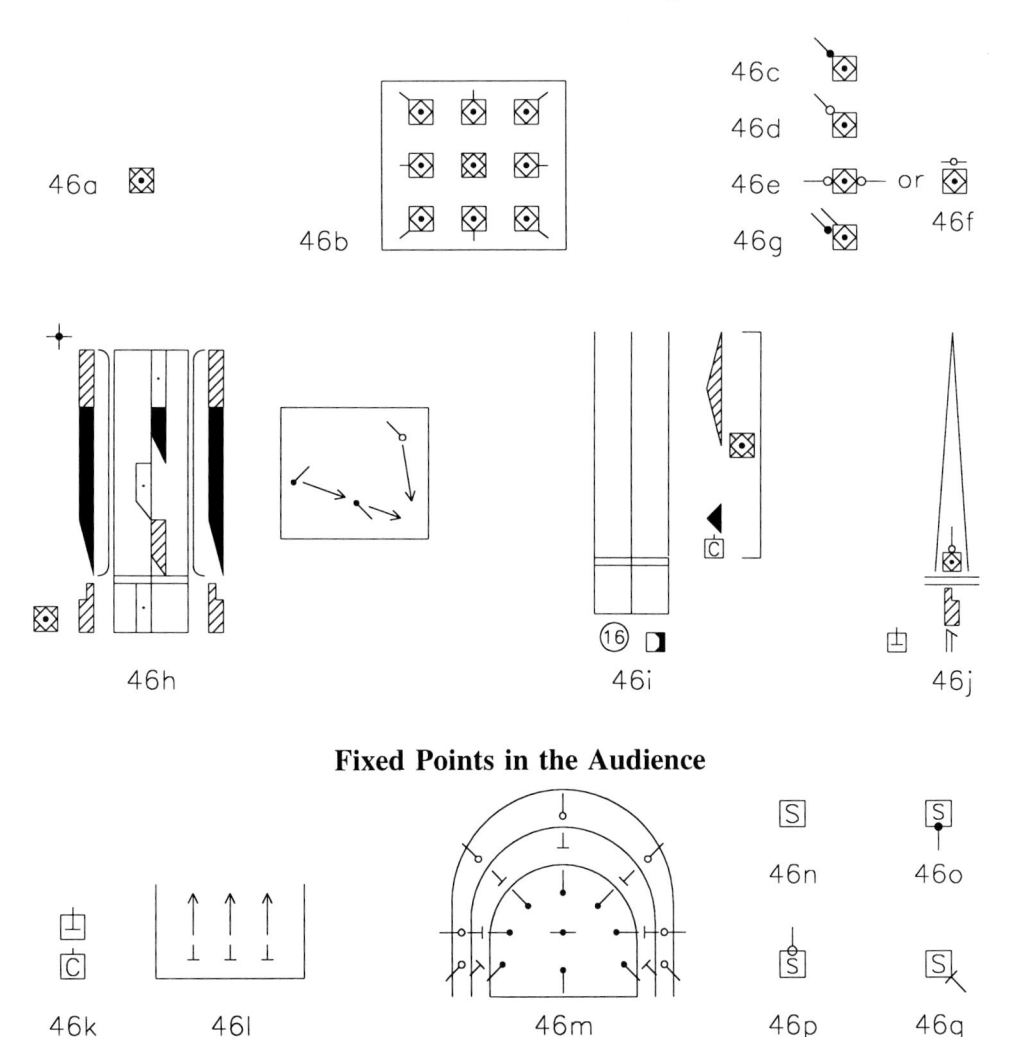

Fixed Points in the Audience

X MISCELLANEOUS

47 Carets, Spot Holds, Same Spot Caret

The purpose of this section is to explore in detail the transitions between positions of the feet, weight on both, weight on one and the difference in meaning according to how these transitions are written.

47.1. **Use of Ordinary Caret.** The basic meaning of the caret is 'the same'. It is used for the same part of the body, the same circling (continuation of a circular path), the same support, and so on. Here we are concerned with its application to support symbols. We will look first at the basic meaning of the direction symbols in the support column, progressing from the simplest to the less obvious, and see how the caret modifies or clarifies the performance.

47.2. **In Place.** In **47a** weight changes from being on the right foot in middle level to being on the left foot in middle level. The manner of performance is clearly to take a step in place. The addition of the hold sign in **47b** indicates that weight is held on the right foot and so the performer ends with weight on both feet. If a change of level must be indicated, a hold sign cannot be used; therefore in **47c** a sinking on the right foot takes place as the left foot closes in to take weight next to the right. The presence of a gap, as in **47d**, indicates a spring, the landing being on both feet in place. The feet are now on either side of the center line where the single right foot support had been.

47.3. Next we explore the transition from two feet to one. In **47e** a hold sign is placed over the right support, thus, from standing feet together, the right foot is retained while the left is no longer supporting. The hold sign gives no timing, but remaining in middle level is understood. At its basic level, the notation of **47f** states "From weight on both feet, weight changes to being only on the right foot." But should a shift to the right take place or should the right foot lift and take a step in place? The same question arises with a change in level, as in **47g**. Because the initial aim in the development of the Laban system was to produce a structured description of the movement, **47f** and **47g** were given the specific meaning of taking a step in place.[98] The idea that a step should take place came from the automatic releasing of the foot to take a step forward, **47h**, or into any other direction except place.

47.4. To indicate only a sinking on the right leg, the two symbols are joined with a caret, meaning 'the same', as in **47i**.[99] A specific statement of releasing the foot could be given as in **47j**. To show a slow release, the duration line can be linked to the release sign, as in **47k**.

Advanced Labanotation

47.5. Closed to Open.[100] A basic statement of the transition from a closed position to an open is given in **47l**; weight is shown to be retained on the left foot, no change of level occurs. With change of level, a direction symbol needs to be written. Ex. **47m** show the motion description for stepping out into 2nd position bending the legs; the left leg sinks in place (where it is) while the right leg steps out. Both of these occur at the same time so that the weight is carried half a step-length to the right.[101] Writing the resulting position, as in **47n**, is visually easier for most people to understand. But **47n** gives no indication as to how the 2nd position is to be achieved. As there is no gap, it cannot be a spring as in **47o**, both feet opening out at the same time.[102] Nor is there any indication of sliding the feet. In **47p** the caret indicates the left foot does not move, the left foot retains the same support, while the right foot steps out. Note that, while 2nd position is featured here, the usage is applicable to any open position.

Use of Ordinary Caret

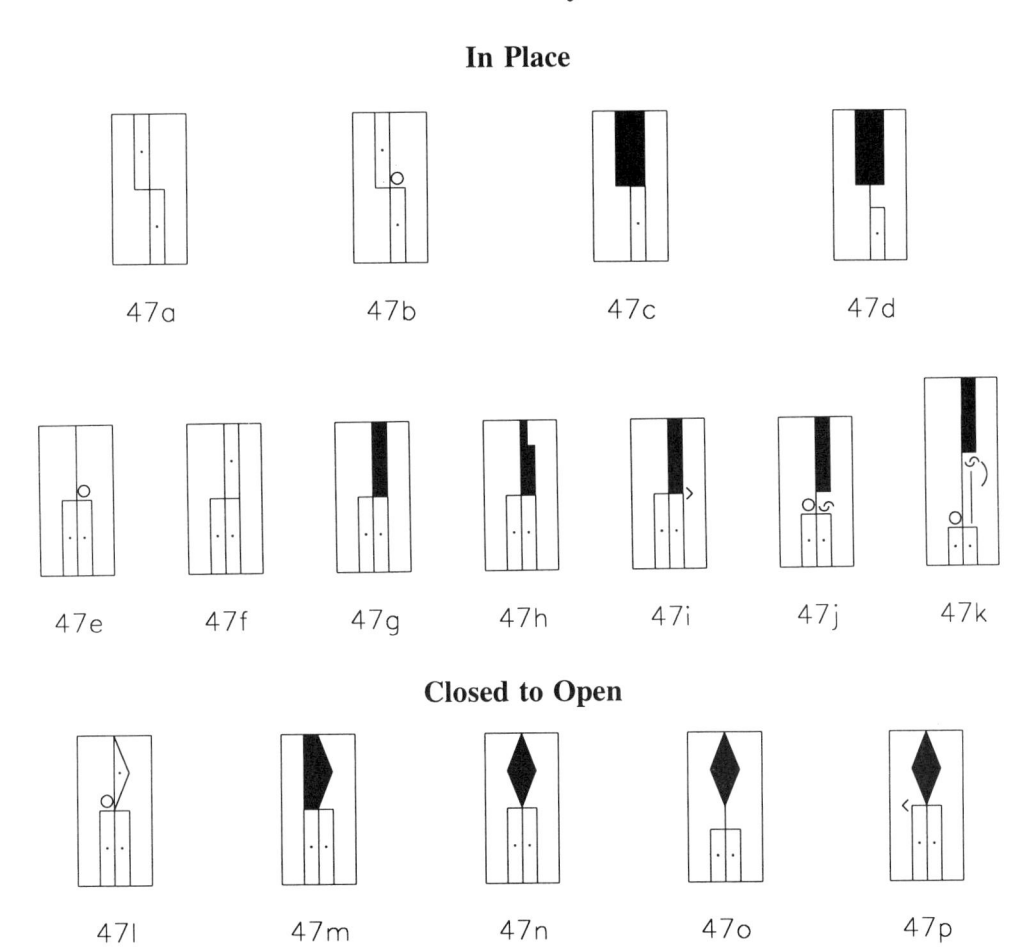

In Place

47a　　　47b　　　47c　　　47d

47e　　47f　　47g　　47h　　47i　　47j　　47k

Closed to Open

47l　　　47m　　　47n　　　47o　　　47p

47.6. **Open to Closed on Two Feet.** The next examples explore changes from an open position to a closed position on two feet. The basic statement of **47q** is a transition from 2nd position with legs bent to 1st position in middle level, but no manner of performance is given (compare with **47n**). In **47r** a spring occurs, thus both feet are brought in to place. Ex. **47s** specifies that the left foot is to retain the same support while the right closes in.

47.7. The addition of a pin, as in **47t**, shows which foot is active, here it is the right foot which closes in to form the 5th position, the caret is not needed in this case. The sideward pin of **47u** can give the same message by producing the same result as **47s**, the right foot next to the left (a sideward relationship). Both feet can slide in at the same time, as in **47v**; to achieve this with weight constantly on the floor, the floor needs to be sufficiently slippery and the performer needs to have strong legs, particularly if the action is to be slow. For a quick action of this kind, a slight lifting of the weight usually occurs, enough to facilitate sliding the feet together, **47w**, in which the short lines in the leg gesture columns indicate weight is lifted, no longer a total support. In **47x** the closed position is achieved by sliding the right foot into place. For this to happen, the weight must be taken onto the left foot. The performance of **47x** may well be closer to **47y**. Here the sliding is shown as a gesture, weight being taken on the right foot only at the end. For the right foot to slide without weight, it is understood that weight will have been shifted onto the left foot, although this is not indicated in **47y**. A caret here for the left foot, **47z**, may facilitate reading, though in terms of movement logic it is not necessary.

47.8. The brief description of **47s** is not converted so readily into a highly detailed description of the actual movement involved. The shift of weight to the left must be indicated separately, **47aa**. What is the timing of this shift before the right foot closes in? Is it rather quick, as in **47aa**? Or slower, as in **47ab**? When does the change in level take place? Is it after the weight shift to the side, as in **47ab**? Or does the level change during the weight shift as shown in **47ac**? The motion description allows for finely detailed differences which may be important, however, they may also not be important, especially when the action is quick. Thus even professional notators make use of position writing when it best serves their needs.

Advanced Labanotation

Use of the Ordinary Caret (continued)

Open to Closed on Two Feet

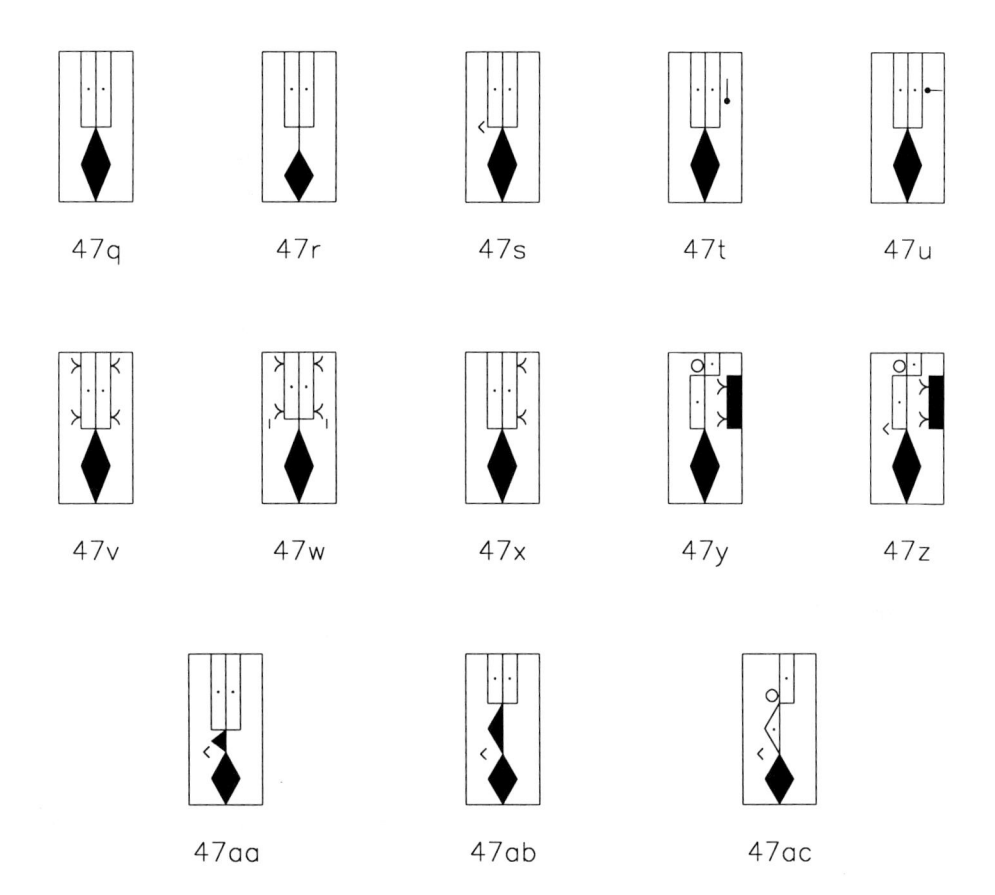

47q   47r   47s   47t   47u

47v   47w   47x   47y   47z

47aa   47ab   47ac

47.9. **From Open Position to Weight on One Foot.** Moving from an open position to weight only on one foot needs careful consideration. If no special rule has been learned, the symbols in **47ad** state: from 2nd position with bent legs, weight changes to being only on the right leg in middle level. If this were to be a spring, as in **47ae**, clearly the right foot lands in place, between where the two feet had been. Ex. **47af** appears the same as **47ad**, but the caret stating 'the same' indicates that the right foot takes weight as the level changes.

47.10. A look at understood but unwritten movements is of value here. In **47ag**, from a 2nd position, the right foot steps across to the left diagonal. To achieve this, the weight must first be transferred (shifted) onto the left foot. Two unwritten actions occur where the arrow is pointing in this notation: the lifting of the right foot and the shift of weight to the left. It is because of these understood but unwritten actions that it can be considered logical to place the release sign next to the end of the 2nd position support sign, as in **47ah**, to indicate the releasing of weight that automatically occurs before a step. With this understood, the notation of **47ah** reads as a step on the right foot in place, next to the left foot. The validity of a symbol often depends on what follows. As we have already seen, shifting the weight and releasing the foot from the floor can both be described in detail when needed.

47.11. **Rise Without Adjusting the Feet.** The need to show that one foot remains where it is, comes up in the following examples, which show change of level in 5th position.[103] In **47ai** the 5th position pin is not repeated, thus a rise into 1st position should result. How this 1st position is achieved can be shown with the caret, **47aj**, here the left foot is not displaced, it is the right foot that closes in to 1st. This statement could also be made with the 'at the side' pin, as in **47ak**. The pin shows the active foot.

47.12. Repeating the pin for the right foot in **47al** shows that the right foot moves to form the 5th position as you rise. In **47am** it is the left foot which moves. Because the pin gives sufficient information, use of a caret for these last two examples is not needed. The small gap in **47an** allows the weight to be off the floor enough for both feet to adjust into the 5th position. A barre exercise usage is **47ao**, illustrated in **47ap**, in which both balls of the feet remain where they are. This produces an untidy, somewhat open 5th position, used in movement exercises.

47.13. **Motion or Destination Description.** In **47aq** the shift of weight to the left foot is accompanied by a resultant right leg gesture touching on the toe. The transition to the left foot is shown as the motion of sideward sinking. Described with position writing, **47ar**, the message becomes more one of sinking

Advanced Labanotation

in place. To complete the position writing, the right leg gesture should also be included, **47as**. A wrong emphasis is given here because the direction symbol usually states an active (rather than a resultant) leg gesture. For quick writing such subtle distinctions may not be important. Because of the step gesture rule,[104] the movement in **47at** will be one of sinking on the right leg, the left foot being freed of weight at the start of the count.

Use of Ordinary Caret (continued)

From Open Position to Weight on One Foot

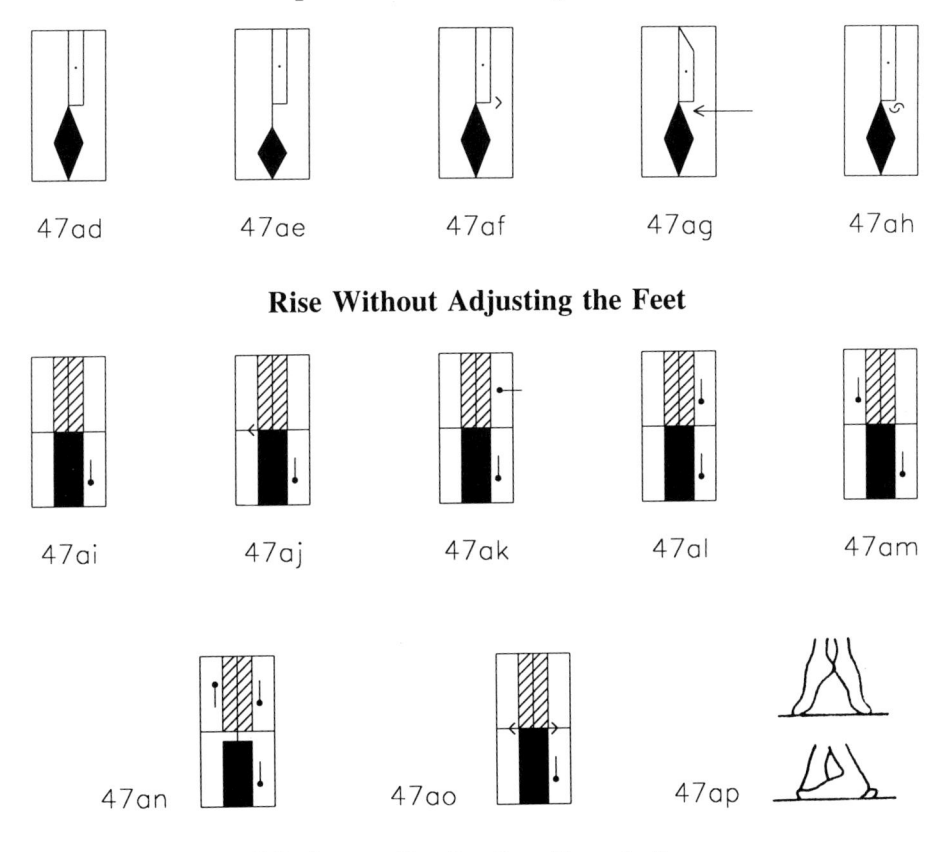

47ad   47ae   47af   47ag   47ah

Rise Without Adjusting the Feet

47ai   47aj   47ak   47al   47am

47an   47ao   47ap

Motion or Destination Description

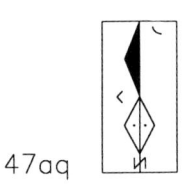

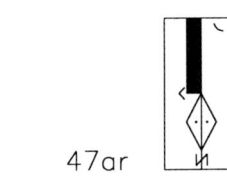

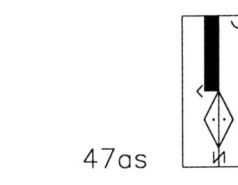

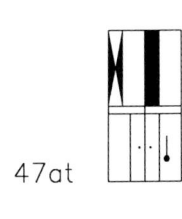

47aq   47ar   47as   47at

47.14. **Zed Caret.** A zed caret[105] links a gesture to a support or a support to a gesture. In **47au** the foot may, or may not, lift and step beyond where it was touching, exact performance is left open. The zed caret in **47av** links the toe touch to the new support, thus clearly stating that the foot does not lift but is placed so that the toe remains where it was. Often an ordinary caret is used here with the same meaning. A new step must occur in **47aw**, because the contact with the floor is released.

47.15. In **47ax** the toe remains where it was in the parallel 4th position, the weight shifting back to allow the toe contact to happen. Note that a different spatial result is produced in **47ay** because the feet are very turned out.

47.16. When a step follows after a free, off the floor leg gesture, the zed caret can be used with the meaning that the free gesture leads into (is connected to) the following step. This modifies the usual performance. In **47az** a 45° forward low leg gesture is followed by a step forward. By linking the two with a zed caret, **47ba**, the purpose of the gesture is different, it will be much lower, leading directly into the step, a preparatory movement, rather than a full gesture in its own right. (See 47.21 for use of the Same-Spot Zed Caret.)

47.17. **Retention of a Spot (Spot Hold).** A survey of the familiar uses of the spot hold sign, **47bb**, will be given first. Note the cancellation sign of **47bc** for a spot hold. The toe touch in **47bd** is to remain on the same spot during the turn to the left. While lying on the floor in **47be**, the left leg is to retain its spot while the right leg circles out to the side, up and across to the other side before returning to its forward starting position. From a squat, the hips slide backward in **47bf** while the feet stay on the same spot. The right hand retains an imaginery spot in the air in **47bg** while the performer walks a half circle around it. This spot hold is released when the torso tilts to the side.

Advanced Labanotation 177

Zed Caret

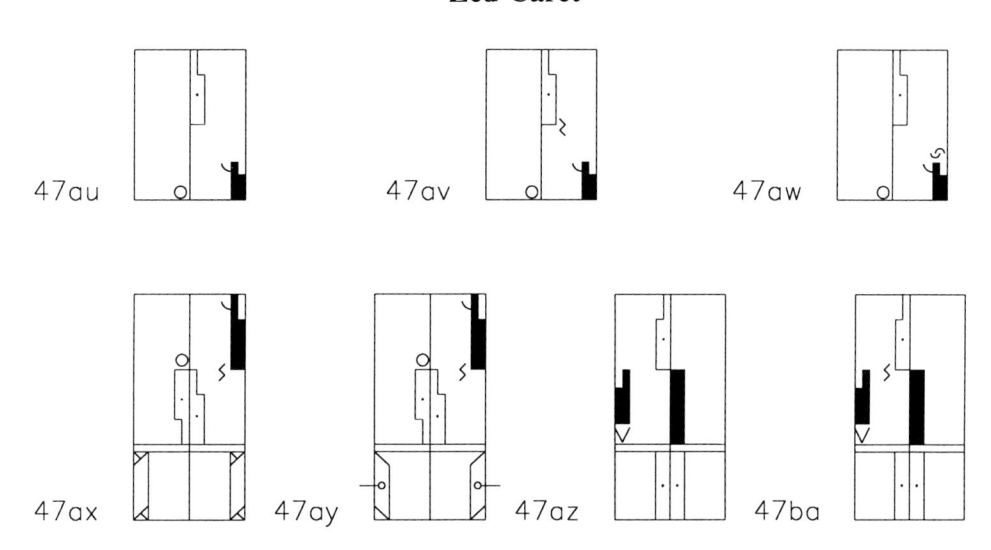

47au 47av 47aw

47ax 47ay 47az 47ba

Retention of a Spot (Spot Hold)

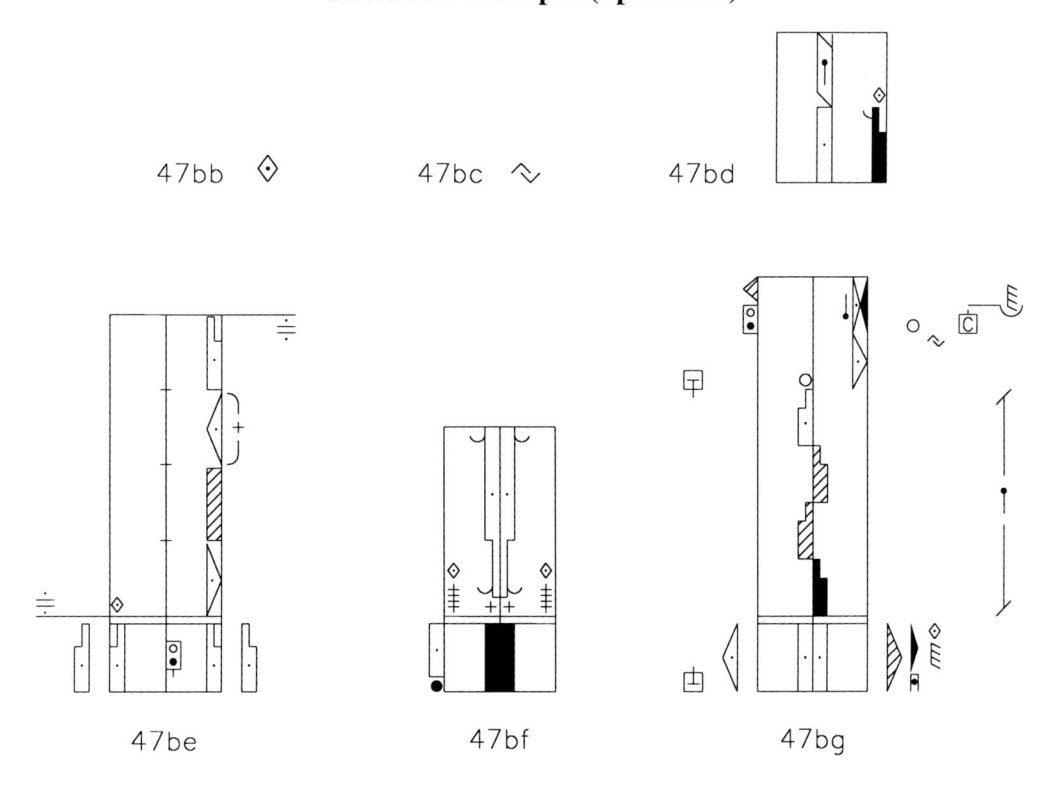

47bb 47bc 47bd

47be 47bf 47bg

47.18. **Same-Spot Caret.** Retaining or returning to the same spot can occur from a support to a support, in particular after a spring; from a support to a gesture; or a gesture to a support. The 'same spot' caret, derived from the spot hold sign, is distinguished by the addition of the dot, **47bh**.[106]

47.19. In **47bi**, from a 4th position, the front foot is released and then steps on the same spot. An ordinary caret is not so serviceable here; the same-spot caret is more definitive.

47.20. The next examples show use of the same-spot caret after springing.[107] Without the same spot caret in **47bj**, the left foot would land in place between where the two feet were located; the same spot caret defines what is meant by the place sign here. It is likely that a preferred description would be **47bk**, which states the sideward motion onto the left foot. The next example is from one foot to two; in **47bl** the same-spot caret indicates how the resulting 2nd position should be reached, i.e. the left foot lands on the same spot. A preferred description may be **47bm** in which the left foot returns to where it had been previously while at the same time producing a 2nd position with the right (the movement description).

47.21. **Same-Spot Zed Caret.** The support-to-gesture same-spot zed caret may be needed after a gesturing leg has been lifted from the ground. In **47bn**, after the spring, the right foot touches where it had been when it was supporting. An example of gesture-to-support is **47bo** in which, after the foot has released, the step is to take place on the same spot where it had been touching. In **47bp** the sideward step is to be placed on the spot on the floor below which the right foot had been extended.

47.22. Landing in place where the other foot was previously may be needed. In **47bq** each foot lands in its own track, next to the other foot. The elongated zed caret of **47br** indicates that the right foot should land where the left foot was, and then vice versa, resulting in landing each time on the same spot. Springing from 2nd position and landing with the right foot where the left foot was previously is shown in **47bs**.

47.23. Use of Direction from Body Part (DBP - see <u>Advanced Labanotation</u> *Floorwork and Basic Acrobatics* can also clarify the relationship of one foot to the other.

Same-Spot Caret

47bh ⟨∙ or ∙⟩

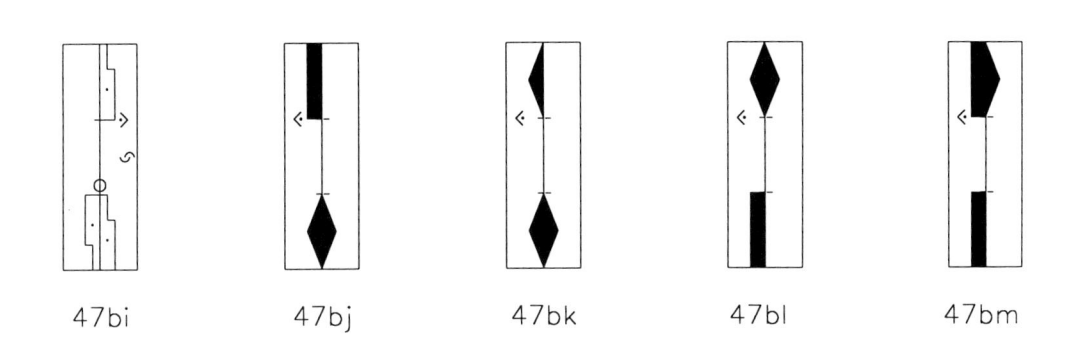

47bi   47bj   47bk   47bl   47bm

Same-Spot Zed Caret

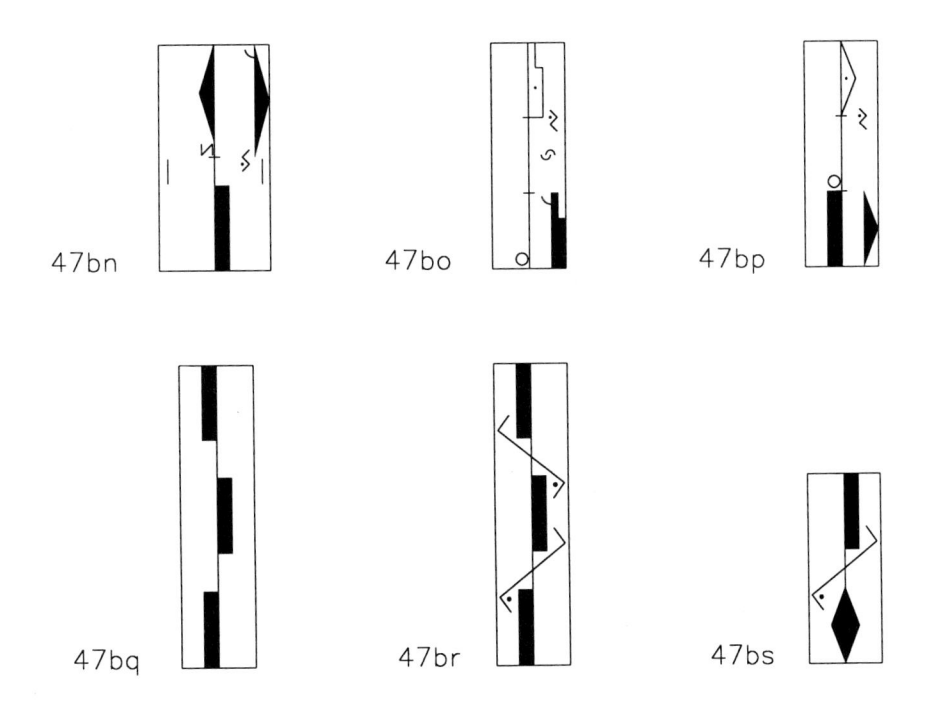

47bn   47bo   47bp

47bq   47br   47bs

47.24. **Foward Reference Caret.** A forward reference caret, (a 'refer forward' caret), **47bt**, is used to alert the reader to what is coming next, this is necessary because the movement that follows will affect the performance of the initial movement. A typical example occurs when one touching leg gesture leads into another, or a touch is followed by lowering to a support. The exact placement of the initial touch may have to be analysed according to what follows. When the leg is place low, contacting the floor with the toe, as in **47bu**, the toe is usually placed somewhere near the heel of the supporting foot; the simple statement does not give an exact placement. This is true for the outwardly rotated legs in **47bu** as well as the parallel stance in **47bv**. This placement is illustrated with an x in **47bw**.

47.25. Ex. **47bx** shows a typical touch and kick hopping sequence; the ball of the right foot being specifically placed directly in front of the ball of the left foot on each touch. In **47by** the touch occurs specifically next to the heel, as indicated by the sideward pin.

47.26. However, if the toe touch of **47bu** is to be followed by lowering the heel, this lowering is impossible when it occurs with marked outward leg rotation as the ankle of the other foot is in the way. With parallel rotation the right foot will end placed backward, rather than in line with the other foot, as illustrated in **47bz**. If it is intended that the lowering of the heel should result in the two heels being together, then the placement of the toe touch must anticipate this ending situation. The 'refer forward' caret is attached to the end of the toe touching gesture in **47ca**, linking it to the lowering of the heel which follows. The same device is used when there is no timing gap between the symbols.

47.27. If the gesture is farther away, as in **47cb**, the heel can be lowered without needing to plan ahead. If the contact is closer, as in **47cc**, the heel may not lower into the correct placement next to the other heel, the distance written needs to be accurate and the performance needs to be correct. For an example of this kind it is clearer to warn the reader by using the 'forward reference' caret.[108]

Advanced Labanotation

Forward Reference Caret

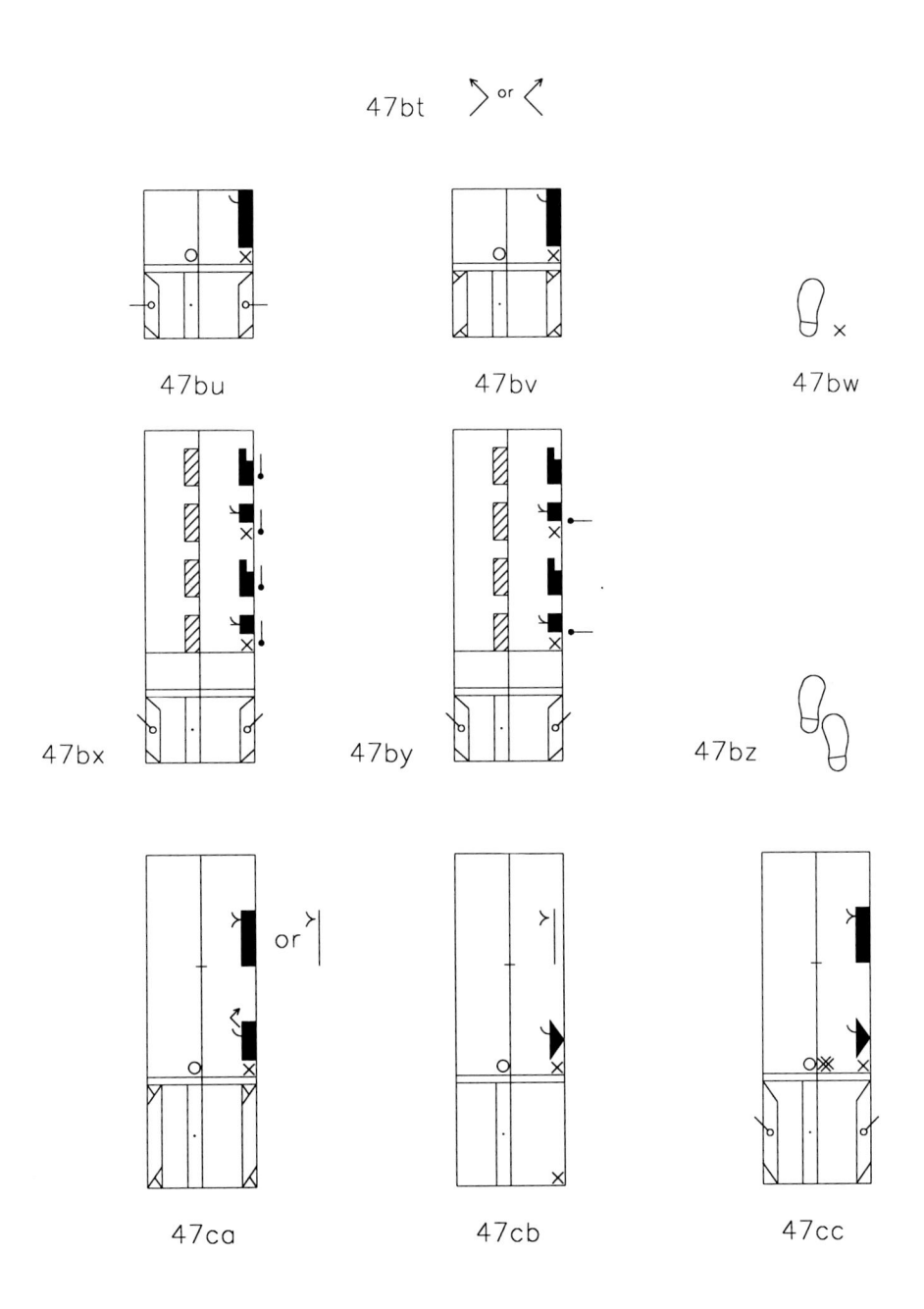

47bt ⟩ or ⟨

47bu

47bv

47bw

47bx

47by

47bz

47ca

47cb

47cc

47.28. **Forward Reference Caret: 'Lead Into' Zed Caret.** For every step (transference of weight) into a direction, other than in place, the stepping foot has to be freed of weight and the leg carried into the stated direction. In **47cd** the forward step occurs on count 3. The preparatory gesture of the right leg will probably occur on count 2, but in this example nothing, no timing or manner of performance is specified. A fairly slow preparatory gesture is shown in **47ce** and is linked to the following step to indicate its relationship to that step. A quick preparatory gesture is shown in **47cf**. Because in structured Labanotation (in contrast to Motif Notation), such an action stroke is understood in Labanotation to indicate a movement appropriate to the context, the simple zed caret suffices to indicate the link to the step.

47.29. A specific leg gesture is indicated in **47cg**. With a sequential movement the leg gestures forward low, arriving at the standard 45° angle before the step is taken. In this case the gesture is important in its own right and should be fully articulated. What is sometimes wanted, however, is simply a stylized preparation for the step; the gesture has the sole purpose of leading into the step, it has no importance on its own. To indicate this particular performance, a forward reference 'leading into' zed caret is used, **47ch**.[109]

Advanced Labanotation 183

Forward Reference Caret: 'Lead Into' Zed Caret

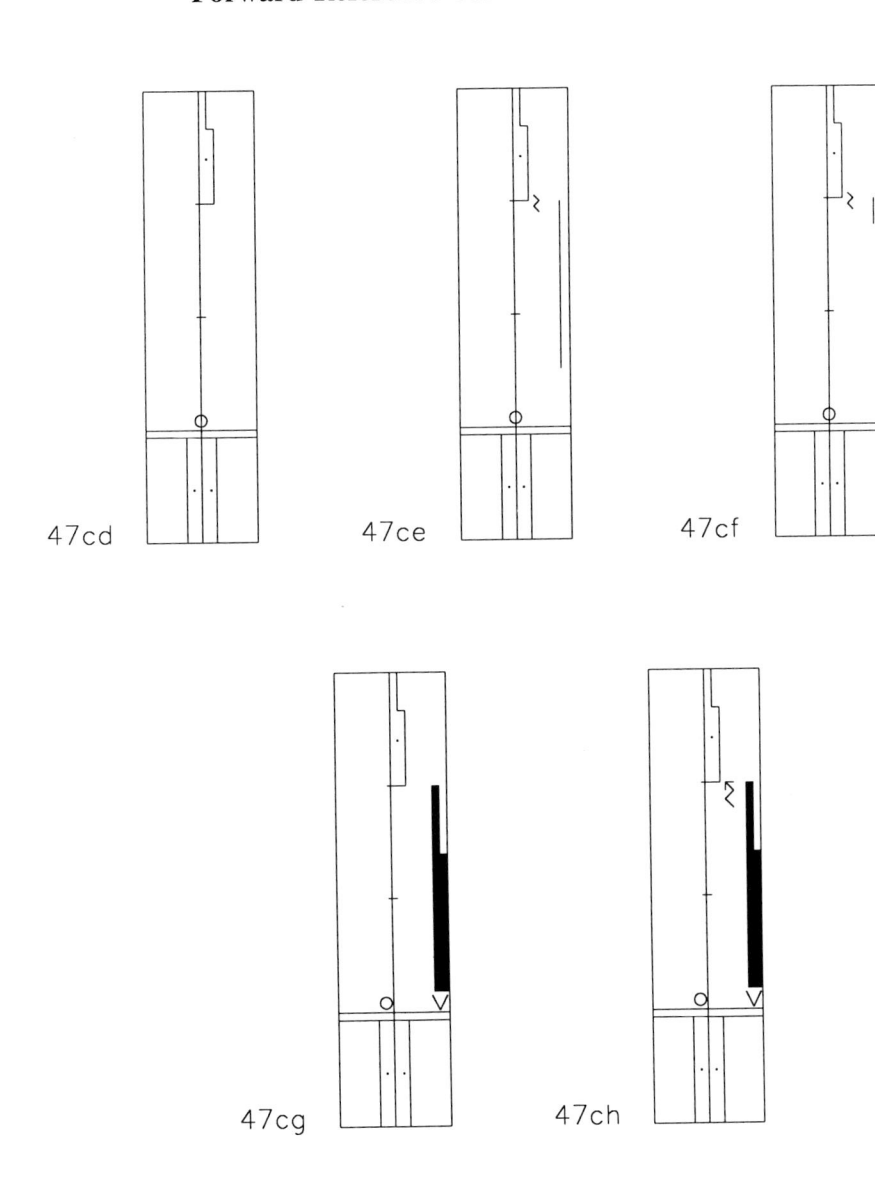

47cd   47ce   47cf

47cg   47ch

48 Reading Examples

Examples of spatial variations occur in a number of scores, no one piece of choreography or notated exercise features one particular aspect. The examples selected here are not presented in any particular order. Because several different usages may appear on one page, it seemed visually more helpful in the following extracts to pin-point each particular incidence through use of circled letters and arrows, reading up from the bottom of the page. Use of these spatial variations contributes to the style of the choreography. Some of explanations given here are to topics other than Spatial Variations, details which may not be generally known.

48.1. **Lark Ascending.**[110] In this excerpt, **48a**, from the Alvin Ailey score, details are taken from the parts for dancers E and H. For E, while his right arm moves forward and up with placement next to the body center line (letter A, see B.22), he is coming out of a turn on both feet which ends with the right foot sliding behind on the toe. He then takes two low steps backward before twisting the torso slightly to the right, the head not included in this twist. At the same time the chest-to-waist leans toward the backward high Stance direction, no degree stated (letter B, see 25.4) and the right arm contracts in its forward middle direction, the back (tip) of the elbow facing Stance-backward (letter C).

48.2. The forward run for performer E is modified to carry him slightly to the left forward diagonal (letter D, see 12.7). Both his arms (letter E) are forward low, one-third toward forward middle (see 1.8). The sign at the start of H's run (letter F), indicates that this run can be started on either foot.[111] This same sign is used for the steps of dancer E after he has caught dancer H in a lift and starts to turn around.

48.3. The direction for E's arms as he lifts H (letter G, see 2.1) is up, slightly forward. Note that the forward middle pin (tack) is linked to the place high sign to indicate that it is not a relationship indication, but modifies the direction. Because of the adjacent ad lib. sign meaning more or less, this direction need not be exact. For the indication of H's entrance on stage (letter H), see 44.4. For the floor plans in this score, the notator has used quarter stage marks (letter I) and also indicates center stage with an 'X' (letter J).

Lark Ascending

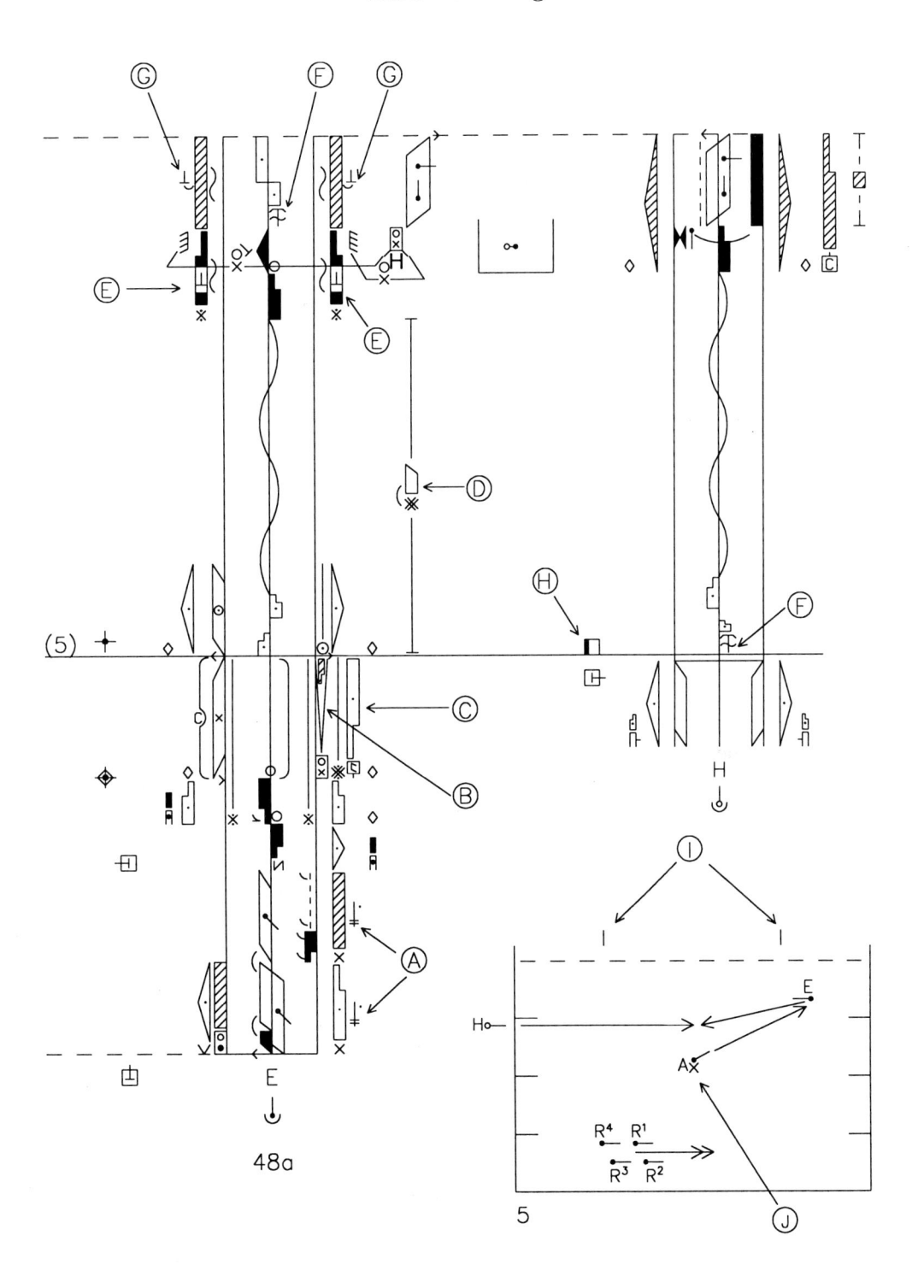

48a

48.4. Measures 57-58 of the *Lark Ascending* score, **48b**, contains three examples of motion toward a direction. Dancer L performs an inward left leg gesture which leads to an arched *arabesque penchée*, during which partner A inclines his torso toward forward high, the exact degree is left open (letter K, see 25.4). L then releases her right hand from partner A's grasp and, as she comes upright, swivelling to the left on a lowering support, her right arm lowers somewhat, i.e. a motion toward place low (letter L, see 25.4); no doubt this is needed to avoid touching her partner.

48.5. During her low half turn to the left, dancer L's left leg gesture lowers in preparation for the step forward, note the linking here of the gesture to the support (letter M, see 47.29). As she changes her relationship with partner A, her right arm moves toward side high (letter N, see 25.5) while he changes to kneeling in preparation for the lift which follows. Her right arm gesture is that of the lark 'raising a wing' as she prepares to place the front of her waist on his left shoulder, taking this arm into a forward *arabesque* line, the left arm balancing it. Dancer A's arms are shown as being forward middle, one third raise to forward high (letter O, see 1.8).

Advanced Labanotation

Lark Ascending (continued)

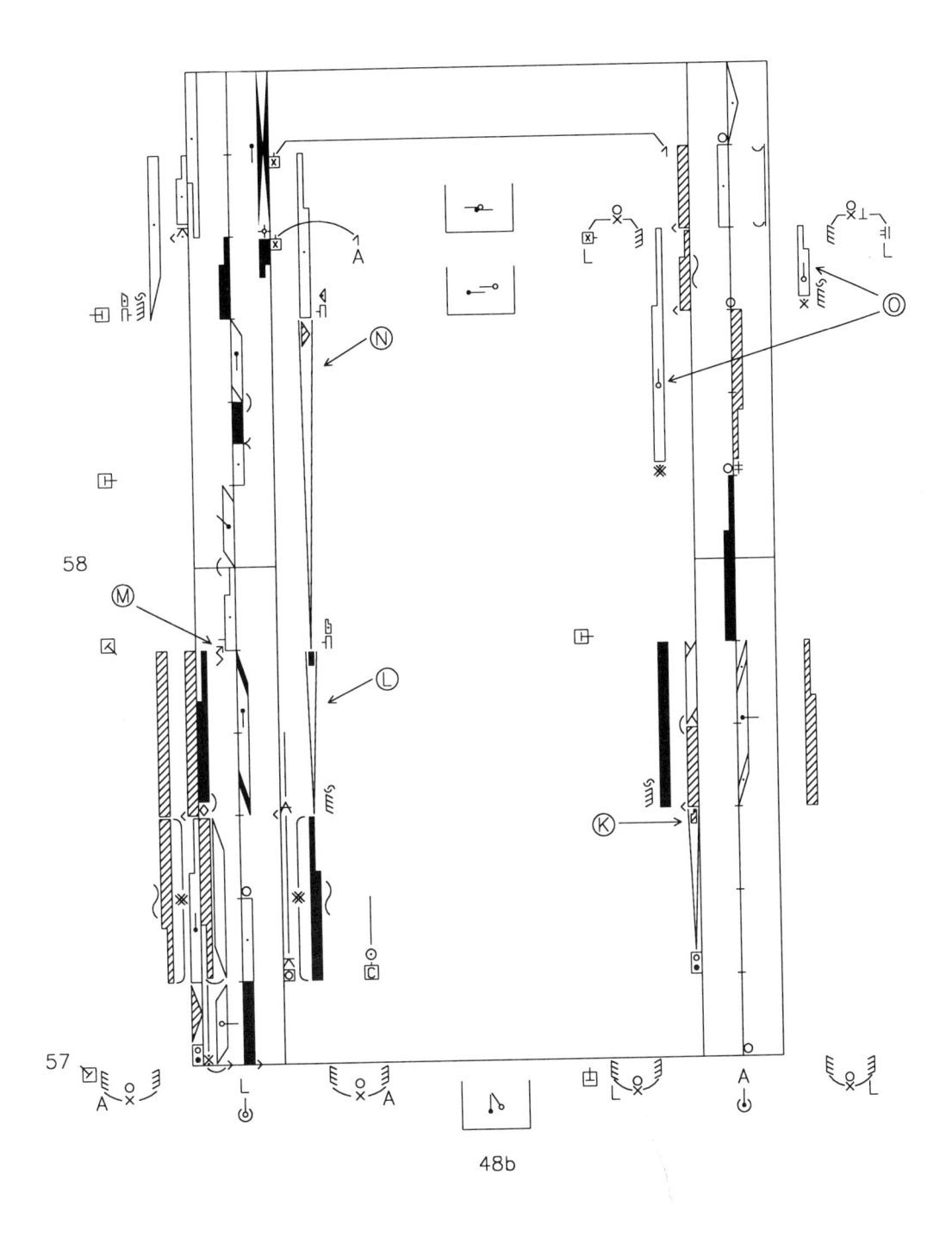

48b

48.6. The next excerpt, **48c**, measure 59, is a continuation from the previous page with dancer A traveling closer to center stage while carrying dancer L. As he adjusts her position and his left hand is shown to be sliding (while supporting) along her waist, dancer A's left arm is shown to be more or less in the intermediate direction of right side middle, one third toward side high (letter P, see 1.9). Similarly his right arm is given a place high direction, slightly displaced backward, (letter Q, see 2.1), which does not require exact performance as his arm slides from supporting both her legs to supporting her waist. While this arm rises, it deviates toward side high, the deviation being judged from the center point of the movement (letter R, see 9.8).

48.7. At the end of dancer L's adjustment - a wheeling and rolling action during which her arms and then her legs cross the center line, as shown by the track pins (letter S, see B.22), she ends with her legs-to-head in a crescent shape (letter T).[112] She is then supported by the back of her waist resting on his neck. Dancer A releases his left hand and supports against her left leg, his arm being in the area of side middle[113] (letter U). Similarly his right arm in the area of side middle (letter U) supports against her left arm. As he travels sideward with her, his arms perform overlapping successions (to represent flying).

Advanced Labanotation

Lark Ascending (continued)

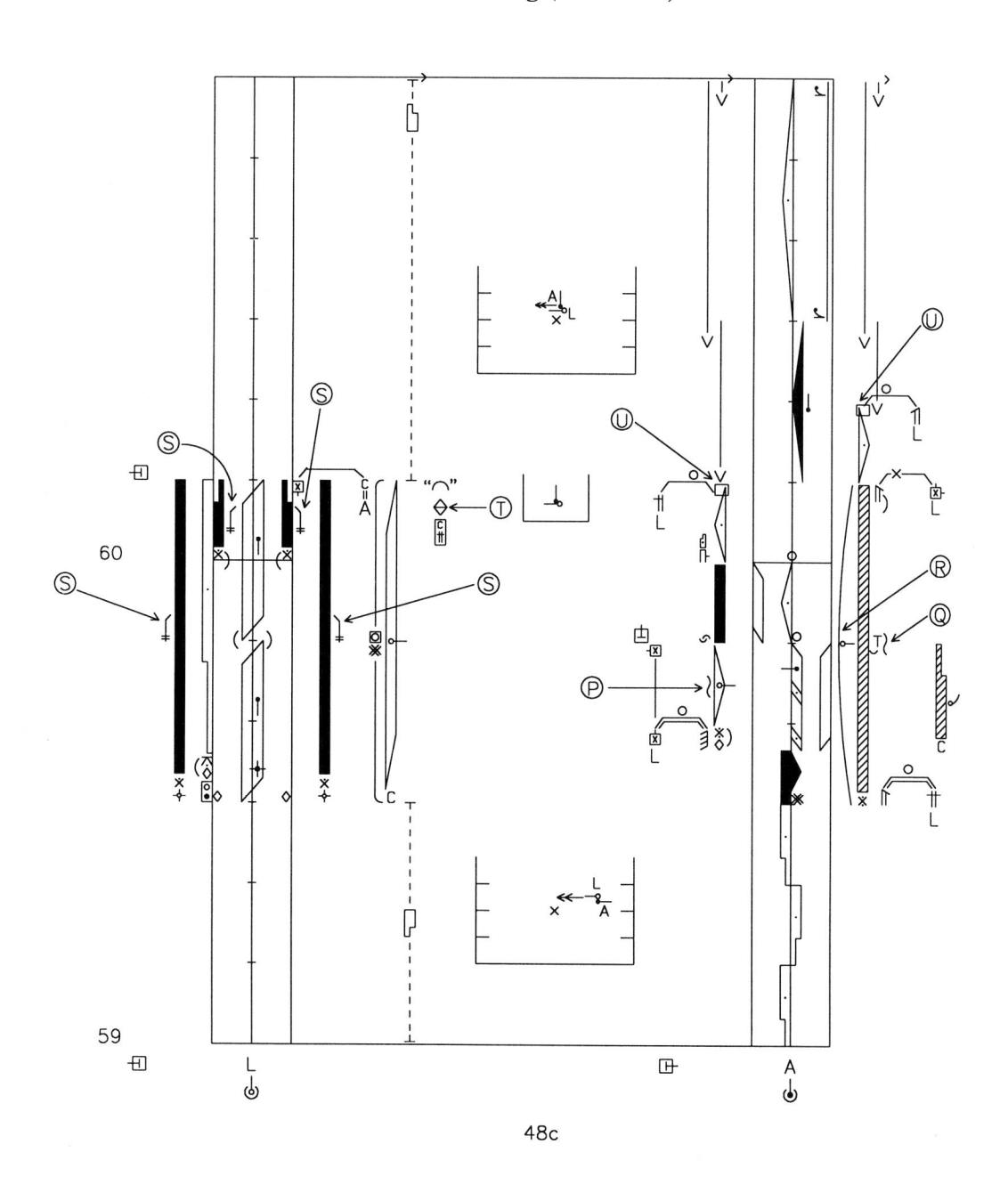

48c

48.8. In this excerpt, **48d**, measures 154-161 of the Ailey *Lark Ascending* score, track pins are used to show that the finger tips are very close (letter V, see B.22). This gesture is performed with a 'gathering' action (letter W), as the torso bends forward, to be followed by a scattering movement (letter X), as the chest-to-waist area inclines to the right and the arms, making a straight path (letter Y, see 4.5) to the side low/side high third-way intermediate points (see 1.8). For these arm gestures the thumb facing indications also require intermediate points (letter Z, see 1.8).

48.9. In measure 159 the finger tips are again close to the center line (see letter V) as, with the chest inclined to the left, the head turns to the right looking under the right arm (letter 'a', see B.6). At the end of 161 the resulting forward low leg gesture is shown by the 'lead into' zed caret (letter 'b', see 47.28), to be linked to the step which follows on the next page. Without this zed caret the left leg would end in a full forward low gesture; with this forward reference zed caret the gesture becomes lower and 'leads' into the forward step. Note that in measure 159 the left foot was already touching the floor, hence the special arrowed zed caret was not needed.

Lark Ascending (continued)

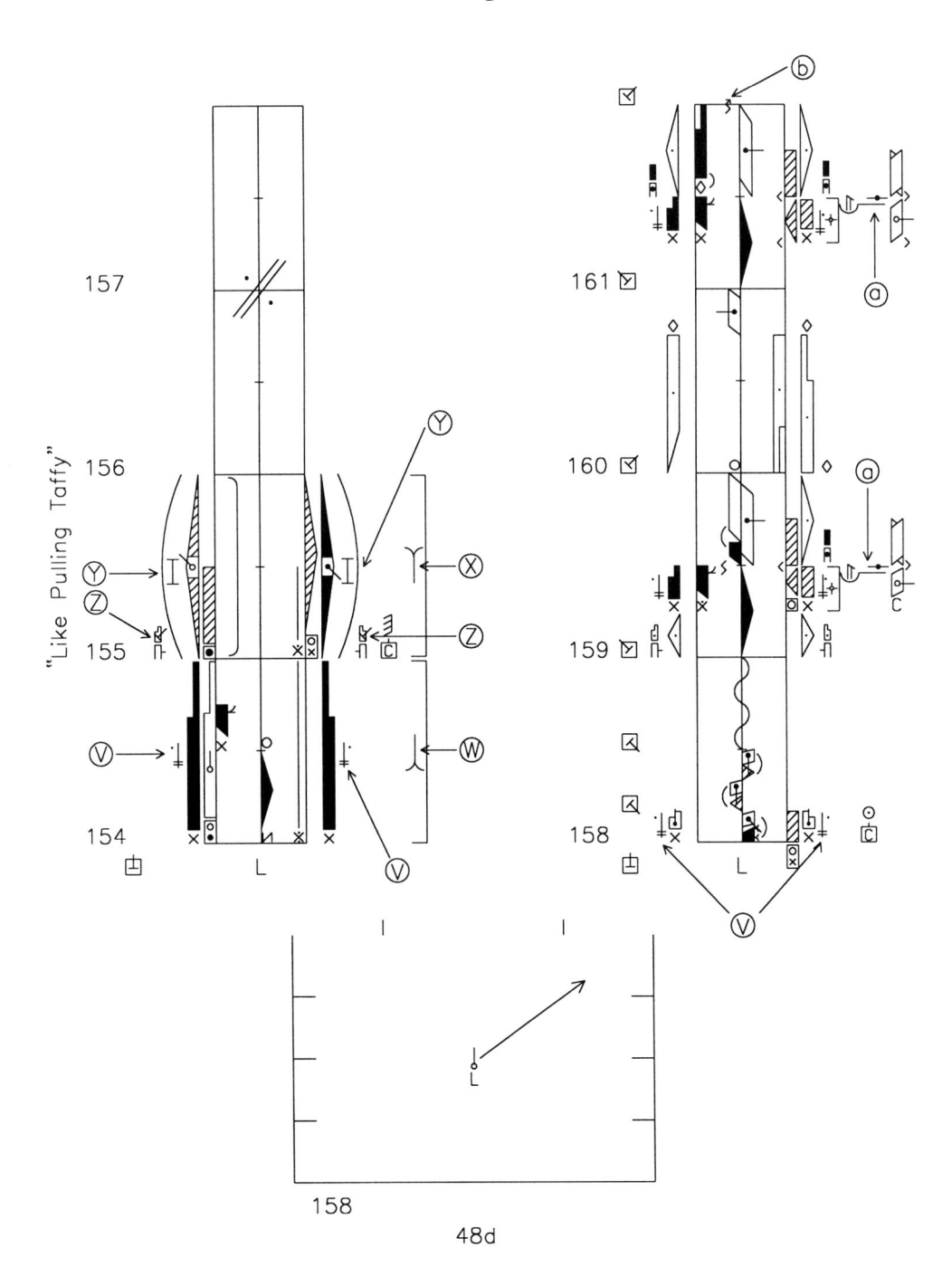

"Like Pulling Taffy"

48d

48.10. This example, **48e**, measures 162-165, a continuation of the *Lark Ascending* score, starts with the 'lead into' zed caret (letter 'b', see 47.28). The finger tips are on the center body line (letter 'c', see B.22), the left arm higher than the right; neither of these directions, however, being exact. As the torso inclines slightly forward, the right palm addresses the heart, the lower arm then makes small rapid backward and forward movements, indicated with distal pins (letter 'd', see 16.8). During this movement there is a slight unemphasized contraction of the torso (letter 'e'). Note the notator's choice of sign to indicate the palm addressing the heart (letter 'f'), this will have been explained in the glossary.

Lark Ascending (concluded)

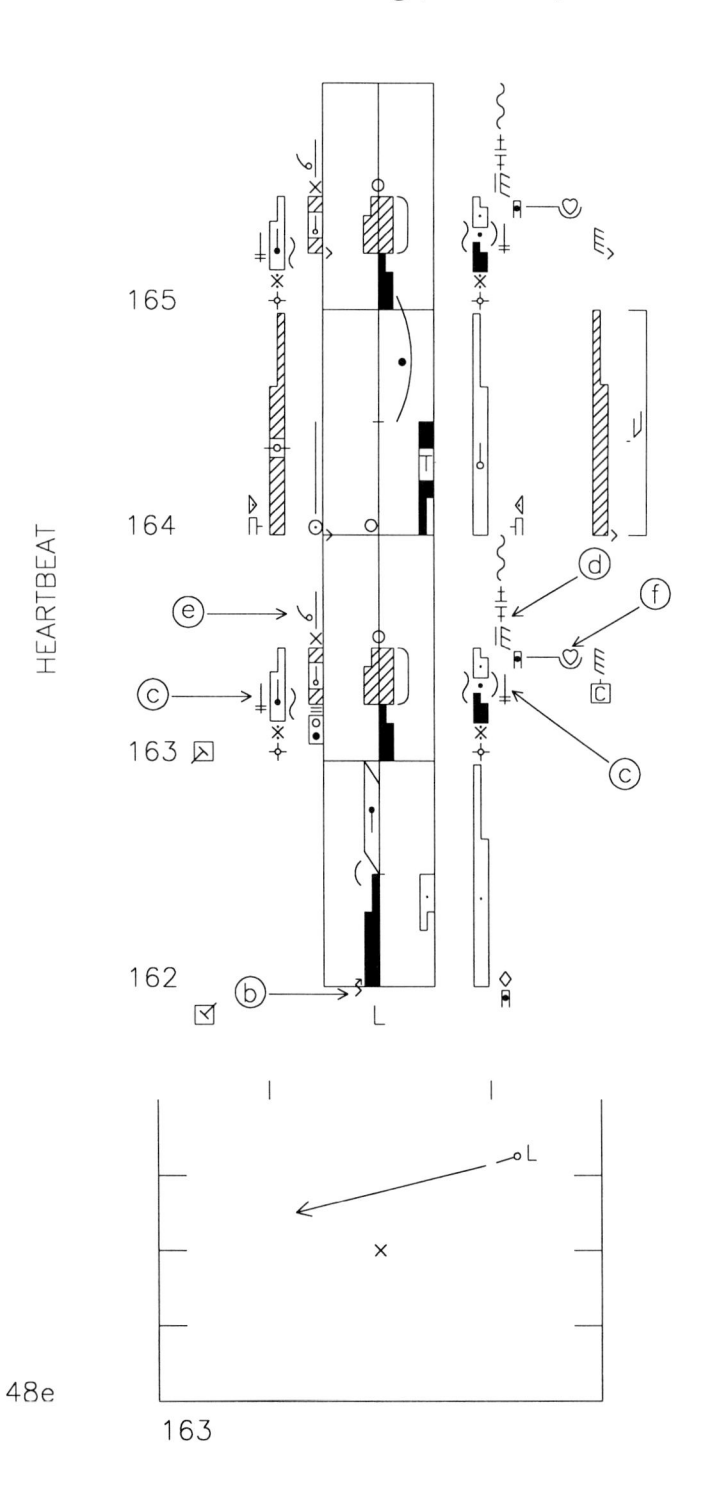

48e

48.11. **Roses.**[114] In this duet for dancers M and D, excerpted from Paul Taylor's *Roses,* Ex. **48f**, the man begins in a comfortable open position, the addition of the horizontal ad lib. sign indicating that it need not be exactly in 2nd position (letter A).[115] The meaning of this detail will have been included in the glossary. The arm direction for male dancer D as he lifts M, is given as a straight path upward, i.e. up from where the hands (the extremity of the arms) were before (letter B, see 24.10, 26.1). The arms reverse this direction (letter C).

Before the lift, dancer M does a preparatory 'step-hop-step' to gain momentum for the 3/8 forward somersault rotation, her legs opening side high as the inverted torso, chest-to-pelvis, rises backward high. As the man turns to the left, M is carried, hence her turn sign is indicated as being resultant (letter D). His revolving on a straight path results in her passively doing the same thing (letter E). This revolving continues into the next measure, however, the next section is not included here. Note the traveling indication (letter F, see 14.2, Ex. **14c**), the direction being taken from the Constant Key.

Roses

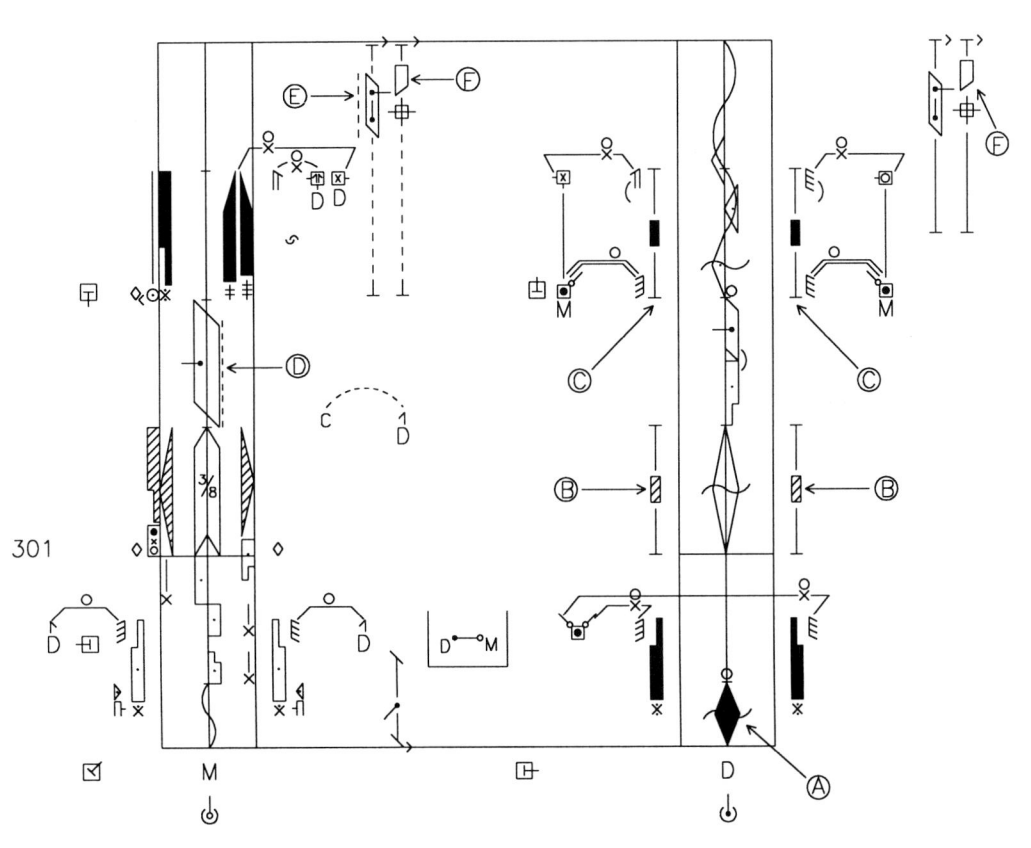

48f

48.12. **Sorcerer's Sofa.**[116] In this excerpt, **48g**, from Paul Taylor's *Sorcerer's Sofa*, dancer R, near the end of measure 845, raises her right arm directly to what will be backward low at the end of the turn (letter A); her aim is to grasp Q's left wrist. The black diamond (space hold sign) indicates an undeviating path. It is comparable to an ordinary space hold sign within a direction symbol, but the direction stated is judged from *after the turn is completed*, rather than before the turn starts.

The overall pattern for the last three measures is for the three dancers to diverge into a straight line. This divergence is written as a slight diagonal deviation of the forward path (letter B, see 12.7, Ex. **12u**) together with the indication for the group becoming smaller. This is stated with a circle representing the body - in this case the body of the group - and the X within it which states a small group. Placed within the toward sign (letter C, see Section 25), it signifies becoming smaller.[117] In this score the notator has also provided the indication for arriving in a file (letter D) as the aim of the closing ranks path.

In addition, small floor plans indicating before and after locations, have been included. While some redundancy could have been avoided here, each detail reinforces the other related indications, often making for swifter interpretation.

Advanced Labanotation

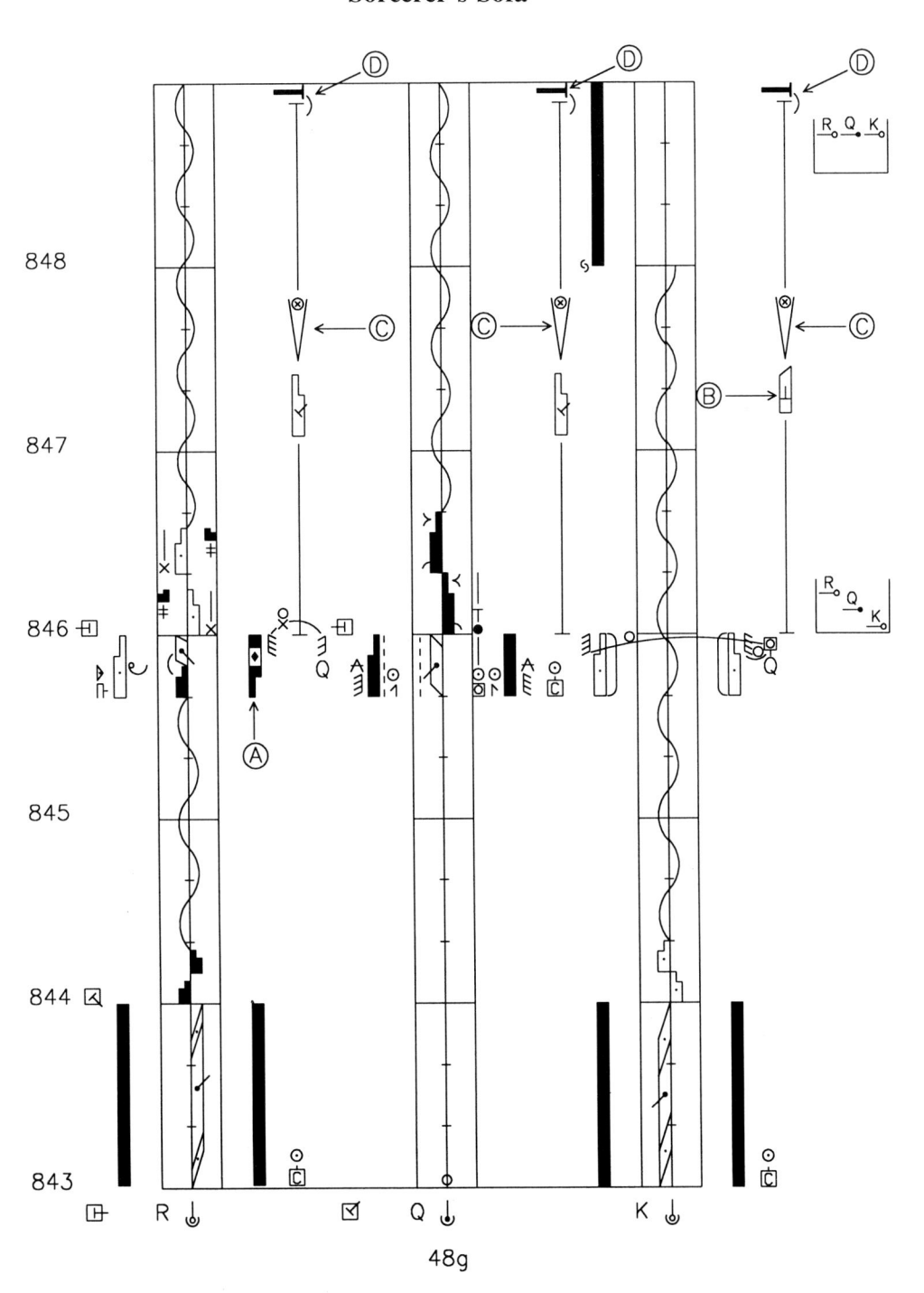

Sorcerer's Sofa

48g

48.13. In this second excerpt from *Sorcerer's Sofa*, **48h**, measures 672-674, the two performers dance in unison after the *pas de chat*-like *assemblé* which lands in a deep *plié*. On this landing the torso bends (folds) slightly forward, but the head is not included in this torso movement, as shown by the exclusion sign (letter A). There is then a rebound spring, but not very high, shown by the very small upward path (letter B, see 12.6). During this spring the legs spread and the arms make what is basically a straight path up to side high (letter C, see 4.6), but with the slight overtone of a curve, hence the upward deviation (letter D, see 4.6).

48.14. The next two landings are not quite as low, and the last is to a normal *demi-plié* level.

Advanced Labanotation 199

Sorcerer's Sofa (continued)

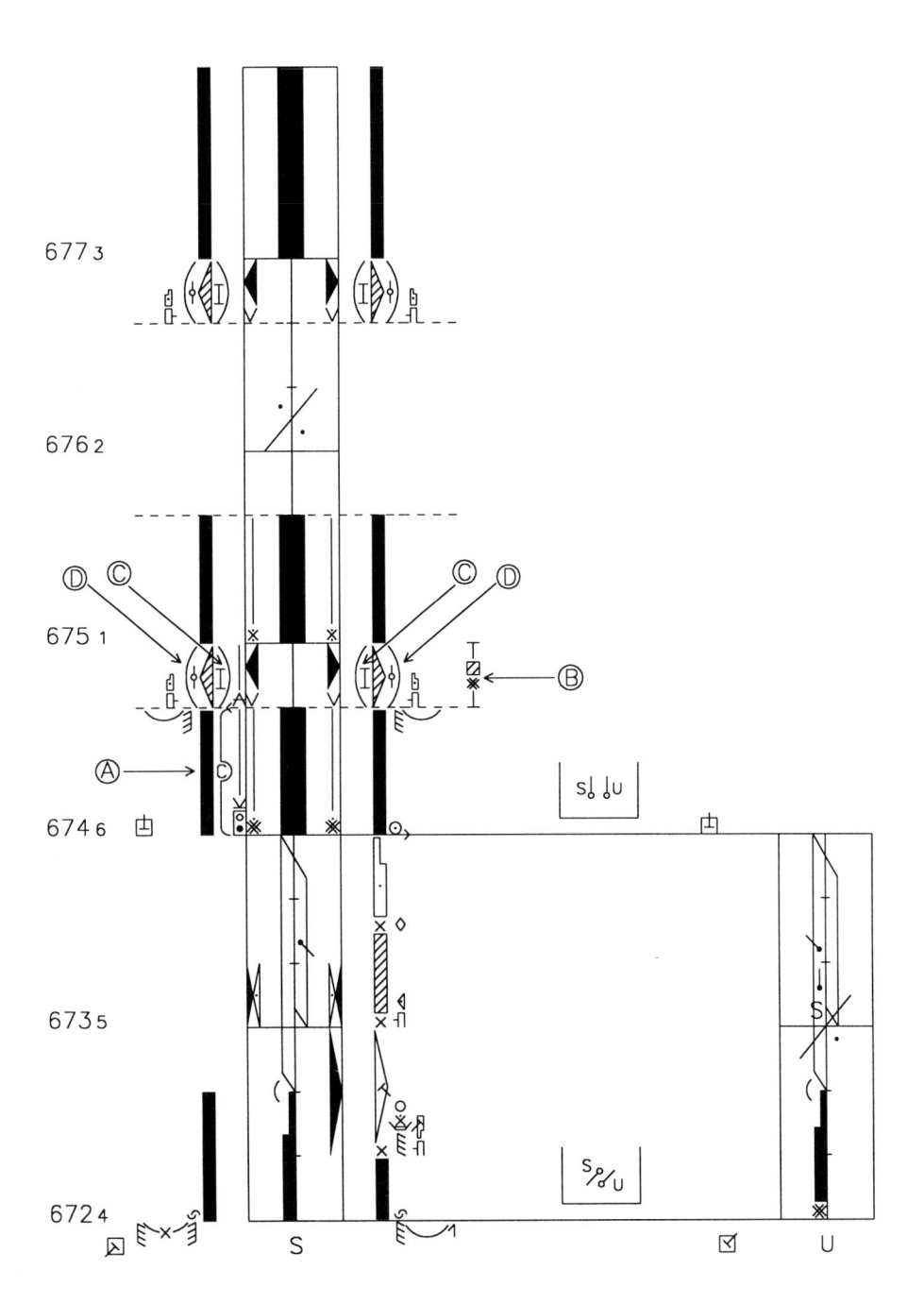

48h

48.15. **Snow Pas.**[118] This extract of a *pas de deux* from Anton Dolin's *The Nutcracker*, Ex, **48i**, makes use of approximate directions (letter A, see 1.8), here needed as the height and placement of the man's hand may vary. At the end of the ballerina's *arabesque penchée*, they both raise their right hands (arms) directly upward (letter B, see 24.10, 26.1), before releasing the grasp. Because of the intermediate direction for her right arm (letter C), the facing indication for the thumb edge of the hand (letter D), must also be an intermediate direction (see 1.8).

48.16. In **48j**, at the start of measure 48, track pins (letter E, see B.22) show that the dancer's right arm gestures are with the finger tips next to the body center line. The 'lead into' arrowed zed caret (letter F, see 47.28) provides the message that the low *retiré* position is passed through as the leg lowers to take the backward step, it is a 'lead into' gesture and not a *retiré* position to be achieved in its own right. The arms make an 'undercurve' deviation (letter G, see 9.8) as they rise during the backward step.

Advanced Labanotation 201

Snow Pas

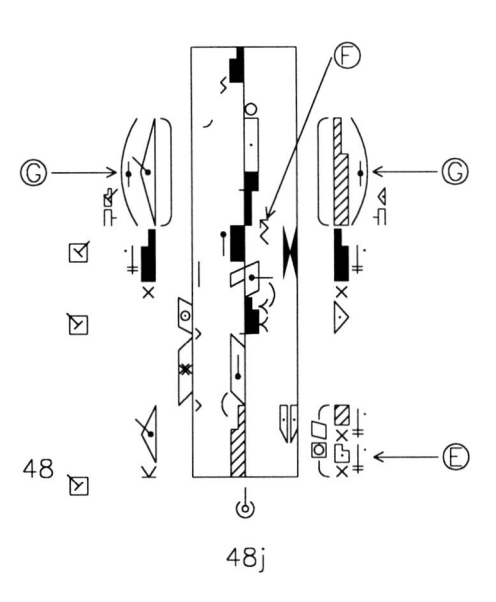

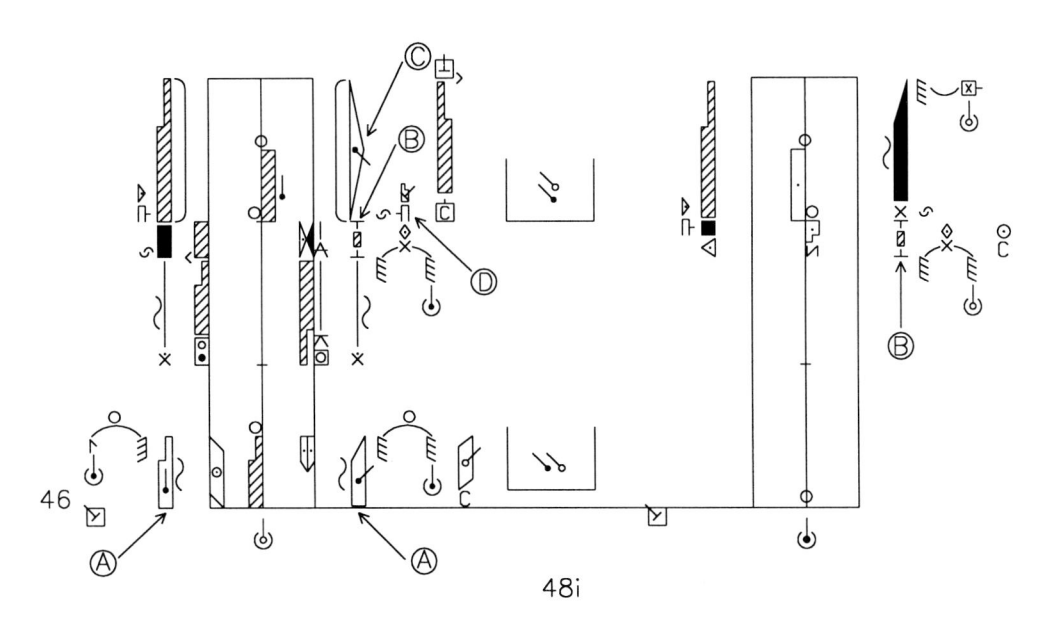

48j

48i

48.17. In measure 49 from the *Snow Pas*, Ex. **48k**, the dancer performs a series of steps as preparation for the *grand jeté*. The small unfolding left leg gesture (letter H, see 47.28) is shown to be linked, i.e. to lead into the diagonally crossed step. Thus, while this gesture must occur, it must not be incorrectly emphasized. Whilst this step pattern has been carefully notated, the inclusion of an ad lib. sign alongside (letter I) indicates that there may be some freedom in personal performance. No doubt dancers have their own preferences for working up momentum for a major leap such as this.

48.18. The arm gestures which occur during the leap follow a straight path (letter J, see 4.6), the arms rising directly to their destination, thus adding emphasis, a flourish. Of importance here is that the dancer should cross the center stage line on that leap. This center line is indicated on a small floor plan sign (letter K), which, for clarity, is included in the glossary for the score. The center line statement generally used in Labanotation is shown in the example of letter L (see 45.8, **45af**).

Snow Pas (concluded)

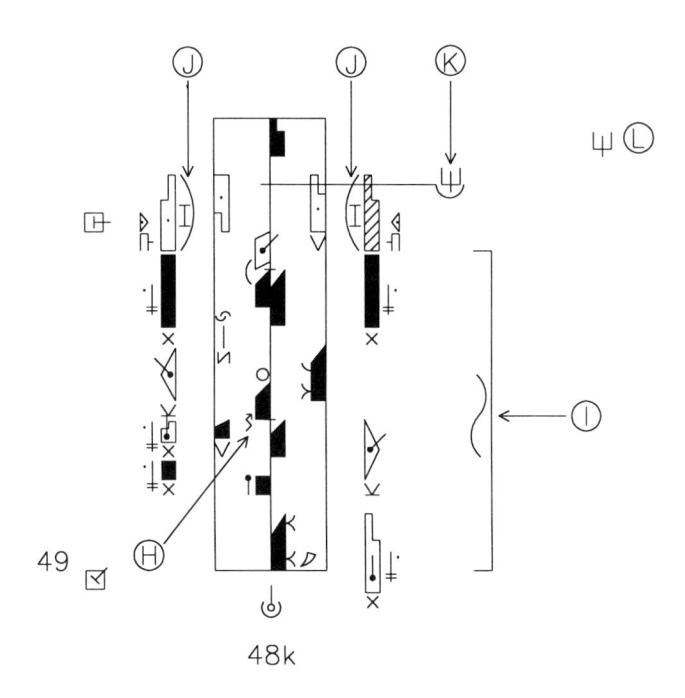

48k

48.19. **Parade.**[119] This, for its time, was a very modern ballet. Created in 1917 by Léonide Massine, it contained many unusual characters and movements. In this first excerpt, **48l**, the American Girl (AG) mimes a sailor pulling a rope, as she leans forward and scoots backward, feet slightly apart (letter A, see B.7). As she raises her right arm which deviates over forward (letter B, see 9.8), her hand spreads and then closes as, 'pulling the rope', her arm lowers. This same arm pattern is repeated one count later for the left arm. During these small backward slides, she deepens the level of her supports while her torso gradually comes back to normal. With her right hand above her left, she makes a circular gesture with her right hand (letter C, the sequence of deviations, see 18.2), twisting her arm inward as the hand stretches and spreads, then twisting it outward as her hand closes into a fist having made a half circle around her left hand, ending below. The end of this 'knot being tied' occurs as both arms take a straight path to their destinations (letter D, see 4.6), the left arm extending higher than the right which remains bent, as before. Note that until the left arm extends, both arms remain contracted three degrees.

Parade

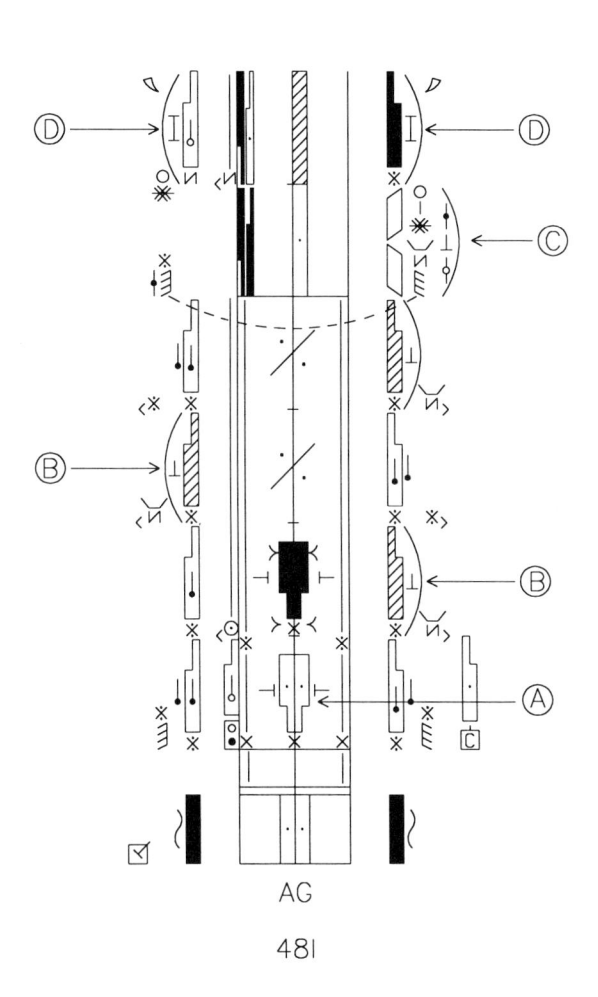

AG

481

48.20. The following antics of the horse in *Parade*[120] are performed by FH (the man who takes the part of the front of the horse) and BH (the man who is the back of the horse). In the starting position of **48m**, BH is shown to be grasping FH's pelvis while FH is grasping BH's hands. Note that for the latter, the hand signs are placed together in FH's staff, it being understood that the outer hand is that of the other (or another) person. During a couple of sliding steps to adjust their position, the torso and head for FH make three 'nodding' movements, FH ending with the torso forward high, a third-way to forward middle (letter E, see 1.8).

48.21. The sideward 'rocking' pattern which follows is performed with the feet not quite closing together (letter F, see B.2), shown by the sideward displacement tacks. During these steps the two men travel slightly forward (letter G, see 37.8). The quality of these steps is shown to be uplifted, buoyant (letter H). In measure 19 the back man lifts the front man. As FH tilts backward during the lift, his thighs are open a third-way to the diagonal from the forward direction (letter I, see 1.8). BH is shown to press his arms upward on a straight path (letter J, see 4.6). As though exhausted from that effort, BH puts FH down and, leaning forward, goes down to his knees (a low kneel), still grasping FH's pelvis. After the lift, FH sequentially extends his right leg diagonally before placing his right flexed ankle on his left knee as he takes his weight slightly backward (letter K).

Parade (concluded)

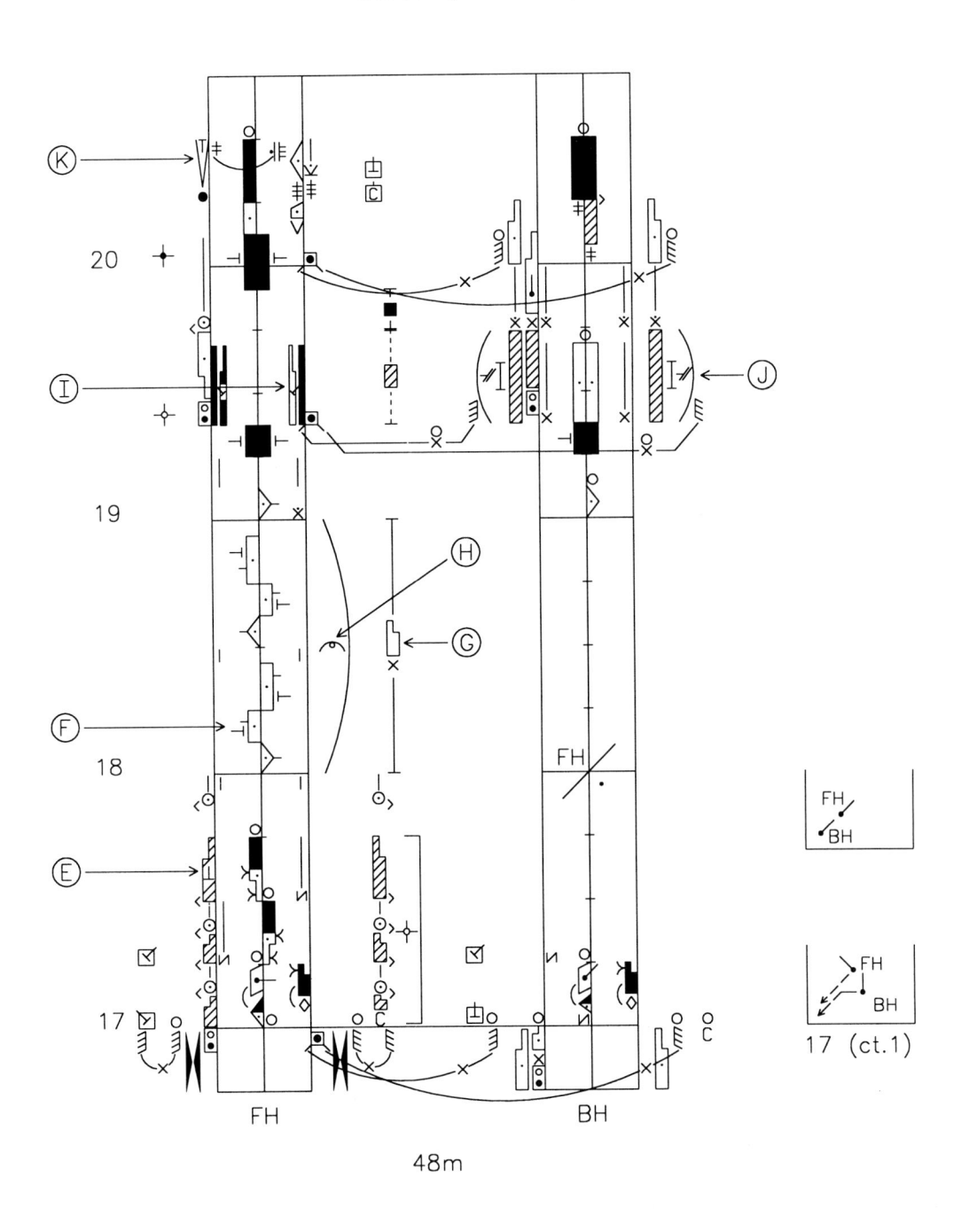

48.22. **Rooms.**[121] This excerpt, **48n**, from Anna Sokolow's study of the human condition begins with performer F sitting asleep on a chair, leaning on the back, hands on the thighs. The head is inclined slightly forward (letter A, see 1.4); the whole position is relaxed (letter B). The words written alongside give the person's thinking or feeling. The sequence starts with an intake of breath (letter C), the lungs being shown to increase before the torso slumps forward with a heavy quality (letter D).[122]

48.23. The slow sinking to the floor is shown to have freedom in timing, in duration (letter E).[123] The large double X sign (letter F), written across the whole staff and coinciding with the turn, indicates a contracting movement for the body-as-a-whole; the body descends to the floor. During this, as the performer rolls to the left, he rolls onto the left knee and then the right, ending on the right side of his torso. Because body part symbols need to be placed in the support columns, for easier reading the rotation sign is placed outside the staff (letter G).

The sign for more-or-less facing stage right (letter H) results from the previous degree of turn (more-or-less $^3/_4$). To return to an exact facing direction (front sign) the destination for the turn, the new front, is described (letter I) rather than the degree of turn.

48.24. With a very strong accent (letter J) the limbs extend strongly and the body contracts over the back. After a slight pause this is followed by a rapid roll, the number of rolls being expressed by the infinity sign (letter K). The rapidity of rolling is shown by the time sign for much speed (letter L). The aim of this rolling is to arrive in the upstage left corner area (letter M, see 25.9, Ex. **25ag**), ending lying on the right side of the body, the legs sagittally separated. In addition to the word notes, the greatest possible amount of stretch in the legs has been written (letter N), the performer thus being urged to strive for that result even if it is not totally possible for each individual. Note use of the Body Key (letter O) for the directions from here on.

Rooms

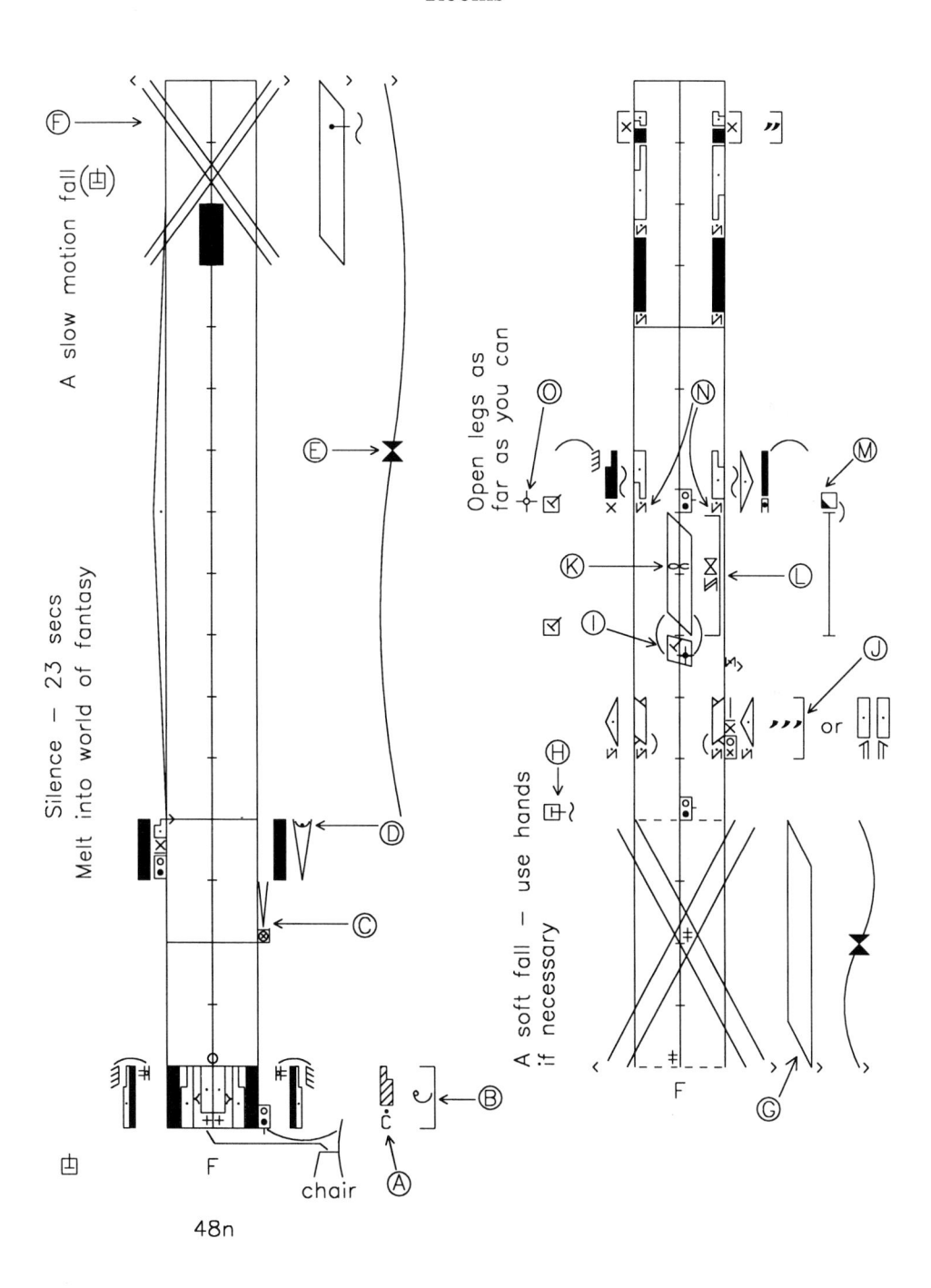

A slow motion fall

Silence – 23 secs
Melt into world of fantasy

Open legs as far as you can

A soft fall – use hands if necessary

chair

48n

48.25. **Spanish Dance.**[124] The following excerpts illustrate certain spatial variations. Ex. **48o**, the *Ceasé y contraceasé andaluz*, features the typical intermediate arm directions used in Spanish dance. In addition the change from one position to the same on the opposite side through a slight sideward deviation is also a characteristic feature (letter A, see 1.8, B.5, 9.8).

48.26. *Paso de tango*, Ex. **48p**, starts in a 3rd position (letter B, see B.2) and features a sideward deviation for the left leg as it prepares to step forward, thus producing a slight *rond de jambe* sliding on the floor (letter C, see 9.8). The ending movement for this pattern is a *coupé* under for the right leg, the left gesturing quickly to a lower than normal forward low position (letter D, see 1.8).

48.27. *Paso de cachucha*, Ex. **48q** begins with the arms (the hands) exactly above the shoulders (letter E, see B.26). It features a higher and larger *rond de jambe* for the right leg (letter F, see 9.8), augmented by the 1/4 turn to the right. The left arm lowers to a rounded 5th position *en bas (bras bas)* (letter G, see B.5). Then, as the left arm rises it is shown to be led by the outer side of the upper arm (letter H). Toward the end of this arm movement there is a one-third way backward tilt of the unit pelvis-to-head (letter I), which is shown to be read from Stance, i.e. the direction of the forward step on the left foot. The right foot comes into place in a 3rd position relationship behind the left leg (letter J, see B.2).

48.28. The *Gorgallata de escuela bolero*, Ex. **48r**, features a small outward *rond de jambe* shown with intermediate directions (letter K, see 1.8) and slight deviations, shown with pins for the lower leg (letter L, see 9.8). A little spring leads into a similar, but inward, *rond de jambe* with the left lower leg. This pattern ends with a slightly larger backward body tilt, this time of the whole torso (letter M). The undeviating path for this tilt is written with the diamond within the tilting indication, an alternate way of producing the same spatial result in terms of direction as with the Stance key used in Ex. **48q** (letter I). At the end of the step forward the right leg comes into a *cou de pied* position, the right foot being placed behind the left ankle (letter N, see B.4).

Advanced Labanotation

Spanish Dance

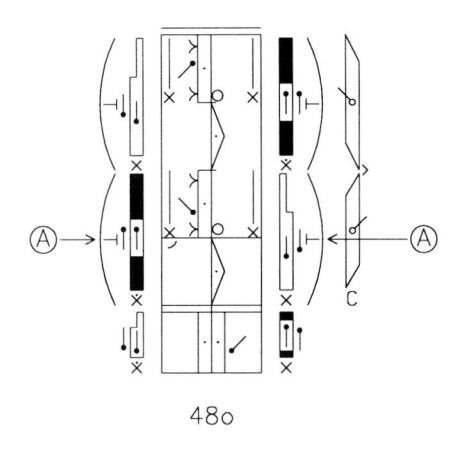

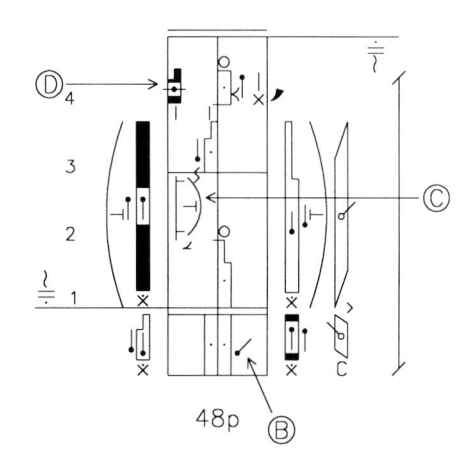

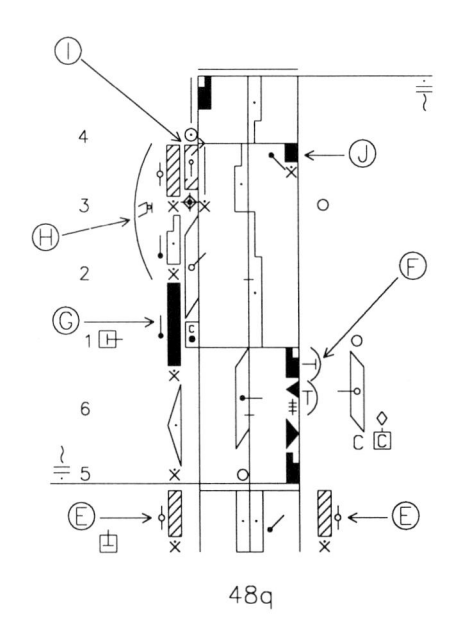

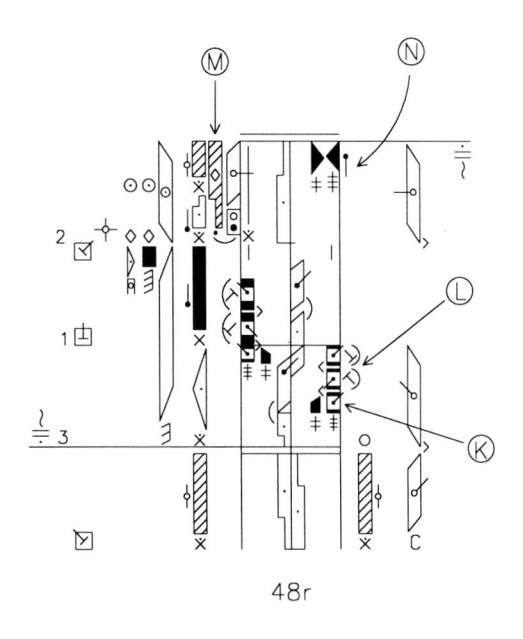

48o

48p

48q

48r

48.29. **Hungarian Dance.**[125] The first couple dance, Ex. **48s**, shows the man and woman each to have their partner at the right forward diagonal placement (letter A, see 41.1). The woman's step in place on the right foot is shown to be in a 3rd position behind, but displace slightly sideward (letter B, see B.2). In addition, her diagonal traveling steps are shown to be small (letter C). Although she is circling, the indication for the length of step was traditionally placed in a straight path sign to indicate that the X referred to the path, i.e. the steps.

48.30. For Ex. **48t** the couple are shown facing each other (letter D, see 41.1). The woman's first step to the left side is on the backward lateral track (letter E, see B.2); this is to compensate for her step on the right foot in the same direction which will be on the forward lateral track. With the spring into a small 2nd position, landing with both legs rotated to the right (letter F), the woman also travels to the left on the curved path during this spring (letter G). During this pattern the man's steps must be very small (letter H). His 2nd position is reached by keeping the left foot where it is and stepping out with the right foot to form the 2nd position (letter I, see 47.5, Ex. **47p**).

Advanced Labanotation

Hungarian Dance

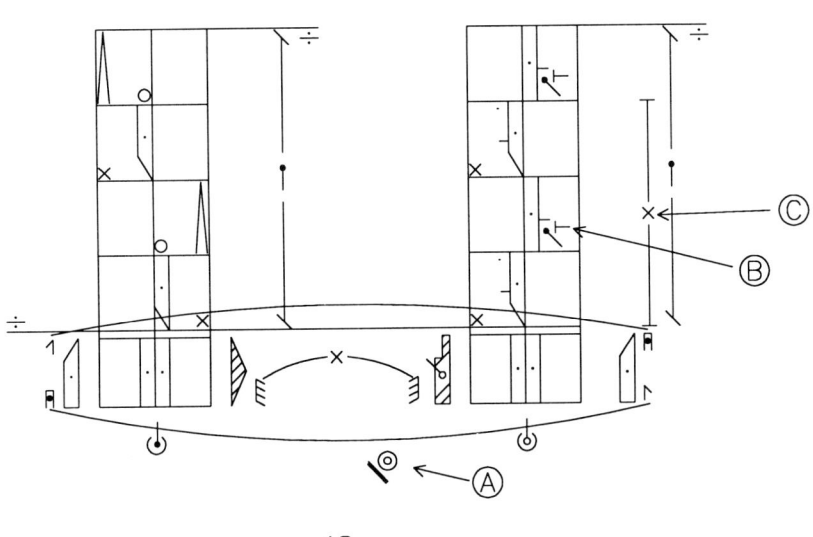

48s

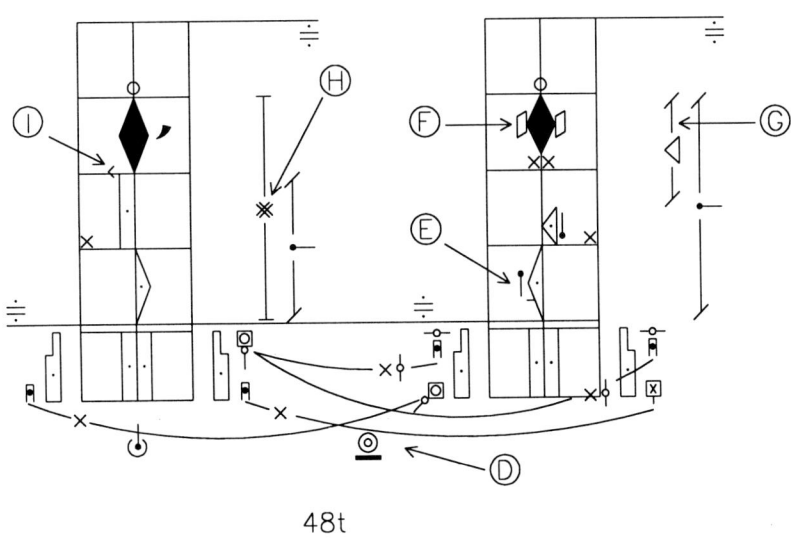

48t

48.31. **Water Study.**[126] The brief excerpt of Ex. **48u** makes interesting use of the fixed point (letter A, see 46.3, Ex. **46h**) as a key to the traveling direction for the dancers. The notated diagonal run is in fact more of a forward run for the performers, but each person's path needs to adjust so that the previously spread group converges in the downstage left corner of the stage, the fixed point direction. Note use of the flat pin (tack) within the turn sign (letter B, see B.12, Ex. **Bbe**) to indicate the destination of the turn in relation to the stage directions (Front signs).

Water Study

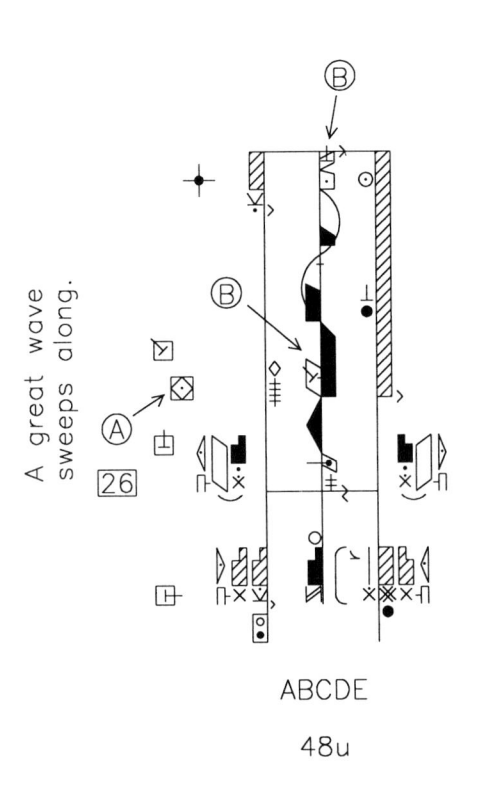

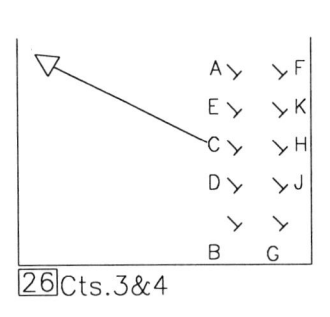

A great wave sweeps along.

26

ABCDE

48u

26 Cts. 3 & 4

APPENDICES

A The Direction System of Labanotation

A.1. In his paper *The Direction System of Labanotation/Kinetography Laban, A Clarification and Proposal*, presented and accepted at ICKL 1993, János Fügedi draws attention to and clarifies the fact that two models exist in the Laban system for judging directions, particular for the analysis of diagonal directions. For facing directions for hand surfaces and edges, he proposed a minor modification of certain intermediate directions to produce a coherent direction system, in which perpendicular facing directions for these surfaces and edges can be stated for all directions in our notation system. The following extract is partly based on Fügedi's paper.

A.2. **Definition of Direction in Labanotation.** Laban originally identifed directions by name only, he did not analyze their relation to each other or the angle of a limb in relation to the horizontal plane or the vertical line of gravity.[127]

As part of his Space Harmony (SH) theory, *Choreutics*,[128] based on mathematical shapes such as the cube, octahedron, and icosahedron, Laban created a directional system in which the center point (place) is identified as the Center of Gravity[129] in the body (usually taken from the waist, the navel). Ex. **Aa** illustrates the place middle point when the person is within a cube. This SH system of reference is a separate study, not to be confused with the spherical model used in the Standard Directional System of Labanotation. Spherical analysis gives each limb/limb segment its own sphere within which to move, the point of reference being at the base (point of attachment) of that limb. Ex. **Ab**, from the Eshkol/Wachmann book *Movement Notation*,[130] illustrates the main directions for the arm, moving at the shoulder. Ex. **Ac** shows the local parallel systems of reference for different body parts, illustrated here are the horizontal circle of directions around each joint.[131]

A.3. The SH spatial points are mainly intermediate points, not the main directions used in Labanotation. Therefore, strictly speaking, SH should always use modified main direction symbols. For example, in **Ad**, the points marked i) are the correct notation for the upper left and right points in the 'door plane', a third-way displacement toward place high. The standard side high direction from this center (place middle) is shown as ii). It has, however, been the practice in SH studies to use the standard Labanotation side-high symbols for the i) directional points. Similarly, the corners of the table plane in **Ae** should be diagonals opened one third-way toward side middle, as shown in iii) and iv).

Advanced Labanotation

Definition of Direction in Labanotation

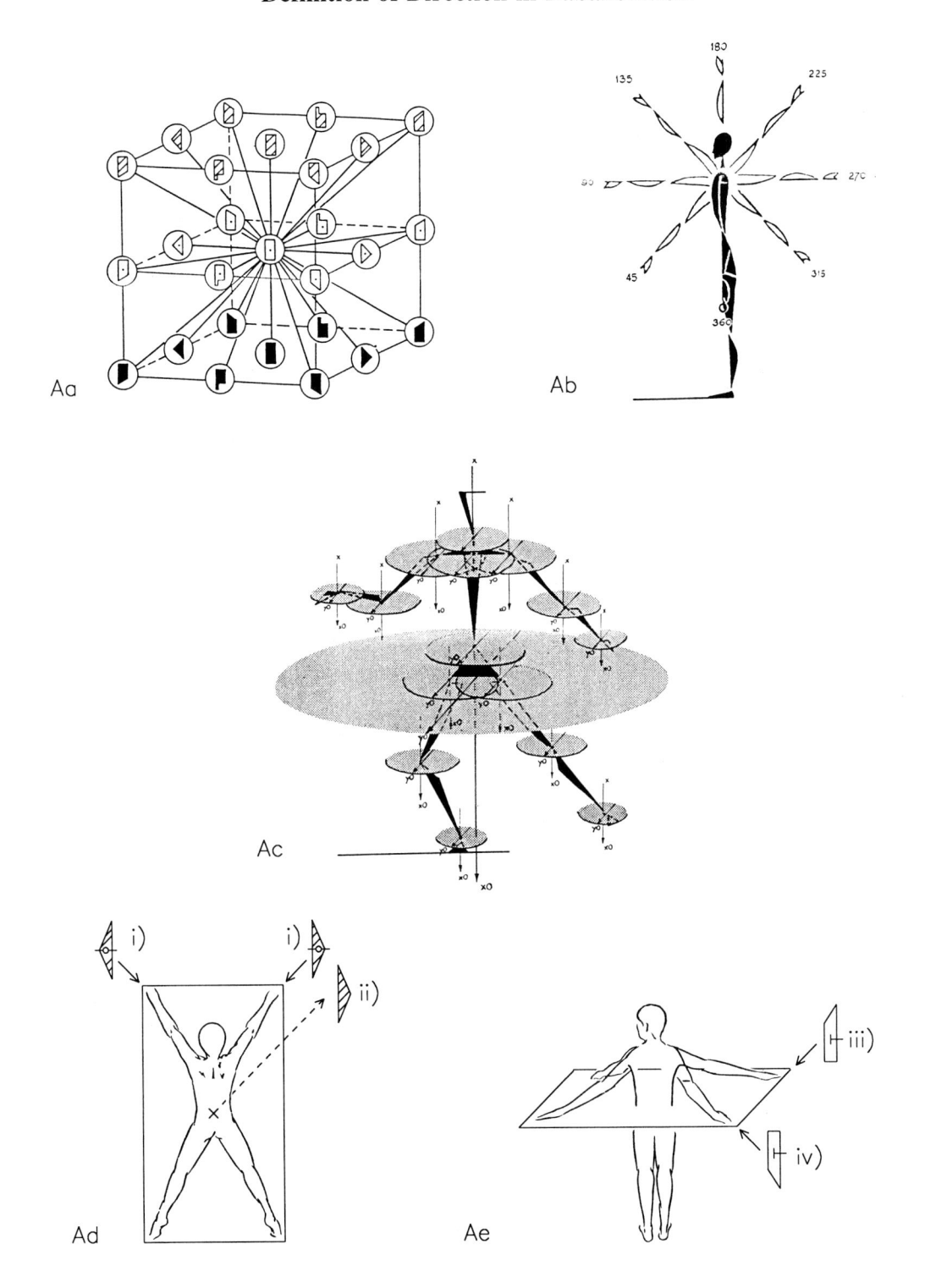

Aa

Ab

Ac

Ad

Ae

A.4. Space Harmony (SH) is initially used mainly in creating *full body movements*. When the SH directions are applied to the arm, for example, it is common practice for the whole torso to tilt (incline) and/or rotate in the direction of the arm to create a more total involvement, the movement flowing out from the center through the arm. Laban's SH four-ring 1-7 is illustrated in **Af**.[132] However, in SH focus is on the directions judged from the center of the body (Laban's 'center of gravity') and, therefore, not on the individual system of reference for each part.

A.5. Many people encountering Labanotation through studying Laban Movement Analysis (LMA), believe that the LMA spatial analysis is the basis for the directional system used in Labanotation. This is not the case. Again, *in SH directions are judged according to a cube, octahedron or icosahedron with, the center of the body as their point of reference, while in Labanotation a spherical model is placed at the joint, the fixed end, of each limb for which all directions are determined.*

It is universally agreed that in LN the fixed end of the limb is used as the point from which directions are judged. However, care must be taken that the cuboid model[133] is not used to determine the directions. This especially becomes a problem in the case of the diagonal high and low directions. In a cube the line from its center to one of the corners makes an angle of approximately 35° with the horizontal plane, **Ag**. In the spherical model of LN the correct angle is 45°, **Ah**.[134]

Advanced Labanotation

Definition of Direction in Labanotation (continued)

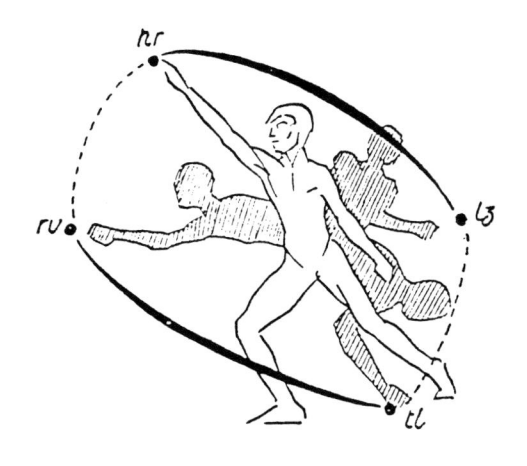

Af Four-ring 1-7

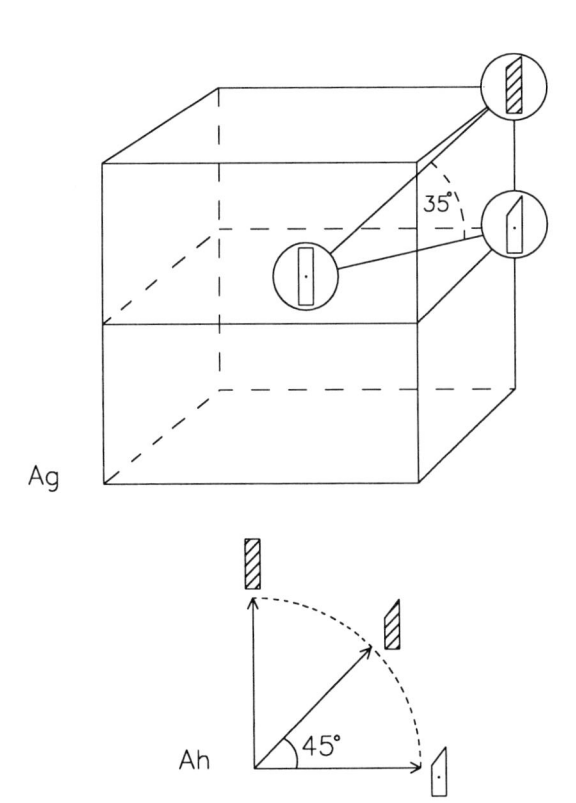

Ag

Ah 45°

A.6. **Intermediate Palm Facing Directions.** A large part of Fügedi's paper deals with the question of accurate statements for intermediate palm facing directions. Fügedi subscribes to the standard palm facing directions established in Labanotation for the main arm directions. If no wrist flexion occurs and only rotation takes place, the palm and thumb-edge facing directions are always perpendicular to the direction of the limb. Thus, when main directions occur for the limb, the palm/thumb-edge facings are always described with main directions.

A.7. Consulting Labanotation scores, Fügedi reveals the problems that were encountered when the arms are in intermediate directions for which perpendicular facings of surfaces or edges cannot be described in the current system. The tendency among notators has been to write palm facing as the nearest standard direction. Ex. **Ai** gives the simple forward direction for thumb-edge facing with the arms side middle. But in **Aj** thumb-edge facing direction is given as if the arms were still at true side horizontal. To perform this statement correctly, there must be a slight folding in the wrist joint. The reader may guess what is wanted but it is not specifically stated. What is expected for **Aj** is, in fact, **Ak**. A similar example is **Al**, indicated here as thumb-edge backward high, in practice often verbalized as 'palms up', which of course, strictly speaking, they are not. The correct indication for **Al** is **Am**.

A.8. These are obvious examples and supplying the additional detail is not difficult. But more subtle degrees are also met and need to be accurately stated. Previously this was not possible for all intermediate directions, therefore Fügedi proposed the following model.

A.9. **The Standard 45° Intermediate Directions.** The spherical model is the basis for Fügedi's analysis of main and intermediate directions. The main directions are defined by increments of 45°, as illustrated in **An**. The intermediate directions are defined by increments of 15°, **Ao**. Only half of the full direction wheel is given here.[135]

Advanced Labanotation

Intermediate Palm Facing Directions

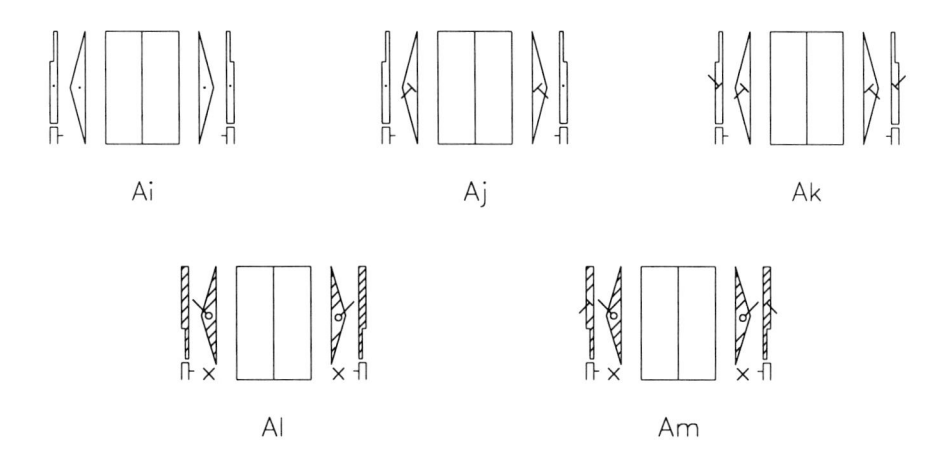

Ai Aj Ak

Al Am

The Standard 45° Intermediate Directions

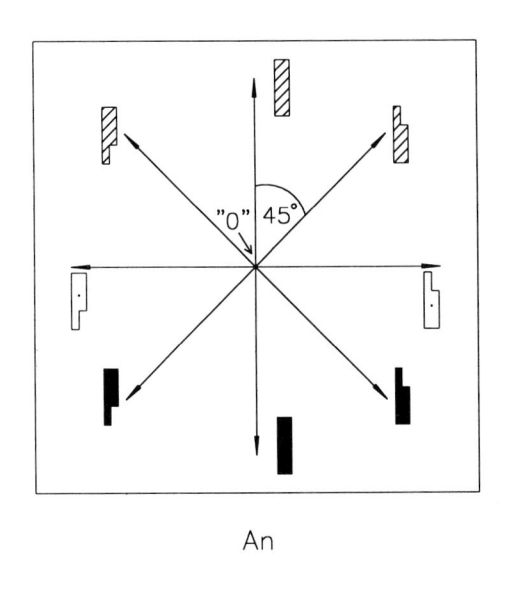

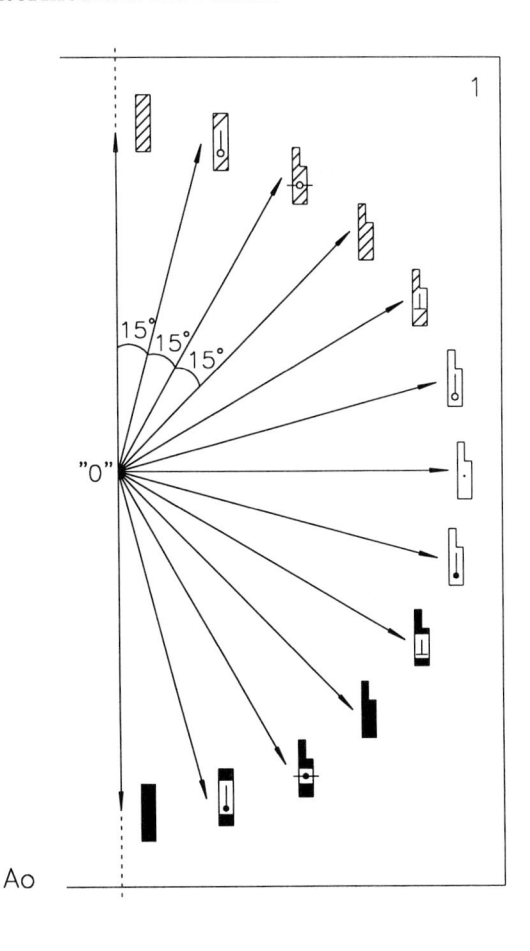

An

Ao

222 Spatial Variations

A.10. The Proposed Intermediate Direction System. If the direction wheel of **Ao** is rotated by 15° to the right, as in **Ap**, all the directions are intermediate ones. The symbols are modified by a pin in accordance with the direction of deviation. The deviations of the main directions are the same as in the present system: **Aq** becomes **Ar**; **As** becomes **At**, etc.

A.11. The new symbol added is a shorter stroke attached to the pin; the pin (the longer stroke) indicates the first deviation, the shorter stroke shows the direction of the second deviation. Ex. **Au** now becomes **Av**; the small stroke being added to the pin, **Aw**.[136] Another example is **Ax**, to which the 15° deviation to the right is added, **Ay**. Note that the additional stroke is much smaller than the pin; the longer stroke indicates the first deviation, while the shorter one indicates the second deviation.

A.12. A further 15° rotation brings us to the chart of **Az**. The small strokes added to the directions in this wheel indicate a *left deviation* from the wheel of **Aaa**. This latter wheel has brought us to the next 45° standard intermediate points. In the wheel of **Az**, the short strokes point 'back' to the previous wheel, towards the forward direction, thus *15° less* than that of **Aaa**.

A.13. Ex. **Aab** shows application of **Ap** and **Az** to a selection of placements, with the commonly used verbal descriptions indicated alongside.

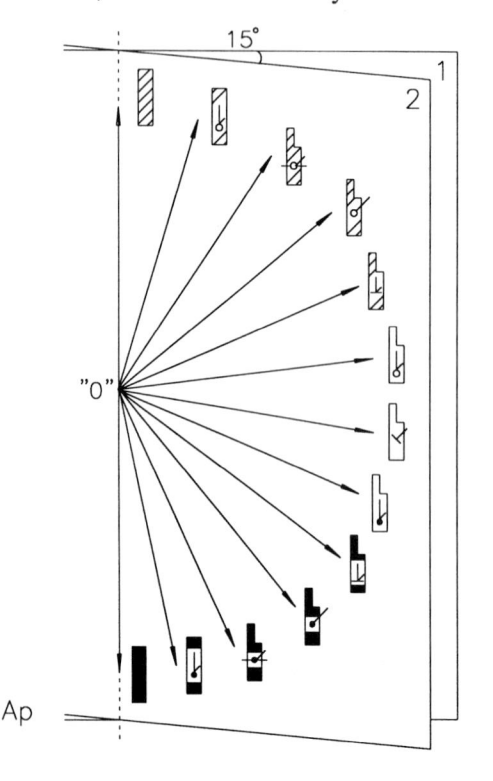

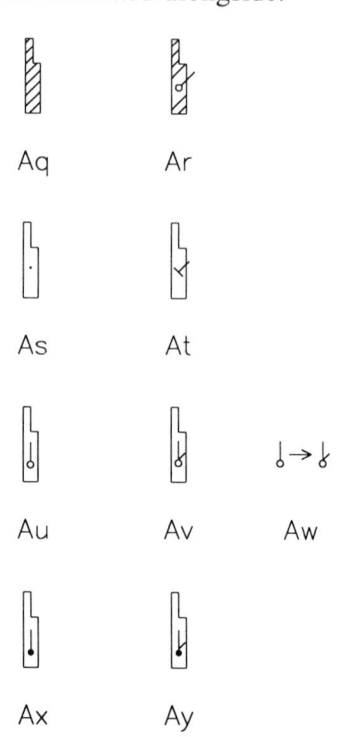

Advanced Labanotation

The Proposed Intermediate Direction System

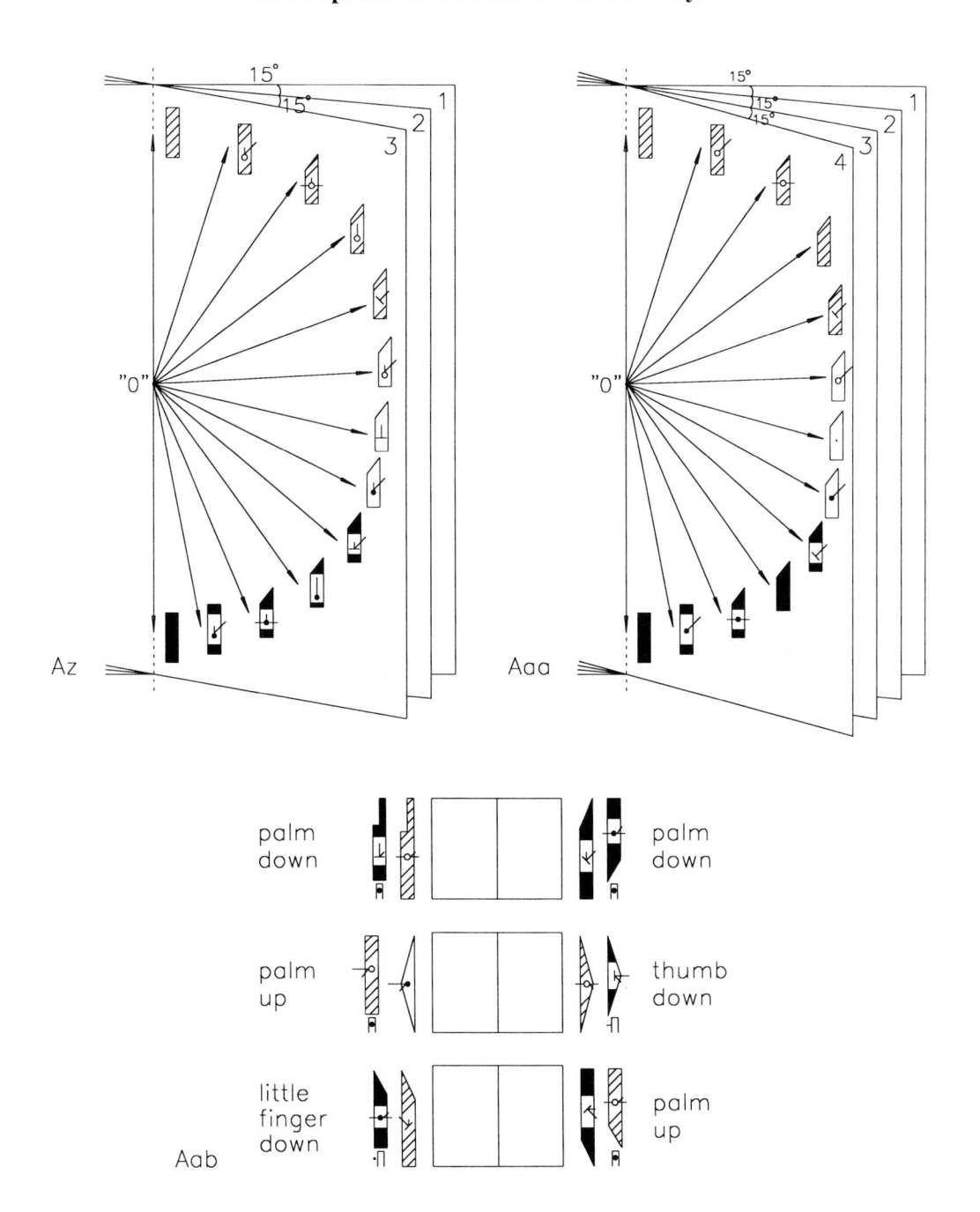

Az

Aaa

Aab

palm down		palm down
palm up		thumb down
little finger down		palm up

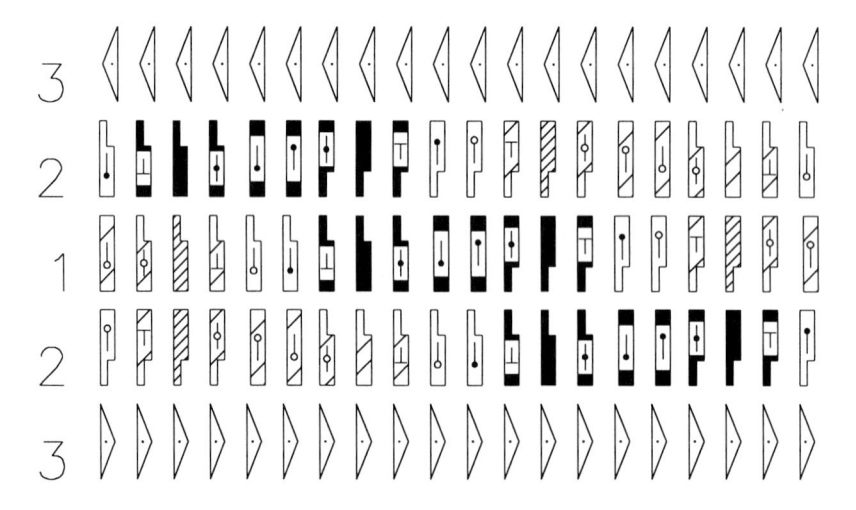

A.14. **Chart of Directions.** Fügedi states: "*In the proposed system all the directions have at least four perpendiculars useful both from practical and rotation reference point of view.*" Indeed, since the directions are defined in increments of 15°, it is apparent that directions, lying 6 x 15° from each other, are at a right angle, i.e. 90°. To spare notators from pondering which exact palm/thumb-edge direction is applicable, Fügedi provides charts which consist of all the directions of the proposed system.[137] The direction at issue is given in the central horizontal line marked '1'. The two perpendiculars in the direction wheel are given in line '2'. Above and below are the two axis directions, marked '3'. One page from these charts is given here as example **Aac**, with **Aad** and **Aae** as one and two increments removed clockwise to that established in **Aac**.

Chart of Directions

1   direction at issue
2   perpendicular on the wheel
3   axis directions

Aac

Advanced Labanotation

Chart of Directions

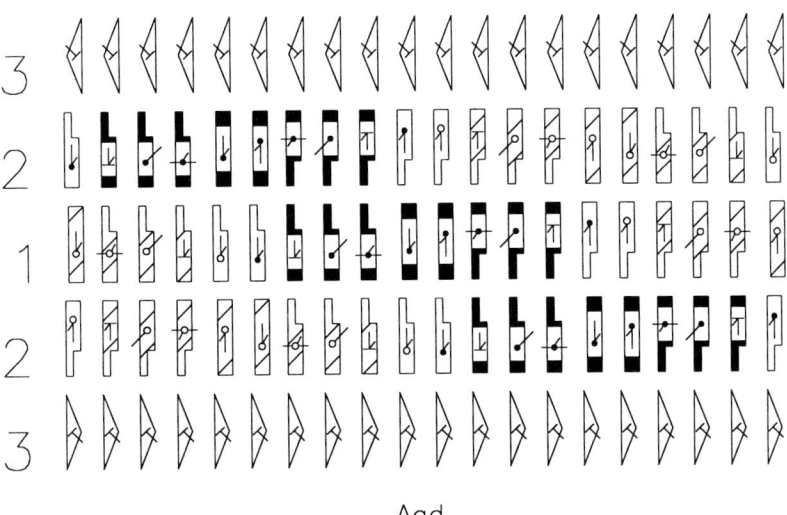

Aad

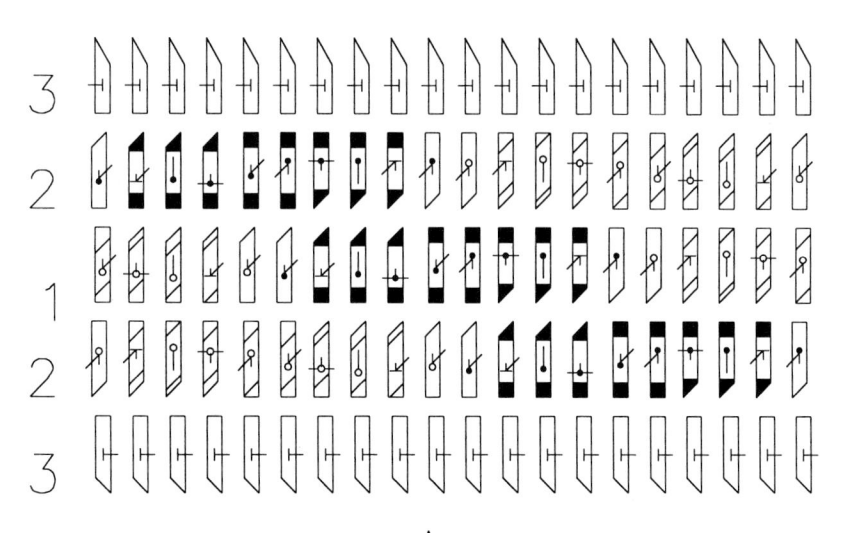

Aae

B Categories of Pins

B.1. In Labanotation pins are applied to a range of needs and the basic logic in the various uses may not be immediately evident. The purpose of this appendix is to give a complete survey of all the different types of pins and examples of how they are used. It does not explain detailed usages of these pins nor describe the rules governing application in each category. Such detail is covered elsewhere in the Advanced Labanotation Textbook Series. Examples given illustrate which pins are used for particular needs.

It should be noted that Appendix B in Advanced Labanotation *Floorwork and Basic Acrobatics* is called "Pins - when Black, when Track, when Tack?". This gives a good comparison between uses of these particular pins.

B.2. **Relationship Pins.** The first use of pins was for positions of the feet; for this reason they were also known as *position signs*. For this need black pins were used as a convention. Ex. **Ba** shows the 5th position of the feet, right foot front. In fact, only one pin is needed for a starting position. In **Bb** 3rd position is shown. When needed, the pin of **Bc** shows closing in 1st, next to the other foot. An intermediate position is shown with a double pin, for **Bd** it is between 3rd and 5th. When the position is with the right foot placed to the left of the left foot, crossing over in front or behind the other leg needs to be stated, **Be**, here the crossing is in front.

B.3. Stepping forward in front of the other foot is shown in **Bf**. After the spring in **Bg** the right foot lands 'under', i.e. on the spot where the left foot was,[138] (compare with 47.22, **47bq, br**). In **Bh** the right foot steps in front of the left and then slides back to be 'behind' where the left foot was. A similar, but smaller, action is shown in **Bi**, the right foot being shown to displace backward as it slides. This description does not relate to the other foot, but to where the right foot was previously.

B.4. Black pins are also used to indicate the relationship of leg gestures to the body. In **Bj** the foot of the flexed right leg is behind the left leg. The forward gesture of **Bk** is in front of the left leg. Beating the legs together, changing 5th positions while jumping, is shown in **Bl**.

B.5. Positions of the arms are also written with black pins, again a convention. The traditional classical ballet arm positions are explored in B.18 - B.21. When an arm crosses the body, it is assumed that it crosses in front and no relationship pin is needed. A pin showing the 'in front' relationship can be added, as in **Bm**. If both arms cross in front of the body there is usually the

Advanced Labanotation 227

need to indicate which arm crosses in front, in **Bn** it is the left arm. In **Bo** the left arm crosses behind the body while the right crosses in front. For **Bp** in which both arms cross behind the body, two pins are needed to show that the right arm crosses behind the body and is also behind the left arm.

Relationship Pins

Supports, Positions of the Feet

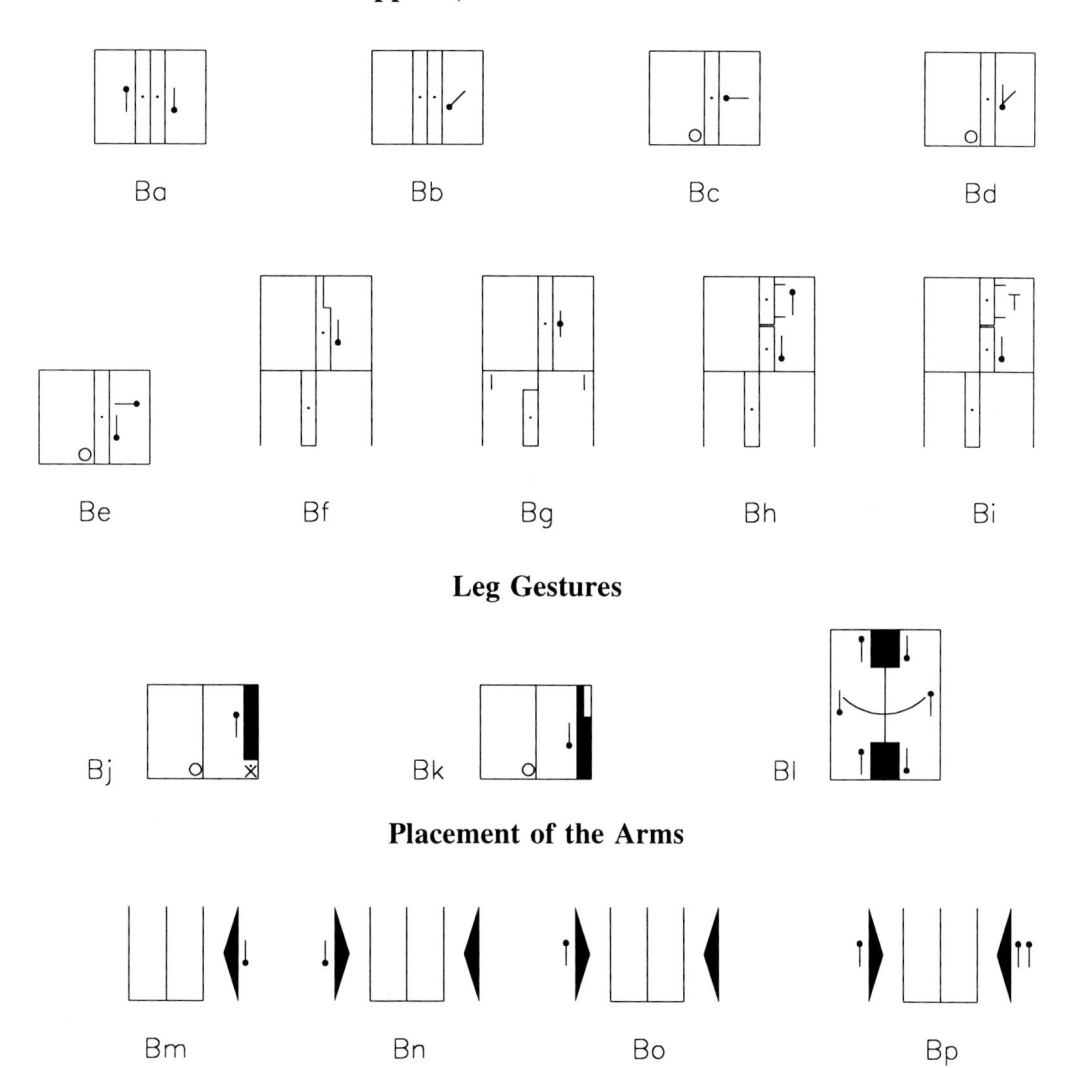

Ba   Bb   Bc   Bd

Be   Bf   Bg   Bh   Bi

Leg Gestures

Bj   Bk   Bl

Placement of the Arms

Bm   Bn   Bo   Bp

B.6. **Relationship Indications.** In determining other forms of relationship the full range of levels for pins - black (low), white (high), and the tack (middle level) may be needed. When the arms cross in **Bq** the right is above the left. Use of the various relationship signs involves the use of pins to be specific. The right hand is under the pot while supporting it in **Br**. The palm touches the pole from the right side direction in **Bs**. The right arm of person H is shown in **Bt** to address person A from above, i.e. the arm is above A.[139] For person H, the meeting line in **Bu** states that person A is below him/her.

B.7. **Minor Displacements.** Pins are used to indicate minor modifications of or displacements from the stated situation (see Part V). In **Bv** the right foot steps slightly apart from the left foot. Walking with feet slightly apart (straddled) is shown in **Bw** (see also **12c**). The 3rd position of **Bx** is shown to be slightly opened sidewards. The right arm is down in **By** but slightly opened to the side; this is comparable to **Bv**. Holding the right arm forward, but slightly below horizontal, is shown in **Bz**. As this is a Distal Center description, the small tick must be added near the end of each pin. Note that, for gestures, to make clear that this is not a statement of relationship with another part, object or person, the pin is tied with a small horizontal bow to the direction symbol. The pin in **Baa** states that the arm is slightly to the right of standard place high. In **Bab** the pin shows the extremity to be slightly backward of standard side middle.

B.8. **Minor Movements.** Minor movements are displacements from a previously established situation. In **Bac**, from the position forward middle, the arm lowers and rises slightly (a small down and up movement, the down movement being accented). The lower arm moves slightly side to side in **Bad**. In **Bae** the head inclines slightly forward and then returns to its normal situation. Because the pins in **Bae** represent a proximal analysis (judged from the point of attachment) there is no need to add a tick to the pin, as is required for Distal Center analysis. A shifting action is shown in **Baf**; the equal sign, used to specify a major shifting action, when placed on a pin, indicates a minor shifting action; here it is a displacement for the wrist, a 'bulging' out of line.

B.9. **Deviations from a Path.** A pin placed within a bow indicates a deviation (a detour) in the path of the movement, i.e. on the way from the starting point to the finishing location (see Part III). In **Bag** the leg makes a slightly outward curve as it prepares to take the step forward. In **Bah**, as the leg is lifted it deviates slightly to the left, producing a curved path. The arm makes a slight undulating movement (up, then down) in **Bai** on its way from side to forward middle. The torso tilt in **Baj** curves slightly forward on its way to right side high. In the middle of the path forward in **Bak** there is a slight deviation to the left, perhaps to avoid a person or object (see also **13b**).

Advanced Labanotation

Relationship Indications

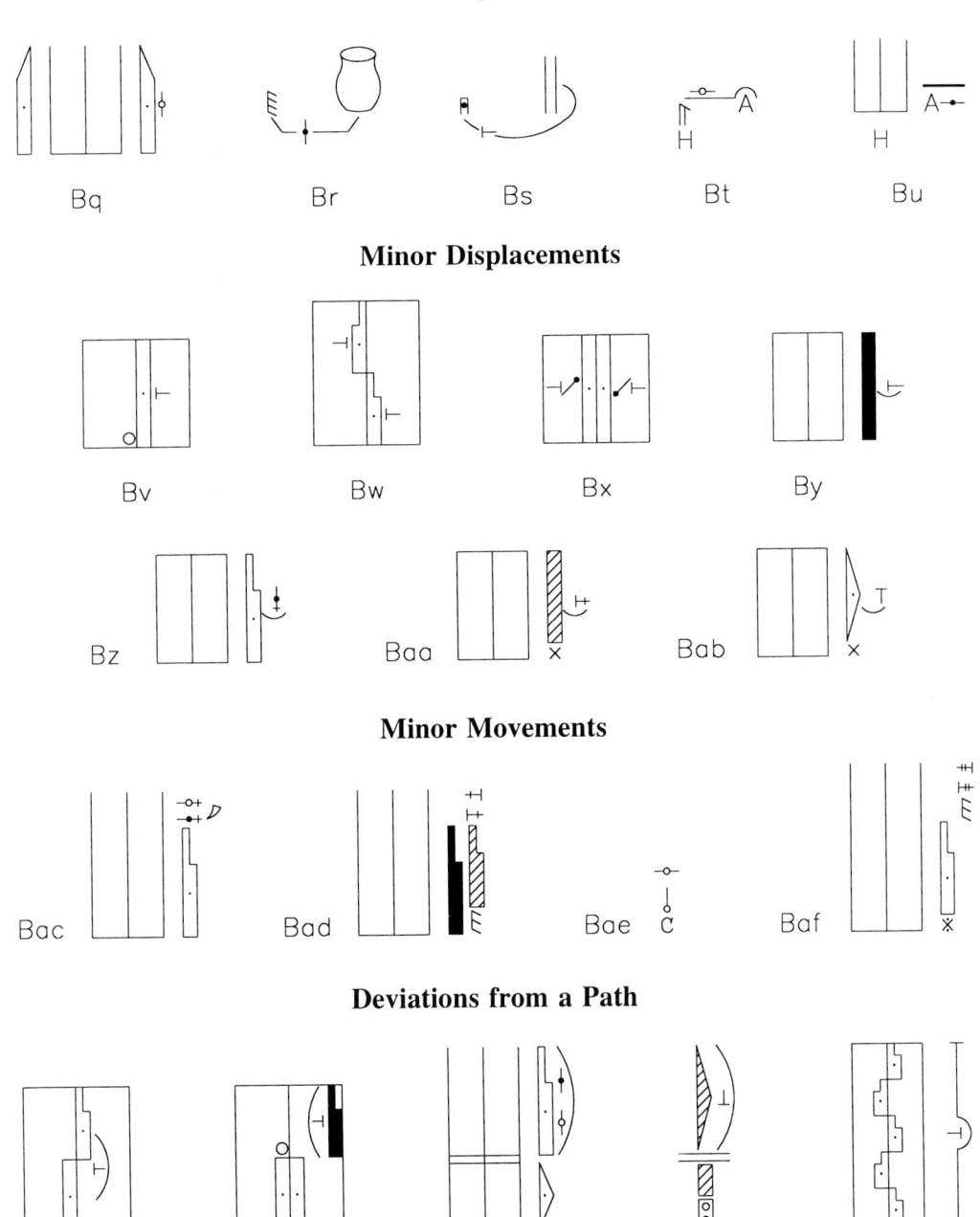

Bq   Br   Bs   Bt   Bu

Minor Displacements

Bv   Bw   Bx   By

Bz   Baa   Bab

Minor Movements

Bac   Bad   Bae   Baf

Deviations from a Path

Bag   Bah   Bai   Baj   Bak

B.10. **Intermediate Directions.** A pin within a direction symbol indicates a $^1/_3$ displacement toward the main direction which the pin represents (see 1.8, 1.12). In **Bal** the direction is $^1/_3$ from forward middle to right diagonal middle. From forward low, the stated point in **Bam** is $^1/_3$ toward forward middle. Ex. **Ban** is similar, but $^1/_3$ toward right diagonal middle. An intermediate point is shown in **Bao** in that, from forward middle, the limb lowers to a point between $^1/_3$ to forward low and $^1/_3$ toward right diagonal low. Another mixed $^1/_3$ way point is shown in **Bap**.[140] From the main direction of right diagonal high, the required point is $^1/_3$ toward place high and $^1/_3$ toward forward high. A less used example is **Baq** which states that the middle level support should be very slightly lower,[141] usually shown with the appropriate degree of leg bend.

B.11. **Specific Parts of the Body.** Different level pins are applied to body parts to show the upper, middle, or lower parts. These will be dealt with in detail in the planned <u>Advanced Labanotation</u> issue on Body Variations. The forward high surface of the chest is shown in **Bar**. The upper right side of the pelvis (the iliac crest) is given in **Bas**. The lower part of the pelvis (the crotch) is given in **Bat**, while **Bau** indicates the diaphragm (the below part of the chest). Various parts of the head are shown with pins, for example **Bav** indicates the forehead, and **Baw** the mouth.[142] For limbs, the upper part of the back of the neck (the limb below the head) is stated in **Bax**, while the lower right side of the left thigh is given in **Bay**.

B.12. **Degree of Turn, Circling.** Black pins show the degree, the amount of turning, $^1/_8$ to the right in **Baz**. For the circular path of **Bba** the amount is $^3/_8$. A black pin is used for a secret turn,[143] **Bbb**. For a particular involved situation, this secret turn indicates the decision to establish a new front, here it is $^1/_4$ to the right of the previous front.

Degree of turn (rotation) for limbs is shown in terms of destination with white pins. These are used for gestures, not supports. The head turns $^1/_8$ to the right from its normal forward looking stance in **Bbc**. Outward rotation of the legs is given in **Bbd**, the zero point being feet parallel and pointing forward. Destination of a turn may also be given in terms of the Constant Directions. The pivot turn of **Bbe** should end facing stage right. Circling to the right ending facing upstage may be indicated as in **Bbf**. This is more commonly expressed as **Bbg**; the aim being indicated at the end of the path sign. A head turn can end toward a stage direction, here in **Bbh** it is to stage left.

B.13. **Axis of Rotation.** Two pins are used to indicate a particular axis for a rotation (see **30d** and <u>Advanced Labanotation</u> *Floorwork, Basic Acrobatics*, Section 16). Ex. **Bbi** shows a somersault forward which is to occur around the right-forward/left-backward diagonal axis, i.e. it revolves diagonally left, halfway between a true forward somersault and a cartwheel to the left. The circular path for the right arm in **Bbj** moves around a forward-high/backward-low axis, i.e. it is performed on a forward-low/backward-high slant.

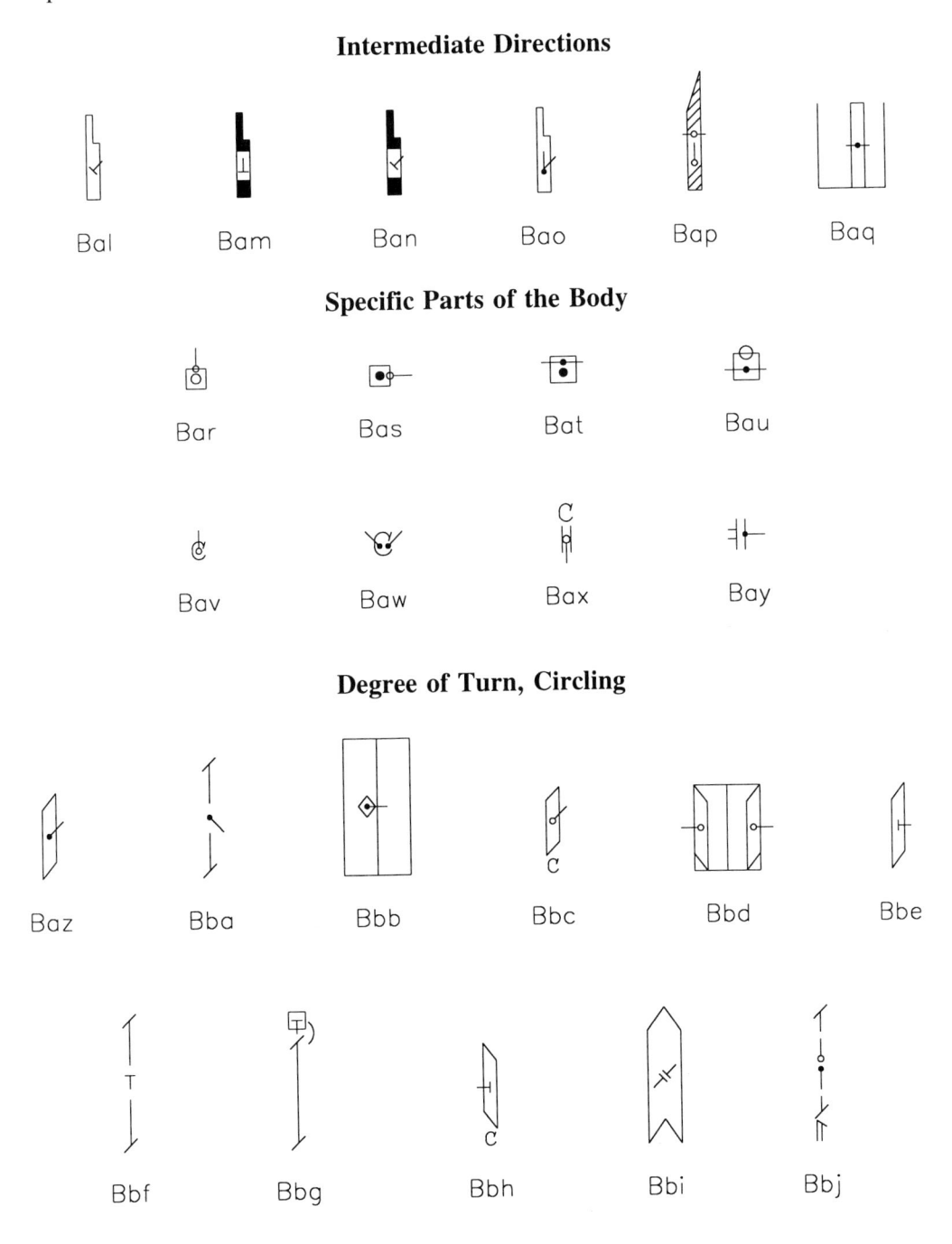

Intermediate Directions

Bal   Bam   Ban   Bao   Bap   Baq

Specific Parts of the Body

Bar   Bas   Bat   Bau

Bav   Baw   Bax   Bay

Degree of Turn, Circling

Baz   Bba   Bbb   Bbc   Bbd   Bbe

Bbf   Bbg   Bbh   Bbi   Bbj

B.14. **Orientation, Front Signs.** From the Constant Key of **Bbk**, the Front Signs, **Bbl**, are derived, using the tack pin. For ballroom dancing the key of **Bbm** provides the signs for Front in relation to the Line of Dance (the Direction of Progression), the Front signs being **Bbn** (see Section 42).[144] The Direction of the Path key (43.2, 43.5), **Bbo**, provides the orientation signs of **Bbp**. An arrow is not strictly a pin, but is included here for comparison. Orientation toward the periphery of a performing area (43.6, 43.8), stated as in **Bbq**, provides the keys of **Bbr**. These are the same keys, of course, as **Bbn**, but statement of this particular orientation will have been clearly given at the start of the score or on the page where it first appears.

B.15. **Track Pins for the Legs.** Section 19 and Appendix A in <u>Advanced Labanotation</u> *Floorwork, Basic Acrobatics* deal extensively with track pins. Steps relating to the center line can be written as stepping in front of the previous support, as in **Bf**, repeated here, but track pins provide a different view for placement of the legs and **Bbs**, stepping in the center track may be a more appropriate description.

B.16. Compare the following: walking forward as though from one 5th position to another, **Bbt**; walking forward as though from a 3rd position, **Bbu**, and walking forward as if from 1st position, **Bbv**. These are a different idea and produce a slightly different result from a similar use of track pins: the forward steps are on the body center line, **Bbw**; the steps are placed on the intermediate line between center and the lateral placement under the hips, **Bbx**; the steps are in line with the hip sockets, **Bby**. Note the difference between this last, in which the feet walk slightly apart and **Bbz**, in which there is a slight sideward displacement from the standard track for the legs in ordinary walking.

B.17. For backward steps or leg gestures, the track pin may be drawn as in **Bca**. Here the left foot steps forward on the center track, the right steps backward on the center track. This instruction could as well be stated as **Bcb**, the use of the forward pointing track pin has the same message, i.e. "on the center track". In **Bcc** the forward and backward leg gestures are to be placed on the center line. For this, the relationship pins of **Bcd** can also be used, the reference being to the other leg.

Advanced Labanotation

Orientation, Front Signs

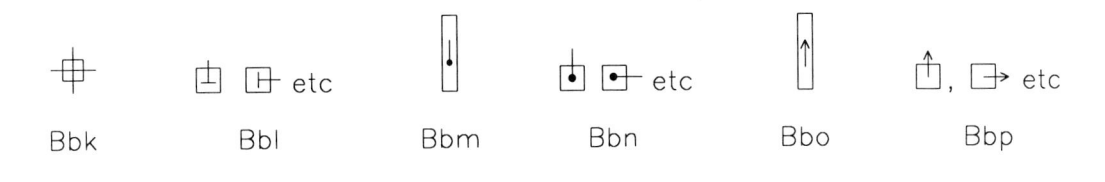

Bbk   Bbl etc   Bbm   Bbn etc   Bbo   Bbp etc

Bbq   Bbr etc

Track Pins for the Legs

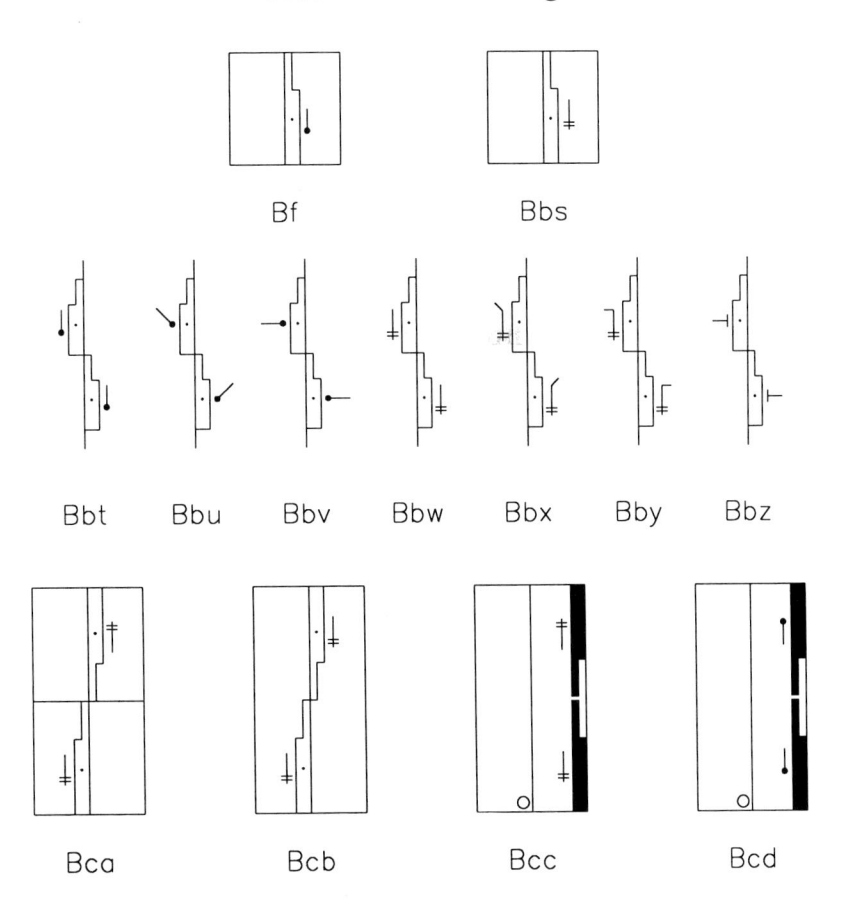

Bf   Bbs

Bbt   Bbu   Bbv   Bbw   Bbx   Bby   Bbz

Bca   Bcb   Bcc   Bcd

B.18. **Black Pins, Positions of the Arms.** One of the applications of black pins, in use since the early days of the system, is to modify arm gestures, in particular to indicate the balletic positions of the arms.[145] For this purpose the black pins indicate relationship to the body (the trunk). The basic position of **Bce** (arms down, slightly rounded at the sides of the body) needs no pins but, were they to be used, they would be the sideward pointing pins shown in brackets. This basic position is changed in **Bcf** to 5th position *en bas* (also known in ballet as low 5th position, *bras bas*) by adding the black pins which indicate that the extremities of the arms, the finger tips, are 'in front of the body'. With the arms forward and rounded these same pins produce 5th *en avant* (5th in front), also called 1st position, **Bcg**. For the arms up and rounded, the 'in front' pins produce 5th *en haut* (high 5th), **Bch**.[146]

B.19. A diagonal relationship to the torso would be indicated as in **Bci**; this is halfway between arms at the sides and extremities 'in front of the body'. The movement of **Bcj** makes use of the sideward pin to stress to the reader that, as the arm moves down to go to the crossed diagonal direction, it should pass through true place low (at the side of the body) and not miss that direction.

B.20. This use of black pins for the sagittal arm positions was applied with a certain freedom with regard to exact placement of the extremities.[147] Placement of the arms in ballet is more subtle than these simple notation examples indicate. The degree of rounding the arm varies from one classical ballet 'school' to another. The distance between the finger tips can vary significantly. It was understood that the reader interpreted the general notation according to the style with which s/he was familiar. When the need arises to specify in greater detail the stylistic differences and identify which is to be used in reading a score or a collection of technique exercises, the track pins are used to express precise placement.

B.21. When directions other than vertical or sagittal are being used, the black pins still indicate relationship to the body, the trunk. In **Bck** the arm is understood to cross in front of the body as it gestures to the left. This relationship can be specifically stated as in **Bcl**. In **Bcm** both arms cross in front of the body, the right arm shown to be in front of the left. The position can be specifically spelled out as in **Bcn**, the second pin referring not to relationship to the body, but the relationship to the other arm. Ex. **Bco** shows the arms crossing behind the body, the right arm being behind the left.

Advanced Labanotation

Black Pins, Positions of the Arms

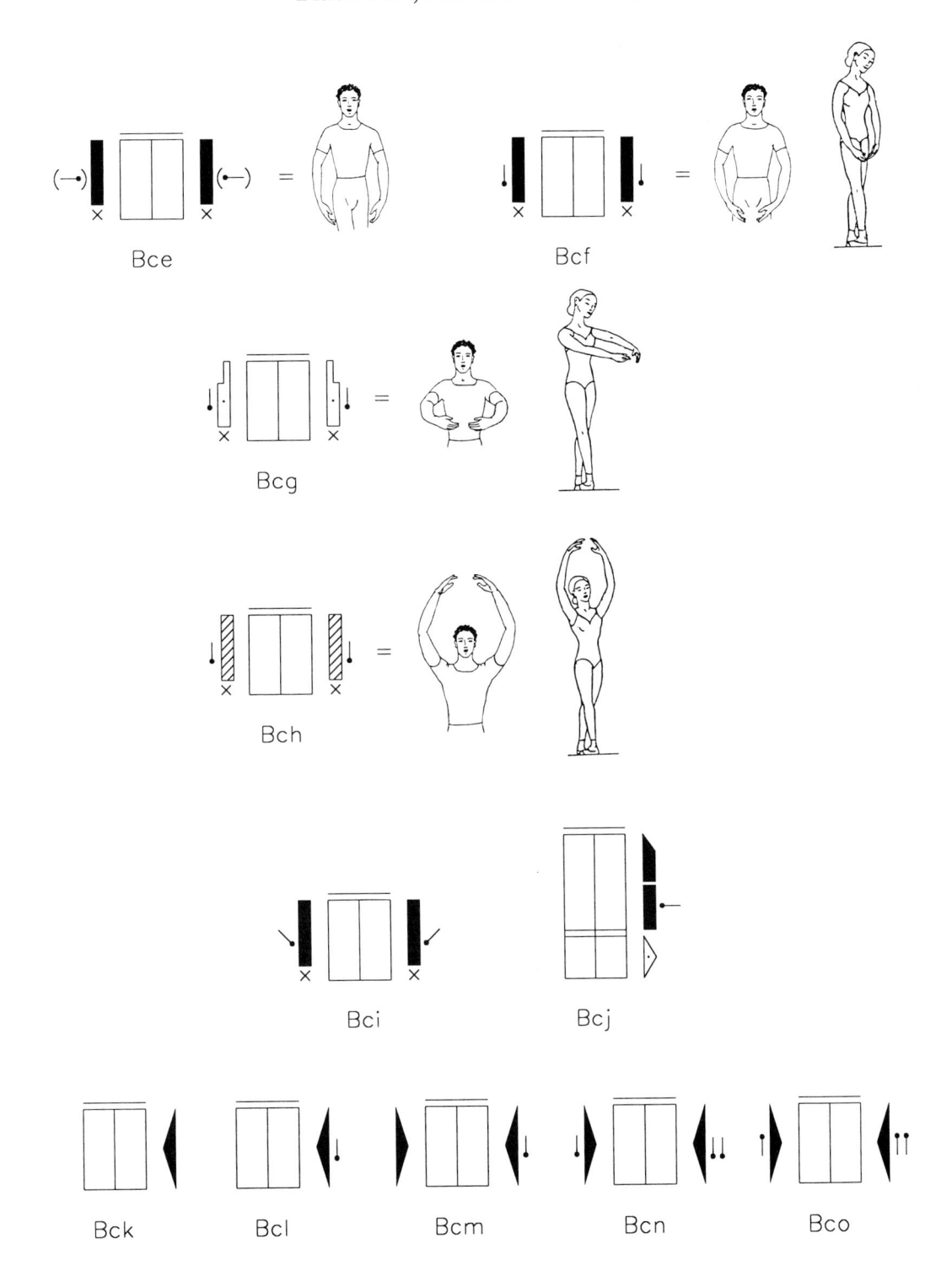

Bce

Bcf

Bcg

Bch

Bci

Bcj

Bck Bcl Bcm Bcn Bco

B.22. **Track Pins, Positions of the Arms.** With the advent of track pins it seemed that they should replace the black pins in showing the positions of the arms in ballet and other styles. Thus many people adopted the usage of **Bcp**, **Bcq**, **Bcr**, etc. However, in these ballet positions, the fingertips are *not on the center line*, but near to it, and how near depends on the 'school' - Italian, French, Russian, etc. Thus **Bcq**, for example, should be written as **Bcs**, finger tips next to the center line. For some ballet styles the finger tips should be slightly more apart, more accurately described as **Bct**. The use of black pins for positions of the arms is intentionally less precise than track pins, thus allowing performance to be open to what the performer is accustomed to.

B.23. Because the 'lateral track' for the forward track pin, **Bcu**, is equal to the standard forward arm placement, i.e. the arm extremity being on a line in front of the shoulder, **Bcv**, the pin statement is not needed here. When both arms are on the center line there is usually the need to indicate the relationship between them. In **Bcw** the right arm is above the left. The arms are up on the center line in **Bcx**, the right arm in front of the left. Similarly, in **Bcy** the arms are down and on the center line, the right in front of the left.

B.24. The track pin of **Bcz** tells the reader that the extremity of the right arm is to be in the normal forward track for the left arm, i.e. in line with the left shoulder. This gives a more body-related description than the diagonal placement of **Bda**. Note the placement of both arms on the right forward diagonal center line in **Bdb**, the left arm bent, the right arm normally extended.

B.25. When grasping the hands with the arms forward, as in **Bdc**, it is understood that the hands meet on the center line, the track pins of **Bdd** are not needed, this redundancy can be avoided. For the arm crossing in front of the body, **Bde**, the usual black pin for 'in front' is appropriate. Use here of the track pin, **Bdf**, is quite incorrect because, what is needed is the relationship of the arm to the body, not a reference to the extremity on the center track.

B.26. Ex. **Bdg** states arms up, above the shoulders. In **Bdh** the right arm is up but in the track of the left arm, the extremity being behind the left arm. Arms overhead (on the body center line), can be written with the white pins of **Bdi**, or the center line track pins of **Bdj**.[148] Note that here the right arm is more bent and so the right hand will be under the left. For tracks overhead, the double pin of **Bdk** may be easier to grasp; similarly, halfway between above the head and above the shoulder can be indicated with the intermediate track pin of **Bdl**. with the pin of **Bdm** to indicate above the shoulder (the lateral part of the vertical track).

Track Pins, Positions of the Arms

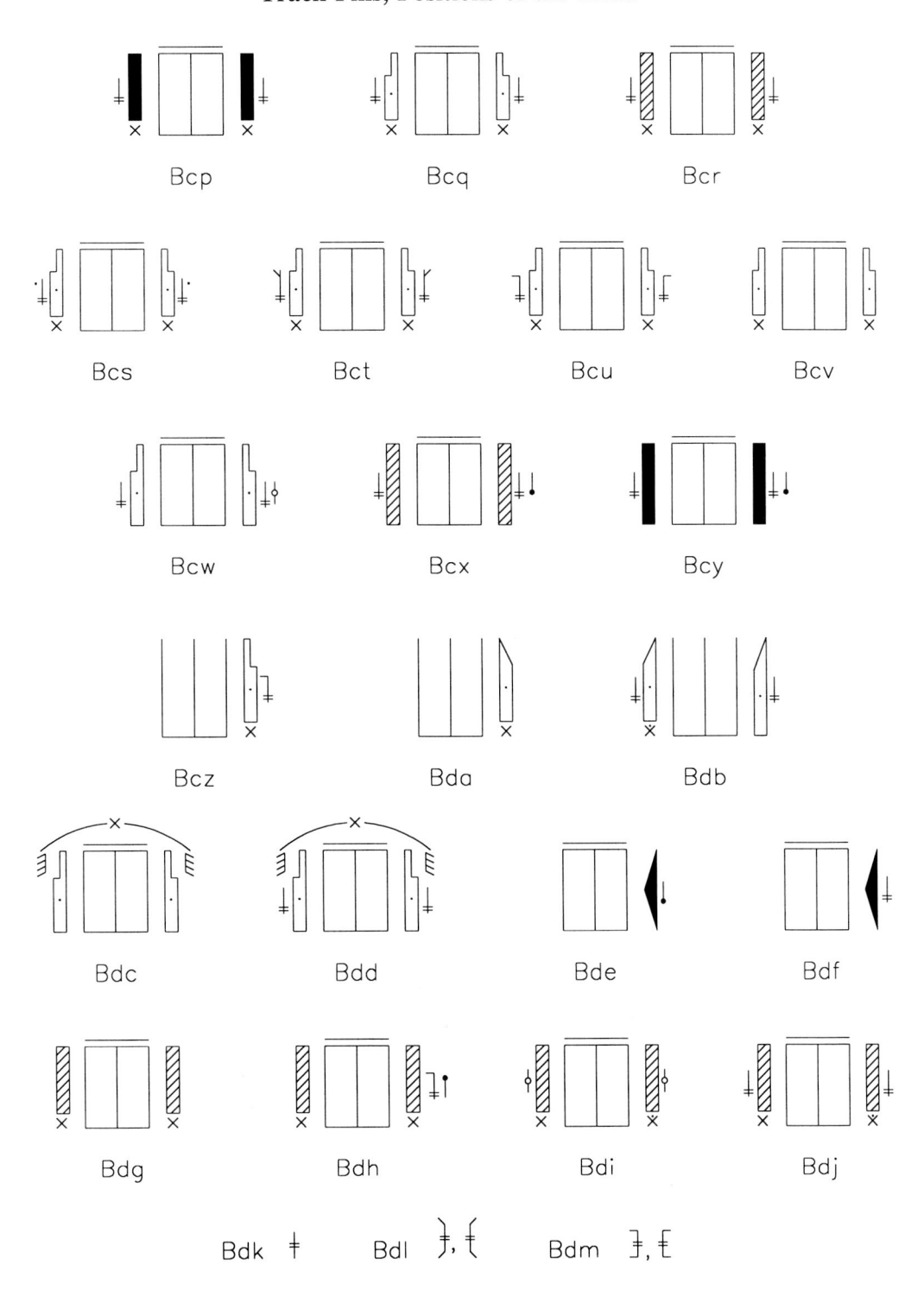

Bcp Bcq Bcr

Bcs Bct Bcu Bcv

Bcw Bcx Bcy

Bcz Bda Bdb

Bdc Bdd Bde Bdf

Bdg Bdh Bdi Bdj

Bdk Bdl Bdm

B.27. **Identifying Performers.** Pins identify performers on stage. Ex. **Bdn** represents a woman, **Bdo** a man, and **Bdp** a person, gender not important or not known.[149] Wedges are used on floor plans to show where a peformer ends, **Bdq** being for the female, **Bdr** for the male with **Bds** meaning a person.[150]

B.28. Indications for performers placed below the staff or in other locations other than on a stage plan are written with a slightly incomplete circle surround, **Bdt**. The advantage is that there can thus be no mistaking the pin for a movement indication. A couple is shown by encircling two pins, **Bdu**. Doubling the circle indicates each, thus here in **Bdv** it states each female. Each couple is indicated in **Bdw**.

B.29. **Surfaces for Design Drawing.**[151] Pins are used to indicate the imaginary surface on which designs are drawn. The sign for a (any) surface is **Bdx**, only the shaft of the pin is used, no level. In **Bdy** the pin states that the surface is as if on the wall in front. The side wall at the right is designated in **Bdz**. The surface is slanting upward toward the ceiling in **Bea**. A curved surface can be specified, as in **Beb**. The curved surface is designated in **Bec** as being above, as on a curved ceiling. In **Bed** it is a curved left wall.

B.30. **Modifying Parts of the Room/Stage.** The room/stage area signs are given more detailed specification by the addition of small strokes (pin shafts) (see 44.15, 44.19). The center part of the general left front corner area of the stage is shown in **Bee**. Specifically the front part of this area is stated in **Bef**.

B.31. **Fixed Points in the Room/on Stage.** The Fixed Points (see Section 46) are located at the outer surface of a defined space. A particular point is indicated by adding the appropriate pin to the Fixed Point sign. In **Beg** it is the front lower left corner. In **Beh** it is upper edge of the right wall. When performers need to look at a particular place in the audience (see 46.6), this can be shown in a way similar to the Fixed Points. Ex. **Bei** states the middle right front of the audience (from the peformer's point of view), perhaps the royal box, the place where the royalty would sit. The lower back part of the audience (back of the orchestra seats) is shown in **Bej**.

B.32. **Pins with Dynamic Signs.** Ex. **Bek** shows that the direction of the pressing action is downward. Indications such as these are often placed within a vertical bow.

Advanced Labanotation

Identifying Performers

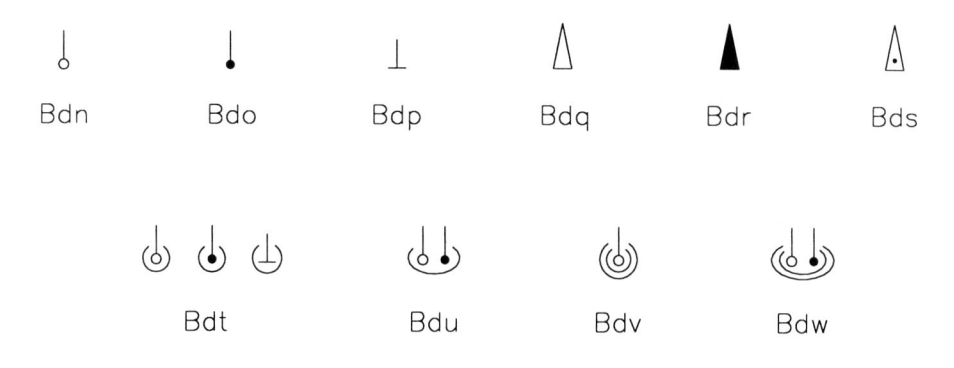

Bdn   Bdo   Bdp   Bdq   Bdr   Bds

Bdt   Bdu   Bdv   Bdw

Surfaces for Design Drawing

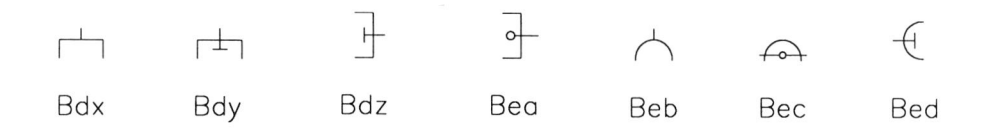

Bdx   Bdy   Bdz   Bea   Beb   Bec   Bed

Modifying Parts of the Room/Stage

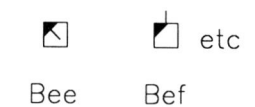

Bee   Bef etc

Fixed Points in the Room/on Stage

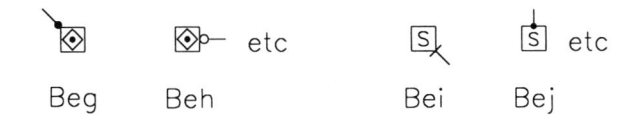

Beg   Beh etc   Bei   Bej etc

Pins with Dynamic Signs

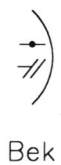

Bek

B.33. **Polar Pins.** As explained in Section 23, unlike standard pins, polar pins have no indication of level. They are based on the idea of a globe, slight up and down movements, **Bel** and **Bem**, being as though on a longitudinal line. Slight horizontal displacements clockwise, **Ben**, or counterclockwise, **Beo**, are on a latitudinal line. Spoke-like outward and inward movements away from, **Bep**, or toward, **Beq**, the central vertical polar line. Wherever the extremity of the limb is situated, these minor movements (displacements) take place as though on a globe concentric with the main global kinesphere. Movements may combine any two or three of these six minor movement possibilities: **Ber** shows rising clockwise; **Bes** states descending clockwise; To illustrate a few, **Bet** indicates an outward and rising displacement; and **Beu** an inward and clockwise minor movement.

Polar Pins

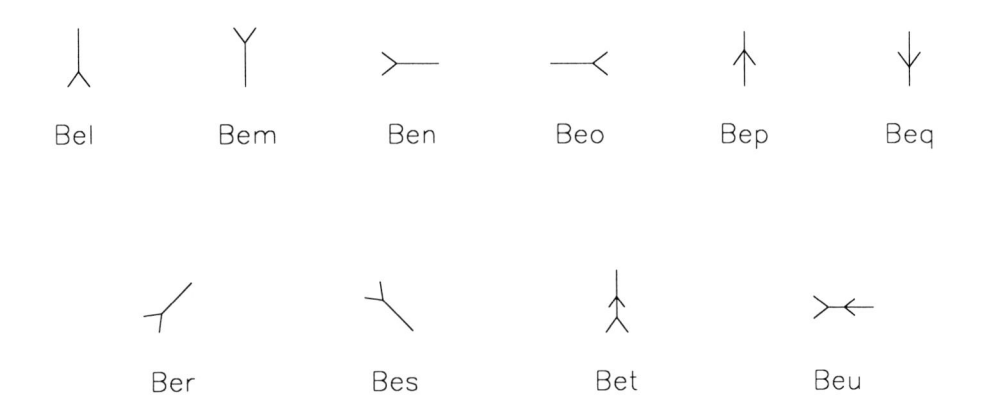

| Bel | Bem | Ben | Beo | Bep | Beq |

| Ber | Bes | Bet | Beu |

C Historical Background on Labanotation Textbooks

The authoritative textbook *Labanotation - The System of Analyzing and Recording Movement*, was first published in 1954. The revised and expanded version, published in 1970 (reprinted in 1989) drew attention to a number of topics which were to be dealt with in greater detail in a subsequent publication, referred to as "Part Two". The need for such statements was high lighted by the reaction of a group in Japan, who, when studying the 1954 Labanotation textbook assumed that it represented the whole system. Since no handling of long sleeves was included, they decided that the system did not meet their needs. It was therefore important to make clear that much more existed. Labanotation did indeed have the capacity of meeting their needs, and in a wider context it was necessary to draw attention to the fact that the system was applicable across the whole spectrum of human movement.

Detailed information on advanced Labanotation usage has not been generally available. Three volumes on advanced topics were published in 1991 and the present series continues the detailed and more advanced material along the same lines.

Labanotation and *Kinetography Laban*, *Motif Description* and *Structured Description*

The above terms may need some clarification. The specific subject of this book is *Labanotation*, the name given in the United States to the system of movement notation originated by Rudolf Laban and first published in 1928. Most European notators and dance scholars refer to the system as *Kinetography Laban*. There are some variances between Labanotation and Kinetography in notation usages, and occasionally in symbols and rules, and since 1959 the International Council of Kinetography Laban (ICKL) has provided an active and successful platform for discussions between practitioners on unification and further applications of the system. Differences are now small so that mutual understanding of scores is ensured. Kinetography rules and usages are catalogued in Albrecht Knust's 1979 Dictionary (see Bibliography).

The aim of the present series of texts is to provide a guide to the *Structured Description* of movement, the highly developed notation offering a determinate description of movement progression by detailing choreographed (or otherwise established) actions. A different and complementary approach is provided by *Motif Description (Motif Writing)*, which uses symbols to represent movement ideas and concepts and provide a general statement concerning the theme or motivation of movements.

The term Labanotation is used in this book to refer to the notation system in general and not to mark a distinction from Kinetography or Motif Writing.

Source materials

Advanced Labanotation contains, whenever possible, systematic discussion of other usages and, where appropriate, comments on the history of symbols and rules and the reason for their inclusion in the Labanotation system. The material presented is based on all available textbooks, on earlier writings of Albrecht Knust and Maria Szentpál, as well as on personal discussions and correspondence with specialists such as Sigurd Leeder, Valerie Preston-Dunlop and members of the Dance Notation Bureau in New York and the Dance Notation Bureau Extension at Ohio University. Another major source of information are the proceedings of twenty two biennial ICKL Conferences.

Much use is made of the comprehensive theoretical account of the system by Knust, summarized in his *Dictionary of Kinetography Laban/Labanotation* (1979), and his earlier publications including his eight-volume encyclopedia of 1946-50 entitled *Handbuch der Kinetographie Laban* (Handbook of Kinetography Laban). The textbook *Dance Notation. Kinetography Laban* by Szentpál, published in Hungarian between 1969 and 1976 is unfortunately not readily accessible to readers outside Hungary, but Szentpál generously provided an English translation for her many colleagues.

In many cases, writing an advanced text of this kind has meant breaking new ground: the intricacies of writing deviations, minor movements and path signs for gestures, for instance, were not adequately covered, and some not included at all in the 1979 Knust Dictionary. Some recent developments in the system such as 'DBP' (Direction in relation to the location of Body Part), track pins and symbols for 'Design Drawing' came too late to be included in Knust's 1979 Dictionary.

The Advanced Labanotation series offers the latest research on the Labanotation system and hence is completely up-to-date as at the date of publication.

Research Involved

A major concern in the research for this book has been the comparison of one rule against another to check applicability in all contexts. Often this has led to discoveries producing new arguments for or against a certain way of writing.

Labanotation is rapidly developing in filling the needs in various areas of movement concern and is being accepted as a tool in recording, in research and in education. Each of these fields has specific requirements. There is a call for maximum flexibility in the notation system, so that it can provide general and simple statements for particular purposes and at the same time be very precise where such specificity is required. In dance research the need for precision has increased to the point where we are obliged to consider questions about the system that only ten years ago did not seem important, let alone when the fundamentals of the system were devised. In this new text we have tried to take these different needs into account while respecting the system as it has been handed down to us and is now used by people all over the world.

Notes

These annotations are mainly of three kinds. Firstly, they identify other major *rules and usages*. Secondly, they mark symbols and rules that have been *recently introduced* or *not described in other sources*, the origins of these being given. And finally, they give the *references for particular notation excerpts*.

On important or controversial issues, a short discussion of rationale is included. Sometimes, old ways of writing are briefly mentioned.

Research of other usages systematically involved *Táncjelírás, Laban Kinetográfia* by Szentpál and the *Dictionary of Kinetography Laban (Labanotation)* by Knust (see Bibliography). Where needed, other sources were also used.

Numbers in parentheses at the end of each note indicate the paragraph in the text to which the note refers. The following abbreviations identify sources; for full bibliographic information see the Bibliography.

References

H70	Hutchinson 1970, *Labanotation, The System of Analyzing and Recording Movement.*
H83	Hutchinson 1983, *Your Move, A New Approach to the Study of Movement and Dance.*
H91	Hutchinson 1991, <u>Advanced Labanotation</u>, Vol. 1, Part 1, *Canon Forms*, Vol. 1, Part 2, *Shape, Design, Trace Patterns*, Vol. 1, Part 3, *Kneeling, Sitting, Lying.*
ICKL	International Council of Kinetography Laban
K79	Knust 1979
LNTR	*The Labanotator*
PD69	Preston-Dunlop 1969
S76	Szentpál 1969-76
AHG	Ann Hutchinson Guest
AK	Albrecht Knust
KIN	Kinetography Laban
LN	Labanotation

1. This subject is treated in some detail in H70. It is presented here in greater detail and with further explanations. (Part I)

2. It would seem that the logical, strictly interpreted meaning of a) below would be: "from the upright position move halfway to side high, marked 1 in diagram b). From there, move halfway toward left side high, ending at a point slightly left of place high (marked here as 2). From this point move halfway toward right side high thus ending at a point which is slightly left of the original point 1 (marked as 3). Should this literal 'halfway' movement be continued, the next point will be slightly to the left of point 2, and so on. As can be seen, if the dot were strictly to mean exactly half-way each time, the result is to arrive at subtle intermediate points which can be calculated on paper but not achieved in movement.

For this reason the following interpretation was established: *when moving from a stated halfway point to another halfway point, the arrival point will be that which is halfway between the nearest cardinal direction passed through on the way to the stated direction.* In a) the head inclines halfway to right side high. For the second movement, the head passes through place high and thus the halfway point to left side high is judged from this cardinal direction; the result is point 4 in b). The third movement will return the head to point 1. (1.5)

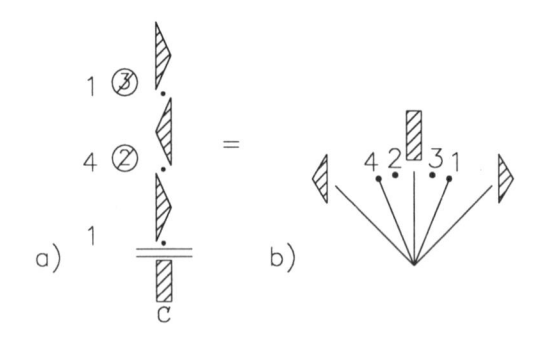

3. To serve the need for finer intermediate direction descriptions, in 1947 Laban advocated the use of additional dots. A presentation of this idea was given in LNTR No. 4, 1959. One dot is shown to mean $1/4$ of the way to the next stated direction; two dots meant $1/2$ way, and three dots meant $3/4$ way. The logic of this was attractive but its adoption would have meant changing the established meaning of one dot. To date it has not become part of the system but could always be used when explained in a glossary at the start of a score. (1.6)

4. A student of AK named Tinkel developed charts in the 1930s showing such relative displacement. These, known as Tinkel's Variations, were considered by the Dance Notation Bureau but discarded in favor of the present usage. Ex. a) here illustrates his suggestion, the pins indicated the relative relationship to the

stated main direction, i.e. 'lower than', 'higher than'.   (1.10)

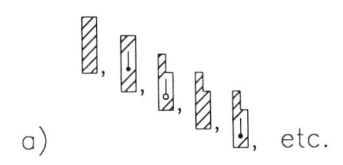

a)   , etc.

5. The original rule in LN was that, for movement to a third degree point, ie. an arc greater than a 90° arc as in a), the 'direct' path was followed, illustrated in b). For this transversal path the arm would unobtrusively bend enough to avoid both the peripheral path and the straight path. To produce the peripheral arc to a 3rd degree point, another direction symbol always had to be added. For the movement of c) this extra direction could be d) or e). The disadvantage of this usage was that, strictly speaking, the choice of direction could slightly change the timing as well as giving some importance to the selected direction. It was examples such as f) and g), which, when performed quickly, decided the original rule that for third degree points the extremity should follow a 'direct' path, as in b). The decision to change the standard performance to c) was taken at the ICKL 1985 Conference (Technical Report I:4). (3.5)

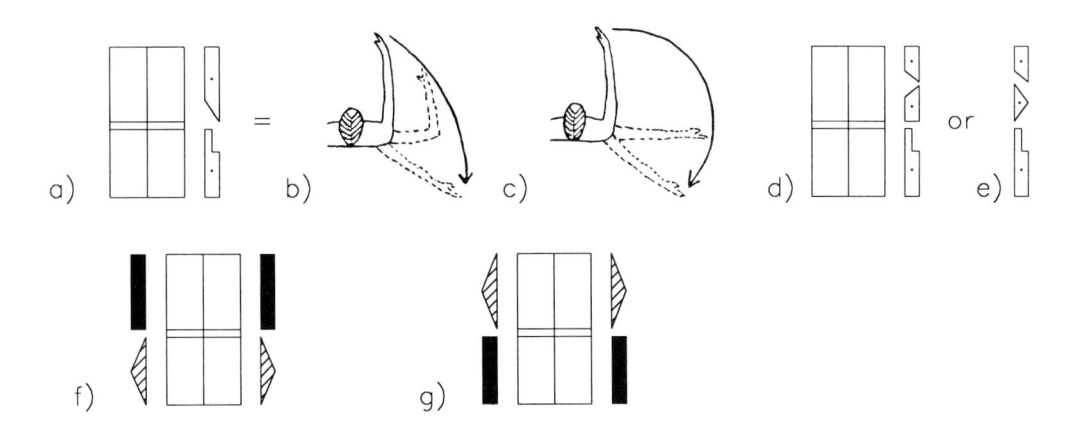

a)   b)   c)   d)   or   e)

f)   g)

6. The term 'Aimed Destination' is a recent replacement for the previous, long-established term *Direct Path*. The LN meaning and performance of 'direct path' had to be learned; it was too often confused with straight path, the word 'direct' being too close in daily parlance to the word 'straight'. In August 2000 the decision was made by the author of this book and advisors to change this term. It is hoped that the new name will convey more readily what has been found to be a general, natural way for the arms to perform these particular movements. (3.6)

248   *Spatial Variations*

7. The idea of an empty direction symbol to clarify a pathway was first put forward by AHG and published in *The Bournonville School*, 1979. (5.3)

8. The categories of *spatially central* and *spatially peripheral* as well as those of *bodily central* and *bodily peripheral* were aspects of Laban's *Eukinetcs* theories, taught in the 1930s at the Jooss-Leeder Dance School. When Laban developed his *Effort* ideas, linked to his early 1940s motion studies, he dropped the 'central' and 'peripheral' aspects and replaced them with *Direct* and *Flexible* (Indirect). Kurt Jooss regretted this omission as he knew that central and peripheral were still much needed in the study of movement/dance. The signs for these aspects and their application were presented in LNTR No. 40, 1985. (6.1)

9. These signs were devised by AHG, first published in the Labanotator No. 40, 1985. (6.2)

10. As discussed in LNTR No. 30, 1980, a phrasing bow is sometimes used to indicate fluent, legato movement. Such legato movement refers to timing, not to the shape of the movement design. The phrasing bow should not be interpreted as the smoothing out of any sharp corners, it provides no direct statement regarding angular or rounded corners. The phrasing bow links movements in terms of the flow of time, or to indicate unity of kinetic 'thought'. (7.1)

11. This development of the 1985 signs (see end note 9) was created by AHG in 1999. (7.2)

12. For Design Drawing see H91. (10.6)

13. Two different understandings have existed in the past:
    1) that use of a small direction symbol relates to the preference in choice of description for a deviation, the size of such deviation being comparable to use of a pin. Discussion on use of a pin versus a small direction symbol appeared in LNTR No. 77, 1994, paragraph 1.6. The interpretation given then was that, in the context of 1f below, 1f and 1g had virtually the same meaning; the pin is easier to draw, but the reader might identify more readily with the direction symbol. The size of the deviation should be the same.

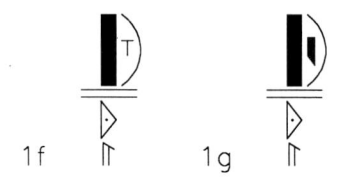

2) that use of a direction symbol indicated a larger deviation. Because direction symbols used for deviations use a different analysis (as distinct from that used for pins) and hence may produce a different curve, it was decided that the system benefited from incorporating this possibility. However, size of deviation should not automatically be larger. Size is always somewhat open and the means exist for indicating size when this is important. (10.9)

14. While use of Standard directions is the norm, i.e. the understood key of a), its counterpart, based on the Body key, b), can also be used when appropriate, i.e. directions centered on a path using the Body Key. In c) the movement is described from the Body Key, the deviation from the path being judged from that key. In the case of d) the Standard key of a) is understood. (10.10)

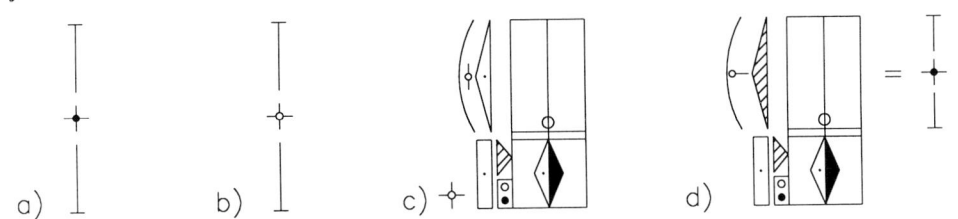

15. A point, which AK observed years ago and explained to AHG in discussion in 1957, is the fact that, when considering deviations from a directional point, the directions of the three-dimensional cross, shown as a) below, each have eight 1st degree neighboring points to which to deviate. Two examples are given here; those for place high in b), those for right side middle in c).

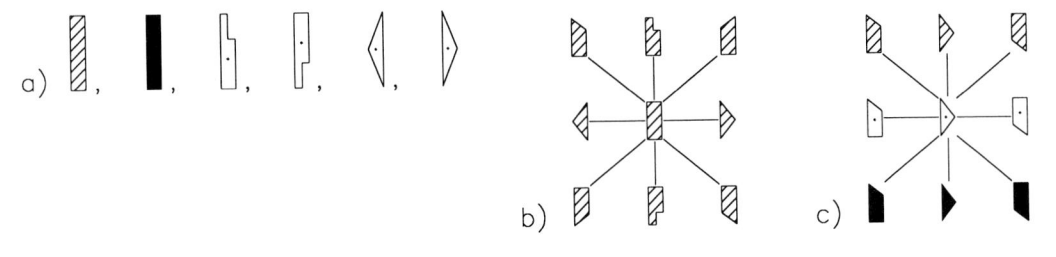

Each of the directions of d) has only six neighboring 1st degree points. This interesting (and unexpected) fact is illustrated for forward high in e) and for right side low in f). (10.12)

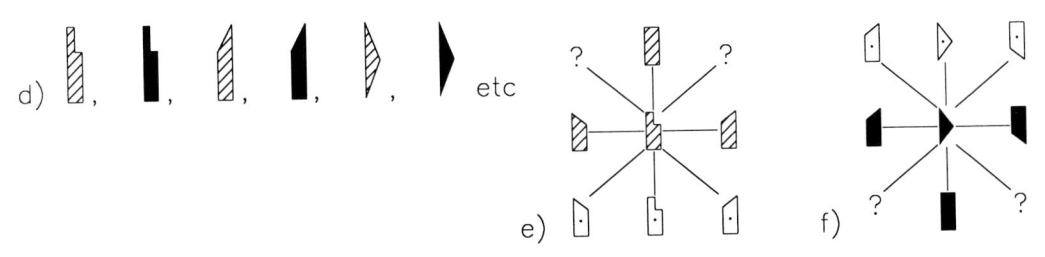

250   *Spatial Variations*

16. From reading professional LN scores it has been observed by the author that many deviations written with pins do not adhere strictly to the established theory. This is particularly true when the line of the movement is three-dimensional. The notator's analysis appears to be based on the path as though it were horizontal. This recently established reference provides a clear statement that this point of view is being used. (10.13)

17. This key was proposed by AHG in 2000 following the logic of indicating a cross of axes based on the spatial path. (10.13)

18. The indication for "See floor plan" was probably invented by Ray Cook in the 1970s. In The Kinetographer, No. 3, April 1974, it was noted that the sign was already being used by notators and the suggestion was put forward that it should be generally adopted. (12.12)

19. Exs. **14e-14k** are derived from K79: 276b, 277a, 277b. (14.3)

20. Example taken from K79: 275b. (15.4)

21. Example taken from K79: 274b. (15.5)

22. These examples are taken from K79: 274c (**15l, 15m**), 276c, d (**15q-15t**), 277c (**15u, 15v**). (15.9)

23. Originally, the term 'Satellite Center' was used to convey the idea of a distant, outside cross of axes. (16.2)

24. It appears that because one cannot see one's own head movements in addition to the short length of the neck which makes the proximal joint (base of the neck) closer, the proximal description for minor head tilts became the choice. (16.6)

25. Proximal Center Analysis for minor displacements was approved for a two-year trial at the 1981 ICKL Conference (Technical Report II:12). This trial was extended in 1983 (Technical Report II:11). (16.7)

26. The Distal Center Key, based on the Standard Cross of Axes, is repeated here, ex. a). Ex. b) is the Distal Center key based on the Body Cross of Axes, while c) is the Distal Key based on the Constant Cross of Directions. (16.7)

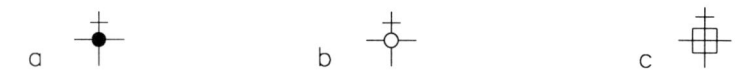

Advanced Labanotation 251

27. **Analysis of Peripheral and Central Displacements.** Because of the nature of the joints of the body, gestures are basically circular. As we know, in moving the arm from side middle to side high (an articulation in the shoulder joint), a slight arc is performed by the extremity, as illustrated in a). For the extremity to follow a straight path, the limb must flex slightly (through articulation in the elbow joint as well as the shoulder), illustrated in b).

Because the peripheral arc is so natural (all tilts and whole limb changes of direction use this form), it is the expected performance of minor movements as well. Thus, displacements away from a point will, in fact, produce a very slight arc, c). Neither the performer nor the viewer is aware that the displacement is on an arc rather than a straight line, as in d). Should there be the need to indicate a very small straight, rather than curved, path, the straight path indication can be added. (see 4.6). (16.20)

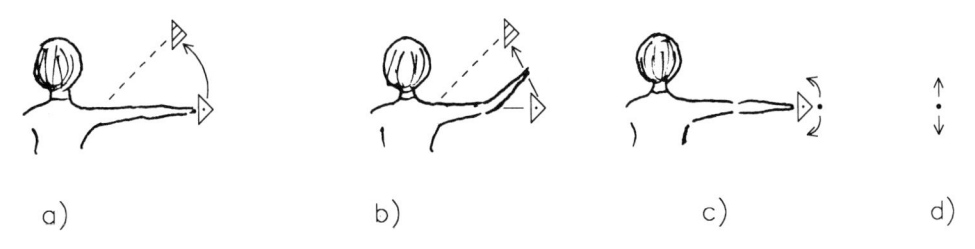

a)   b)   c)   d)

28. For her needs in Hungarian dance Maria Szentpál always used the method of a) below, or b), the pins indicating the direction of circling starting with the general first displacement. Ex. c) shows a set of pins moving in the opposite direction. This practical solution can be seen as a shorthand which gives an immediate message about the desired movement. (18.3)

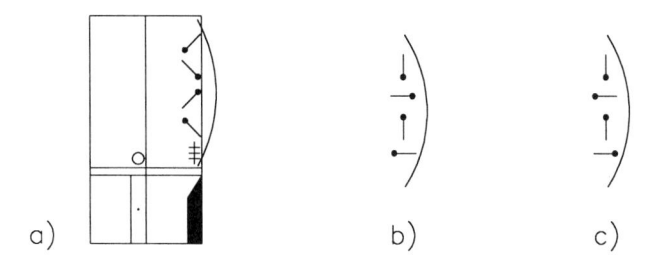

a)   b)   c)

29. Indication of the equal sign for shifting being placed on a pin was first published in *The Kinetographer* No. 10, June 1976. (19.1)

30. In K79: 148b, 330 this head shift is written with the head upright and middle level pins showing the direction of the displacement (the shift). (19.2)

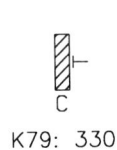

K79: 330

31. This phrasing bow should not be confused with a 'passing event' bow (formerly called the 'passing state' bow). For the latter one main action (usually a direction symbol) has to occur and the passing modification affects the performance of that one movement. A vertical bow connecting a series of direction symbols is a phrasing bow. Without a main movement, a series of pins within a phrasing bow indicate minor displacements, the bow indicates the continuity as well as the overall timing. (21.1)

32. Note that the toward sign indicates **motion,** the destination should be approached but not reached. Because the movement is small, in practice there will not be much difference between a pin followed by a duration line or one placed in a toward sign.

It is important to note the following: In KIN the toward sign (called the 'increase' sign in KIN) combined with a pin, as in a) here, was originally used to indicate timing for a minor movement; it was a destinational statement. AK agreed to adopt the increase sign for motion for space measurement signs, but in K79: 151c it is clear that he retains the destinational meaning of a). KIN uses a duration line to show the timing, followed by the pin, the two being linked by a resultant bow, as in **21h**, here repeated as b). Note that a place high (above), middle (in center) or low pin (below) can be drawn horizontally or vertically. When used in a toward sign, it may be more space efficient to draw this pin vertically as shown in a). (21.2)

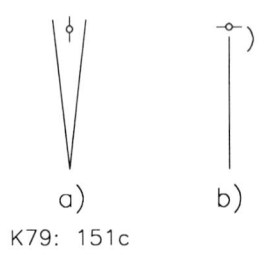

33. For Time Signs see ICKL 1991 Technical Report I:1. (21.3)

34. Used predominantly by KIN. (21.6)

35. Intermediate pins for minor movements are shown by combining two pins, the same device used to indicate intermediate degrees of rotation and intermediate Front signs. Ex. a) states 1/16th of a turn (rotation) to the right. The Front sign of b) indicates facing between the right forward diagonal and the right side of the room. Ex. c) is a minor movement between forward low and right diagonal low. In d) the reverse direction is given, a minor movement between backward high and left backward high diagonal. (23.1)

36. The forerunners of Polar Pins were Monopins, presented by AHG at the 1979 ICKL Conference. The idea of Monopins was that they had no indication of level but operated as though on the surface of a sphere (as Polar Pins). This concept was derived from the Eshkol-Wachmann notation system. Monopins came in three shapes to relate to the different systems of reference: the pins of a) were based on the diamond (representing space) and used the Standard System of Reference, b). The pins with a round base, c), were based on the Body Key, d). The pins of e) were used for the Constant Key, f). The need for Monopins was first recognized by Jane Marriett who collaborated with AHG in presenting a single set at the 1985 ICKL Conference with the name changed to Polar Pins, thus relating them directly to the spherical 'world' with its longitude meridians and latitudes. These Polar Pins were approved by ICKL in 1985 for a two-year trial (see Technical Report II:6 and Appendix C). (23.2)

37. Initially people commented that the rising and sinking pins, which point forward and backward on the horizontal sheet of paper, conflict with the established meaning of pins and other indications pointing into these directions. This valid point was given serious consideration. However, the pins presented here were found to be the easiest and most logical set to deal with. In order to relate to the indications of rising and sinking, the reader must mentally hold the paper vertically. (23.6)

38. This difference - description in terms of motion for supports in contrast to a destinational description for gestures - exists also in most other movement notation systems. (Section 24)

39. First presented at the 1975 ICKL conference (Technical Report, pp.12-13, Paper A). (24.4)

40. In general practice the dot is often not indicated, middle level being assumed. However, to be precise it should be included as omission may indicate 'any level'. (24.6)

41. K79 refers to the V and inverted V signs as increase and decrease signs. For the movement indications dealt with here, the meaning is the same as the LN

toward and away signs. The signs originally came from music where, placed horizontally, they indicate *crescendo* and *diminuendo*. (25.1)

42. This small sign, derived from the three-line staff representing the body, was contributed by Laban in 1947. (25.7)

43. For KIN practitioners the meaning of **25am**, repeated as a) below, is a quick movement to one degree of contraction followed by 'any action'. This is because the two indications are not linked by a small vertical bow, as in b). Such a bow could easily be added in LN but is not considered needed as it is also not needed in c), where the contraction and the direction symbol are seen as a unit. In both KIN and LN c) is interpreted as one movement and not as a quick one degree contraction followed by a movement to side middle. When there is no spatial change, the duration line (which is not interpreted as 'any action' in LN) is used instead of repeating the direction symbol, its length giving the timing, the duration of the contracting action (hence the name 'duration line'). (25.11)

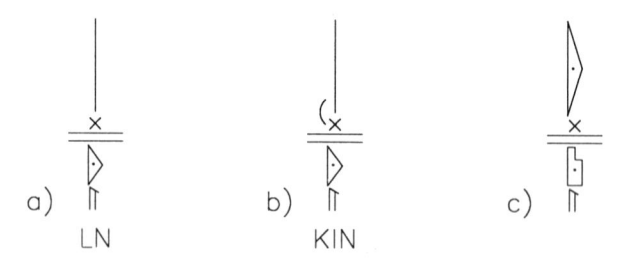

44. The destinational statement of **25ap** is the usual way of indicating movement to a one degree contraction in KIN; this form of the statement is available in LN, when the added emphasis on the destination is desired. There is an interesting 'before and after' view for such indications. By placing the flexion or extension (space measurement) sign at the start, one tells the reader at once what kind of action is to be done, the duration line gives the timing. By placing the indication at the end, one is stating the moment of arrival, the destination, the duration line indicating when this action should start. (25.11)

45. K79: 671 states: "Space measurement signs placed in an increase sign indicate the action of contracting, bending, or stretching, without specifying to what degree this action should be performed and without stating the result of the action." This was the accepted interpretation in Labanotation until further refining of meaning in 2001. In K79: 672, repeated here, AK states: "the first two changes of space measurement are written in the usual way with space measurement signs below the direction sign they modify..... Beside the example

the same changes of space measurement are represented as 'motions'. One can see from this that the first movement is an increase of contraction, whereas the second is a decrease, that is, a motion of extending."

It should be noted that the single 'X' in the increase sign is not given any value, AK does not consider that it is a one degree increment, as is the meaning given to it by some present-day Kinetographers.

In K79, however, there is a use of the increase sign to indicate duration of a destinational statement. This occurs in K79: 675a given here; in 675b he shows the result in a detailed destinational description.

If the meaning of **25ar** should be to contract **one increment** on the 6/6 scale, then statement of this usage must be indicated at the start of the score or on the particular page where it occurs. Alternately, for this purpose, the notator may devise a special indication, different from **25ar** or any other established indication. (25.12)

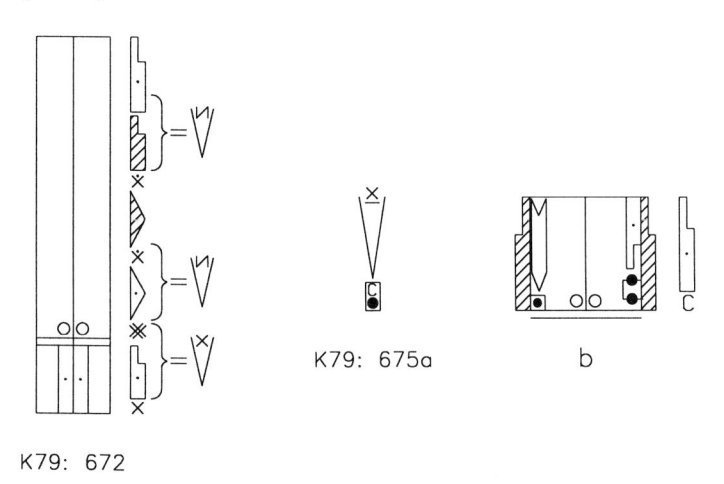

K79: 672   K79: 675a   b

46. Note the difference between the central, vertical placement of the ad lib. sign within the X, a) and the indication of b) which states more or less one degree of contraction. For this the ad lib. sign can equally be placed at the side of the X, as in c). (25.15)

a)   b)   c)

47. This usage was established as a result of discussion between Ilene Fox, Lucy Venable, Sheila Marion, Janos Fügedi and Ann Hutchinson Guest, July, 2001. (25.15)

48. The idea of describing gestures in terms of paths was first brought up by

256   *Spatial Variations*

Sigurd Leeder during discussions with AHG, 1956-57. LNTR No. 8, 1961, presented the use of circular paths for limbs. The topic was then brought up at the ICKL 1985 Conference (Technical Report IV:18), where it was discussed and deferred. Since then, though not officially accepted, the paths for gestures have been found useful in Motif Notation as well as in Labanotation. (Part VII)

49. A long rope used by cowboys to control cattle. (VII Path Signs for Gestures)

50. This usage was described in LNTR No. 57, 1989. (29.2)

51. Such paths are also discussed for the body-as-a-whole in the <u>Advanced Labanotation</u> issue *Floorwork, Basic Acrobatics.* (30.1)

52. The signs of a) and b) have been suggested by AHG for circling around the left forward - right backward diagonal, a) indicating forward direction and b) backward direction of circling. The forward circling of a) has been written out in c). Circling over the right forward - left backward diagonal could be shown by the sign of d). The backward version of this movement could be indicated using e). (30.2)

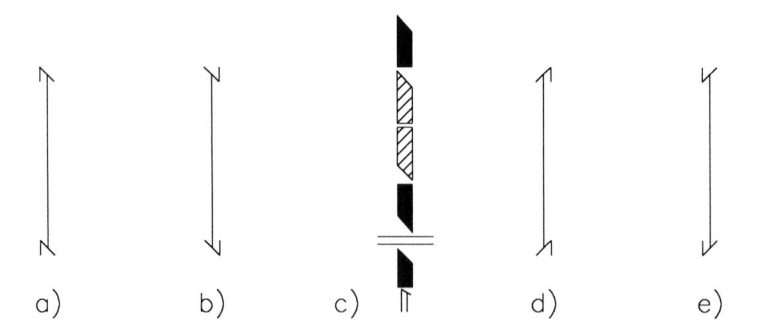

53. This indication of the diametral point was devised by AHG in response to Rob van Haarst's concern in 1990 that the previously suggested indication, which involved a direction symbol, would have been too easily confused with other usages. (31.2)

54. **Indication of Coordinates for Vertical Circles.** In the Eshkol-Wachmann movement notation system a vertical path is indicated by the coordinate in which it lies. While that system uses numbers for the coordinates, we could adopt this

idea, making use of our existing direction signs.

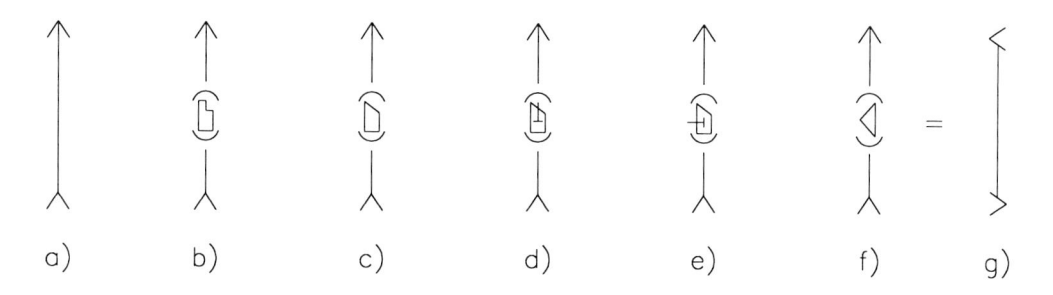

a)   b)   c)   d)   e)   f)   g)

Ex. a) indicates a forward sagittal circle moving along the standard forward coordinate; this is specifically indicated in b). A left front diagonal coordinate is stated in c), with d) and e) showing the intermediate coordinates. The sideward coordinate of f) is, of course the equivalent of g). By showing the appropriate coordinate, Eshkol reduced all such paths to two basic forms - those that are in a positive direction (rising) and those which are negative (descending).
    This idea has not been further explored for LN; with the various means already at hand in our system, it may not be needed. (31.3)

55. A reminder of the difference between a spiral and a helix: a spiral changes in width, a helix has constant width. So, a 'spiral' staircase is, in fact, a helix because the staircase does not become narrower or wider. (32.8)

56. See Advanced Labanotation, *Shape, Design, Trace Patterns*, H91. (33.1)

57. *Shawn's Fundamentals of Dance*, published 1988 by Gordon & Breach, No. 2 in the Language of Dance Series. (34.4)

58. This example is from *Jagdtanz*, a hunter dance from the Chia-rung people from Szetchuan, China, notated by Liu Feng Shueh and Albrecht Knust, 1971. Copyright Liu Feng Shueh, 1972. (34.5)

59. See Advanced Labanotation issue *Hands, Fingers*. (35.1)

60. See Advanced Labanotation issue *Handling Objects, Props*. (35.1)

61. For Time Signs see ICKL 1991 Technical Report I:1. (36.8)

62. The sign for 'a step', 'stepping' is used in Motif Description. It was first published in H83. The derivation is given below: a) indicates an action resulting in a new support; b) shows a step of some kind; c) states a step on either foot; d)

is a step on the left foot; e) a step on the right foot. (37.4)

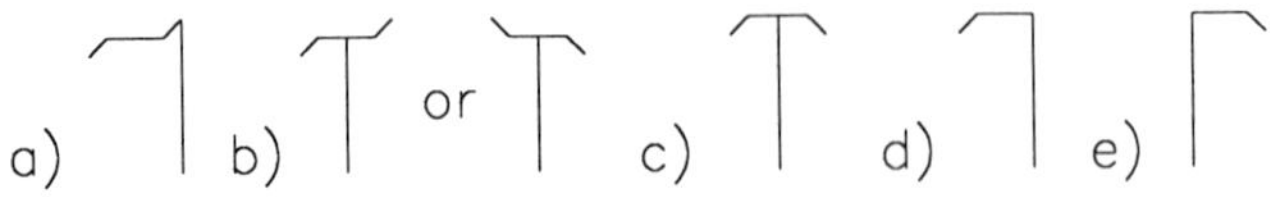
a)
b)
or
c)
d)
e)

63. Specific analysis of length of step was undertaken by AK and AHG in 1957 in Essen-Werden. (37.6)

64. The 8.8 scale for limb contractions or length of steps is as follows:

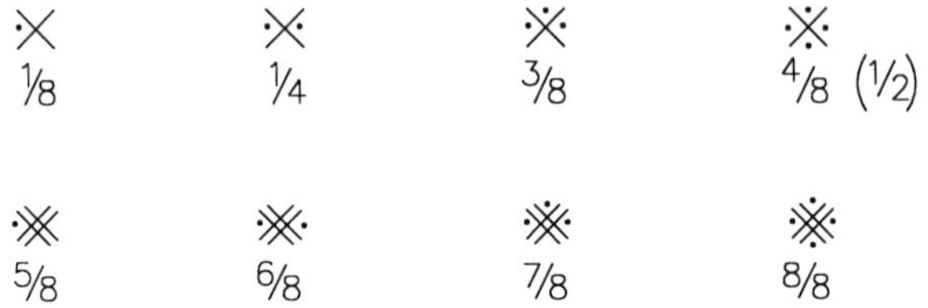
1/8
1/4
3/8
4/8 (1/2)
5/8
6/8
7/8
8/8

The placement of the dots in this scale is distinct from those used in the 6/6 scale, thus the scale being used is immediately identifiable. (37.6)

65. K79 mentions two different specific scales for the extension signs in front of step symbols. To indicate how to interpret the signs, a statement needs to be added. Ex. a) indicates an increase of 1/3 step length with each degree, this is illustrated in c), (K79: 650). Ex. b) shows the key for an increase of 1/6 step length with each degree, illustrated in d) (K79: 651). (37.7)

a)
= 1 1/3
b)
= 1 1/6

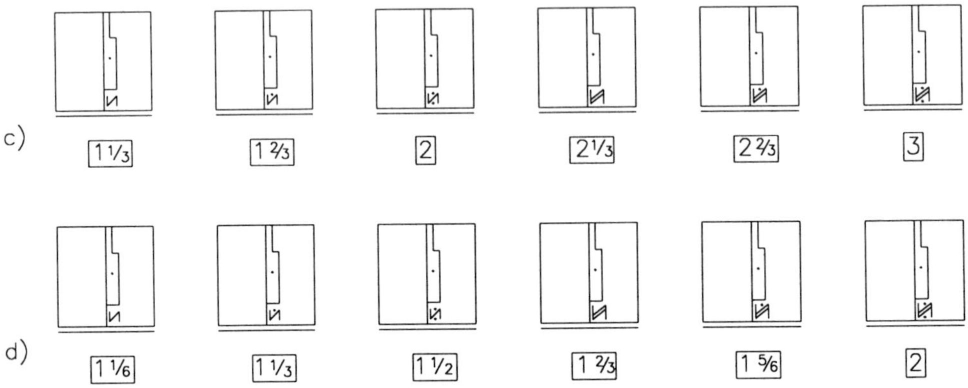
c)
1 1/3
1 2/3
2
2 1/3
2 2/3
3
d)
1 1/6
1 1/3
1 1/2
1 2/3
1 5/6
2

Advanced Labanotation 259

66. This distance sign was established by AK (K79: 653c). (38.1)

67. First published by Valerie Preston-Dunlop in *Practical Kinetography*, 1969, Ex. 376. (38.4)

68. Because Laban's concepts of movement were so space oriented, he did not differentiate between distance of a step, a new support, and the distance of the extremity of a limb from the body center, i.e. the physical state of a gesture. The concept of the physical movements of flexion and extension were not given separate consideration. The signs used were called 'space measurement' signs, space being the mode of measurement. In examining actual present-day use in the system, it has been found that these 'distance' signs are applied predominently to flexion and extension of gestures. While placement of these signs before a step quite clearly describes distance, when used to modify a gesture, as in **39k-n**, the switch in meaning can be confusing. For this reason the diamond indicating spatial aspects is added to state clearly that distance is being described. This usage is illustrated in the next few examples. (39.4)

69. In H70: 245a-d distance from center line was described with the narrow and wide signs. The change was made when it was realized that the same method was being applied to two unrelated needs - distance of leg gestures from the floor and distance of leg gestures from the center line of the body, the latter being the action of separating (abducting) and closing (adducting). Such indications have no relation to distance from the floor, although both could occur within one movement.

The signs for abduction and adduction were introduced by AHG at ICKL 1961 (Technical Report, pp. 7-8) and adopted by AK at ICKL 1967 (Technical Report, p. 10). Use of lateral spreading and closing symbols for distance of leg gestures from the center line was first recommended for trial at ICKL 1971 (Technical Report, p. 11, Paper D). It was included in K79: 981i, j (Appendix II: other usages). Presented in LNTR No. 43, February 1986, it was discussed again at the 1997 ICKL conference (Technical Report II:3, paper by AHG). Ex. a) showed the legs to be closer to the center line, whereas in ex. b) they should be more separated.

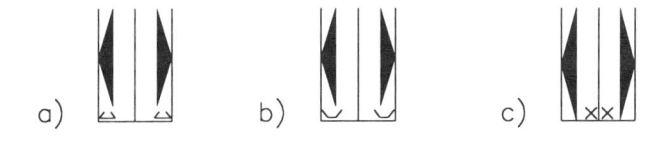

This placement of the signs was incorrect, as these modifying signs did not relate to the state of the leg (the leg is not to change its shape, whereas in c) the X does change the state of the legs). Hence the decision to place the lateral expanding and contracting signs across the center line. (39.9)

70. This sign was devised for Motif Description by Charlotte Wile, 1998. (40.3)

71. This is the same sign as for center of weight, the focal point in the body. Context will always make clear which meaning is intended. (41.1)

72. Usage of the meeting line with the focal point for orientation is an idea that has been considered since 1967 and was put on two year trial at the ICKL conference of 1973. Since then it has been used by notators. It was officially accepted in ICKL 1989 (Technical Report I:8). Ex. a) shows AK established the use of the composite turn sign to show orientation for a starting position, a) states facing the focal point; in b) the performer starts with the focal point at his/her right. In c) the ending aim for the pivot turn is designated with the focal point and the resulting orientation is stated outside the staff to the left by using a small version of the same turn sign.

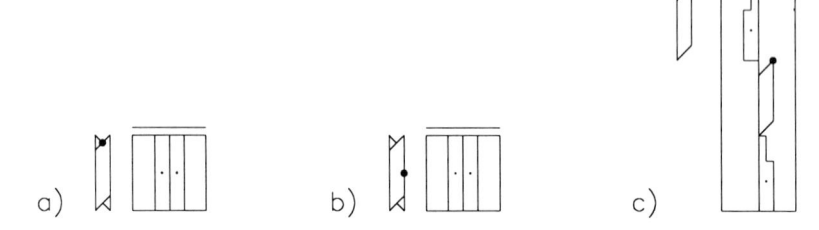

Originally LN used these AK indications, until people questioned why a movement indication was being used for an orientation statement, orientation being a *result*, not a *movement*. This persuaded people to drop the use of the turn sign as an orientation sign and, instead, to use the meeting line. The turn sign with focal point is still used within the staff (see 41.2). (41.1)

73. This example is drawn from K79: 290d. Note indication within a circle of the number of people involved. (41.2)

74. In certain dance choreography, instructions are given in terms of "end facing stage right" or "end facing upstage". In such instances the destination is clear but the degree of turn can only be known from the previous front. Because a different energy and preparation is needed in relation to the degree of turn, the performer may want to know whether a significant amount of turn is to take

place or just a minor change of Front. Therefore, it is good writing practice to state both the degree of turn and the new Front. This usually takes the form of a), the new front being placed near the end of the turn sign. (41.3)

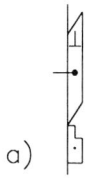

75. Because it is, in fact, the surface of a body part which faces into a certain direction, it is assumed in **4lo** and **41p** that the front of the chest or head 'faces'. These descriptions are seen as shorthand devices. Alternative descriptions which do not raise this question use the addressing sign, as in a) or b). In c) the turning action for the head is given as well as the destination for the face, which is shown to be addressing the focal point at the end. (Dance Notation Bureau discussions, Jane Marriett, January 1984) (41.4)

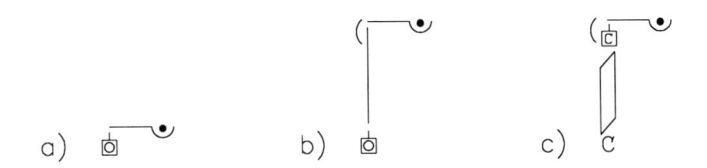

76. This system of reference key was proposed by AHG in LNTR No. 30, February 1980. (41.5)

77. Originated by AHG, this sign was first published in The Labanotator No. 30, 1980. (41.6)

78. First published in The Labanotator No. 30, 1980. (41.8)

79. Such addition of the focal point sign to direction symbols is an exceptional use in the system in indicating the key to be used. It has the advantage of being eye-catching and thus directly stating the key. Use of this device should be stated in a glossary. (41.8)

80. The term 'Line of Direction' was also used in H70. K79 and S76 also mention the 'General Direction of Progression' (GDP). (42.1)

81. These indications, Ex. a), were AK's old way of writing Front Signs to show orientation according to the Constant Cross. At ICKL 1965 (Technical Report, p.

Spatial Variations

3) he changed to the present Front signs, Ex. b), and his old way became available to indicate orientation in relation to the Line of Dance (GDP). (42.3)

a) ⌐, ⌐, ⊞ etc.   b) ⊞ ⊠ ⊞ etc.

82. This and the next example are taken from Maria Szentpál's unpublished book on the Alex Moore English Style of Ballroom Dancing. In this she has described the individual steps, the spatial adjustments and the performer's relationships in great detail. (42.5)

83. K79: 860. (43.6)

84. In 1983 Carl Wolz submitted to ICKL a proposal for a Revised and Expanded System of Symbols for On and Off-stage Areas (Technical Report II:13 and Appendix C). These were based on his experiences in observing and recording Asian dance forms in which use is made of 'offstage' areas as well as circular and other performing areas. His proposal was approved for a two year trial. It was not officially adopted because there was no immediate need. His ideas will, however, be of value in the future when notators are encountering such performing areas and need indications other than the standard ones. (44.1)

85. This example is from K79: 869b. (44.7)

86. Stage area signs developed by Knust, see K79: 863e-h. (44.11)

87. Example taken from VPD69: 380. (44.16)

88. The basic sign for an area, given in **44a**, Ex. a) here, can be given the general statement of being particularly related to space by placing the diamond outside, as in b). For a more defined usage, placement of the diamond inside the box, c), designates an established area. For the parts of the room or stage, the signs of d) represent the specific parts.

a) ☐   b) ◇   c) ⊠   d) ◆, ◪, etc.

For the general sign of a body area, a circle is placed outside, ex. e). Placed within the box, the circle indicates a particular body area, f), this being

Advanced Labanotation 263

the familiar sign for the chest. Other body area signs, the pelvis, g). the head, h), are indicated in a similar way. The area of any joint can be specified by placing the joint sign within a box, i) indicates the area around the right elbow. (44.19)

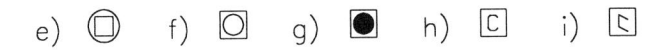

e)   f)   g)   h)   i)

89. Example taken from PD69: 378. (44.20)

90. These examples of areas above or below stage level are taken from K79: 871a-d. (44.21)

91. From K79: 872a-c. (44.22)

92. PD69: 376. (44.23)

93. These indications devised by AHG, date uncertain, not presented in LNTR. (45.5)

94. The original sign for the body-as-a-whole was derived from the three-line staff. In 2001 the new sign, based on a modification of the whole torso sign, surrounded by a circle, was adopted by Motif notation practitioners. (45.8)

95. Derived from Keith Lester's floor plan indications for his Dance Education Syllabus for the Royal Academy of Dancing, 1974. (45.13)

96. Example taken from K79: 890b. (46.3)

97. From the ending of *Night Shadow* by George Balanchine (1946), in which the sleepwalker, holding the candle, gradually mounts the stairs within the building. *Elegie*, measures 25-35. Notated by AHG, 1959, at which time the idea and signs for Fixed Points had not yet been devised. (46.4)

98. This decision was made by AK in the 30s and later, in the 40s, adopted into LN there having been no thought at that time of the future need for open statements. (47.3)

99. The staple was the idea of Sigurd Leeder, circa 1950s. It was used to mark which foot did not move, a) below, the foot being 'stapled' to the floor. First published in LNTR No. 1, 1957. For a time the staple was used specifically with Position Writing (the statement of the position to be reached) as in a), and the

caret was used for Motion Description, as in b), the direction of the weight shift being stated, hence the movement description. In c) the same movement is written as an ending position, hence use of the staple. Many people found it confusing to know when to use a staple and when a caret. Because it is *the direction symbols used* that indicate the difference between a position description or a motion description, it was realized that the caret could equally well serve both. Thus use of the staple was dropped from this application. Use of the caret as replacement for the staple was accepted at ICKL 1987 (Technical Report I:1). (47.4)

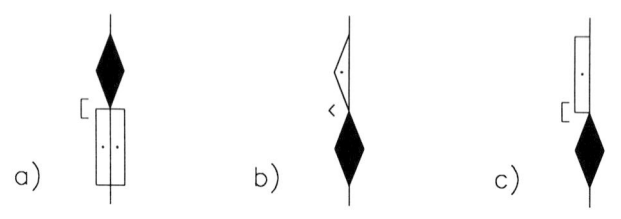

100. A closed position is when the feet are together, in classical ballet these are the positions 1st, 3rd, and 5th. An open position is when the feet are apart in a lateral, sagittal or diagonal placement; in ballet they are 2nd position, 4th position and the open or crossed 4th positions, the diagonal placements. (47.5)

101. For people who have difficulty in interpreting this notation, the advice is to perform the actions for each leg separately, as though the other did not exist, and then to blend them together. (47.5)

102. Examples such as the ones below are understood in KIN to include a springing action although no gap or other weight lifting indication is given. Both a) and b) are understood to be *échappé* actions. However, if the change is from an open position to a support on one foot in place, as in c), Knust maintained the performance was not the same as b), because the ending is on one foot instead of two. AK established the rule that c) should be a step in place next to the other foot. (47.5)

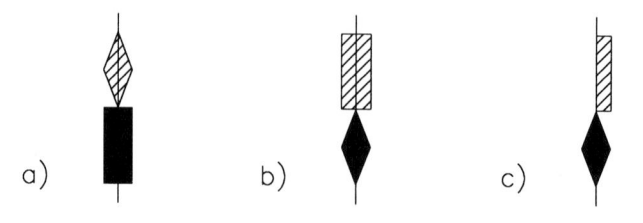

103. These examples were all originally written with staples. H70, p. 68. (47.11)

104. The Step-Gesture Rule is as follows: a transference of weight onto one foot and a leg gesture for the other cannot occur at the same time. Enough weight has to be transferred to the stepping leg for the other leg to be free of weight in order to start the performance of the gesture. (47.13)

105. In British English the letter Z is called 'zed', hence the name given to this Z-shaped double caret. The zed caret is used to connect a gesture to a support, or a support to a gesture. An elongated zed caret is also used to connect one support to another support, particularly after a spring. The zed caret was officially accepted at ICKL 1989 (Technical Report I:4). (47.14)

106. First published in LNTR No. 32, 1980. (47.18)

107. It was Sigurd Leeder's use of the staple for landing from springs which negated the original meaning given to it, that of 'don't lift the foot'. (47.20)

108. Maria Szentpál, who specialized in notating Hungarian dances where many subtle foot contacts near to the other foot occur, relied on accurate statements and performance. For her each such foot contact automatically anticipated the next lowering. Needing a more direct message to the reader, the device of the Forward Reference Caret was presented by AHG and discussed with Szentpál in 1977. With no immediate need among Labanotators for such accuracy in writing this type of movement, the Forward Reference Caret has not yet been officially presented. (47.27)

109. An arrow connected to a zed caret, evolved by AHG, 2000, has the meaning of 'leading into', the one movement having the specific purpose of leading into the next. The gesture has no importance in its own right. An ordinary zed caret does not give such a specific meaning. See Ex. **48d** (letter b) and **48j** (letter F) for other instances of such usage. The idea of this usage was first put forward at the 1989 ICKL conference. Report No. 17, example 17a. (47.29)

110. From *Lark Ascending* by Alvin Ailey (1972) to music by Vaughan Williams. Notated by Sandra Aberkalns, 1993 (Opening p. 9; measures 57-60 and 154-165). (48.1)

111. The sign for 'step on either foot' comes from the Motif sign of a) indicating stepping, combined with b), the sign for 'either', to produce c) which indicates either right or left step. (48.2)

a) ㅜ   b) ㅗ   c) ㅍ

112. For shape indications see H91, <u>Advanced Labanotation</u> on *Shape, Design, Trace Patterns*. (48.7)

113. One aspect in experimenting with directions from the broadest use to the very specific is that of the area around a directional point. The movement may end or take place within such an area. Such usage is found in dance cultures where impusive movements cause the limb to move into the area of a directional point, but with no exact, planned destination. See the book *Your Move*, pages 61, 62, 1995 edition. (48.7)

114. From *Roses* by Paul Taylor (1985), notation by Sandra Aberkalns completed 1999. (48.11)

115. This use of the ad lib. sign across a standing position was contributed by Ray Cook, circa 1985 when, for partnering, the man's exact foot work was not important. (48.11)

116. From *Sorcerer's Sofa* by Paul Taylor (1989), notated by Sandra Aberkalns, 1989-92 (measures 843-846 and 672-677). (48.12)

117. The indications for opening and closing ranks were evolved by Knust (K79: 279a,b). (48.12)

118. As staged by Diana Byer, *Snow Pas* is a *pas de deux* from *The Nutcracker*, choreographed (or a recreation of Ivanov's choreography) by Anton Dolin (circa 1950), notated by Sandra Aberkalns, 1996. (48.15)

119. From *Parade* by Léonide Massine (1917), notated by Jocelyne Asselbourg, 1982 (The American Girl, measures 422-423). (48.19)

120. Starting with measure 17. See previous note. (48.20)

121. From *Rooms* by Anna Sokolow (1955), notated by Ray Cook, 1967, finalized in 1975. The use of words here is important because the individuals' movements may be close to what is written in the notation, but need not be exact. Because of this freedom, some of the actions which could have been spelled out in the symbols, are given in words, thus allowing more leeway. (48.22)

122. For Dynamics see Labanotator No. 40, 1985. (48.22)

123. For Time Signs see 1991 ICKL Technical Report I:1. (48.23)

124. From Matteo, 1990, notated by Jane Marriett. (48.25)

125. From S76, Part 2, Lesson XVIII: 35, 41. (48.29)

126. An excerpt from *Water Study* by Doris Humphrey (1928), notated by Odette Blum, 1966, revised 1978 (measure 26). (48.31)

127. *Schrifttanz* by Rudolf von Laban (1928, 1930). At the Jooss-Leeder Dance School, 1936-39, no mathematical analysis was introduced with LN, but the model was, and always has been, the same as that which is clearly presented in the diagrams of *Movement Notation* (Eshkol/Wachman 1958). The E/W system uses numbers to represent the points on the spherical model; in Labanotation visually based symbols are used, however, the directional analysis is the same. (A.2)

128. *Choreutics* by Rudolf Laban (1966). (A.2)

129. At that time Laban did not have an accurate understanding of the facts concerning the body's center of gravity. In his early books it was equated with the pelvis, rather than being a point of balance which could, in fact, be momentarily outside the body. (A.2)

130. *Movement Notation* by Noa Eshkol and Abraham Wachmann (1958). (A.2)

131. This illustration, entitled "The Main and Private Systems of Reference" is from *Movement Notation* (see note 130). (A.2)

132. Example taken from Laban's 1926 book *Choreographie*. (A.4)

133. This use of the cube model is described in writings by Valerie Preston-Dunlop (PD69, p. 30, **64**) and Sally Archbutt (MPhil thesis, Major Dance Notation Systems: Implications for Art, Education and Research). (A.5)

134. Prior to the 1989 ICKL conference, Janos Fügedi and Maria Szentpál sent out a questionnaire for their paper *The Direction System in Labanotation*. In it they asked what the angle between the diagonal high and low directions and the horizontal plane should be. Most people agreed it should be 45°. However, it appeared that many participants did not realise the difference in determining directions between use of a cuboid model or a spherical model. At the 1993 ICKL conference the spherical model for LN was officially recognized. (A.5)

135. Fügedi states: "According to the derivation principle of intermediate directions, an intermediate direction is defined as deviating from one main direction to another while the distance (Knust 1979: 16), the way toward a neighboring principal direction (Hutchinson 1977, p. 439) or the angle (Szentpál 1965) is halved or divided into three equal parts."
      A history of the intermediate direction symbology was published in LNTR No. 67, April 1992. (A.9)

136. The idea of the small stroke was originated by Maria Szentpál. (A.11)

137. These charts were presented at the 1993 ICKL conference. (A.14)

138. A device introduced by Albrecht Knust, not now commonly used. (B.3)

139. When a relationship bow is short, it can be more practical to place the relationship pin just above the bow, as in Ex. **Bt**, or it can be placed between the body part and the start of the relationship bow. (B.6)

140. A rarely used sign, but a very characteristic holding of the body in authentic (not stage) folk dances, according to János Fügedi, specialist in Hungarian dances. (B10)

141. This level of support has been used by non-trained folk dancers whose knees are almost never stretched. When really stretched, it is so intentional that it must be specifically indicated. Note from János Fügedi. (B.10)

142. This sign is part of a series of signs developed by AK (see K79: 344). (B.11)

143. A special form of turn sign contributed by Knust, K79: 219c. See detailed explanations in <u>Advanced Labanotation</u> *Kneeling, Sitting, Lying*, H91. (B.12)

144. The front sign of **Bbn** is also used in folk dance notation when the dance has no specific orientation. For example, some couples are dancing, but it cannot be said that the dance is performed toward an audience - they dance just for their own pleasure, as in a club. In such cases it is usual to take the camera (when working from film) as front, or often the music band can be regarded as the focus for determining dance orientation. Note by János Fügedi. (B.14)

145. Because of a difference in identifying what is considered to be the extremity of the arm, the 5th position of the arms is written in K79: 144e with

Advanced Labanotation

diagonal pins, as in a), instead of with the 'in front' pins of b). Originally, AK considered the wrist to be the end of the arm; indeed, when the finger tips are in front of the body, the wrist does have a diagonal relationship to the trunk. Later AK changed the definition of the reference part to 'the bulk of the hand', the lower part of the metacarpus. This change did not affect his use of the diagonal pins for the balletic 5th position. (B.18)

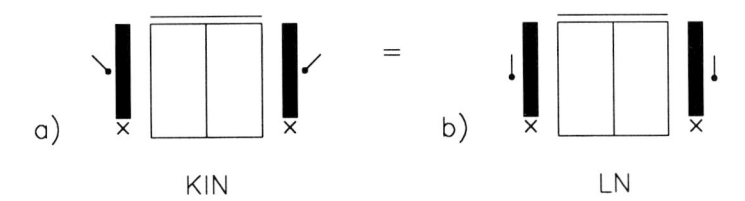

KIN LN

146. Terminology for the basic positions of the arms varies between the established 'schools' of classical ballet (the *danse d'école*). In addition, the precise performance of these positions varies. The black pin provides a general indication for these positions; exact performance is spelled out, when needed, through use of track pins, intermediate directions and the appropriate 8/8 degree of arm flexion. (B.18)

147. At one point in the development of LN, it was considered logical that, for low arm positions black pins should be used; for middle level directions the tack would be more appropriate; and for arms in high level white pins should be used. But trial of such usage only led to confusion. Therefore the convention was adopted that *all standard balletic positions of the arms should be shown with black pins*. However, for the arm extremities directly above the head a) can be used, while b) can indicate the point halfway between the shoulder line and over the head. Track pins are now more generally used. In the 1979 ICKL pin problems paper, *Paper 1, Categories of Pin Usages* by AHG, (Technical Report I:4), example b) here was written as c), also given in K79: 144g. (B.20)

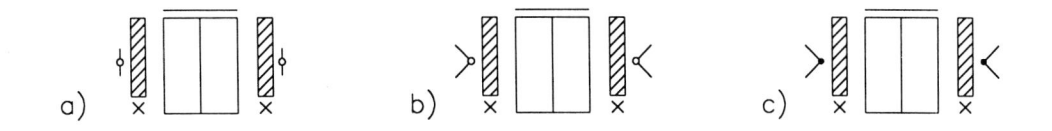

148. Formerly written with black pins, see K79: 144 e, f, g. White 'above' pins are still used, see K79: 144 h. (B.26)

149. Formerly in LN a) could also mean a person. Furthermore, tack pins were used as an alternate set: b) being a woman, c) a man, and d) a person. At ICKL

1989 (item 6, pp. 30-31) the set of **Bdn**, **Bdo** and **Bdp** was adopted. (B.27)

a) b) c) d)

150. The wedge signs of **Bdq-Bds** were officially adopted at ICKL 1989 (item 6, p. 30). However, another wedge sign used for a person, shown as a), was based on the middle level tack of b). Also used was c), based on the pin of d) meaning a person. (B.27)

a) b)
c) d)

151. Full details on indications for surfaces is given in <u>Advanced Labanotation Shape, Design, Trace Patterns</u>, H91. (B.29)

Bibliography

Eshkol, Noa and Wachmann, Abraham. *Movement Notation*, Weidenfeld and Nicholson, London, 1958.

European Seminar for Kinetography (ESK) Discussion Papers, 1985-1989 (unpublished). Available from the Centre for Dance Studies, Les Bois, St. Peter, Jersey, Channel Islands. Great Britain.

Fügedi, János. "The Direction System of Labanotation / Kinetography Laban, A Clarification and Proposal", proceedings of the ICKL 1993 conference, pp. 27-60.

Hutchinson, Ann. Notebooks from Jan. 1936 - July 1938, while at the Jooss-Leeder Dance School.

Hutchinson, Ann. *Labanotation, The System of Analyzing and Recording Movement*, Theatre Arts Books, New York, 1970. (1st published 1954; revised 3rd edition published in 1977)

Hutchinson Guest, Ann. *Your Move, A New Approach to the Study of Movement and Dance*, Gordon and Breach, London, 1983. (3rd reprinting with corrections in 1995)

Hutchinson Guest, Ann and van Haarst, Rob. Advanced Labanotation, Vol. 1, Part 2, *Shape, Design, Trace Patterns*, Harwood Academic Publishers, 1991. Part 3, *Kneeling, Sitting, Lying*, Harwood Academic Publishers, 1991

Hutchinson Guest, Ann. *A History of the Development of the Laban Notation System*, Cervera Press Publication, London, 1995.

Proceedings of the Biennial Conferences of the International Council of Kinetography Laban (ICKL), 1959-1999.

The Kinetographer, bulletin, Language of Dance Centre, London, Nos. 1-11, 1973-1976.

Knust, Albrecht. *Handbuch der Kinetographie Laban*, (Dictionary of Kinetography Laban), unpublished manuscript (8 vol.), written mainly between 1945 and 1950.

Knust, Albrecht. *Handbook of Kinetography Laban*, translated by Valerie Preston, unpublished (1 vol.), 1951.

Knust, Albrecht. *Abriss der Kinetography Laban*, 1956, published by Tanzarchiv, Hamburg.

Knust, Albrecht. *Handbook of Kinetography Laban*, 1958, published by Tanzarchiv, Hamburg.

Knust, Albrecht. *A Dictionary of Kinetography Laban (Labanotation)* (2 vol.), MacDonald and Evans, 1979. Second edition 1997, Poznan, Poland.

Laban, Rudolf. *Choreographie*, Eugen Dietrichs, Jena, 1926

Laban, Rudolf. *Schrifttanz, Methodik, Orthographie, Erläuterungen*, Universal Edition, Wien, Leipzig, 1928.

Laban, Rudolf. *Choreutics*, Macdonald and Evans, London, 1966

The Labanotator, bulletin, issues 1-25 published 1957-65 by the Dance Notation Bureau, New York; issues 26-77 published 1978-1994 by the Language of Dance Centre, London.

Matteo. *The Language of Spanish Dance*, University of Oklahoma Press, 1990.

Preston-Dunlop, Valerie. *Practical Kinetography Laban*, MacDonald and Evans, London, 1969.

Ralov, Kirsten [ed.]. *The Bournonville School. Part 4 Labanotation* (Recorded by Ann Hutchinson Guest), Marcel Dekkler, Inc., New York and Basel, 1979.

Szentpàl, Maria. *Táncjelírás. Laban-kinetográfia* (Dance Notation. Kinetography Laban), Népmüvelési Propaganda Iroda, Budapest, 1969-76 (3 vol., vol. I 2nd. ed., 1st ed. 1964).

Index

1.3, 5.2 etc. refer to paragraph numbers
1e, 6a etc. refer to example numbers
*S*1, *S*2 etc. refer to section numbers
*n*1, *n*2 etc. refer to end note numbers
p.1, p.2 etc. refer to page numbers

- replaces the entry word(s)

In the longer listings, the more relevant references are placed first, separated from the others by a semi-colon (;).

Abbreviation of signs
- cartwheel, 28.5
- spatially central or peripheral, 6.2

Abduction
- lateral spreading, 39.9
- sagittal spreading, 39.11
- sign for, 39.9, *n*69

Accent
- at moment of arrival, 21.6
- on outward movement, 16.10
- strong, very, 48.24

Accented hand displacement, 23.19

Action
- of flexion described, 11.2
- of polishing a mirror, 32.3
- stroke linked with destination, 21.6

Active foot indicated with pin, 47.7

Ad lib. sign
- across standing position, *n*115
- as a front sign, 43.5
- for anywhere in area, 44.23
- for approximately center stage, 44.23
- freedom of distance traveled, 38.1
- modifying front sign, 44.23
- placed at start of circling sign, 12.12

Adduction, sign for, 39.9, *n*69
- lateral closing, 39.10

African dance, actions occuring in, 16.10

Ailey, Alvin, 48.1, *n*110

Aim
- dotted line on floor plan, 15.9
- of arriving at particular destination, 14.5
- of circular path, 15.8
- of path, 12.9, *S*38
  - ,relative location for, 38.3-4
- traveling toward part of the room/stage, 15.9

Aimed destination, 3.6, 4.1-2, *n*6
- ,indication of, *S*4

Amount (see degree)

Analysis
- of circular paths for gestures, *S*27
- of deviations, *S*9
- of peripheral and central displacements, *n*27
- of spoke-like displacements, 23.13-17

Angular performance, 7.2

Any number of people, sign for, 43.3

Approximate distance in path sign, 26.6

Apron of stage, sign for, 44.10

Area/s
- above or below stage level, 44.21
- ,anywhere in, 44.23
- ,approximate, 44.23
- arrival point at end of traveling, 44.3
- ,arrive at stage, 12.9
- closer to center of stage/room, 44.9
- designated focal point, 44.3
- ,detailed signs combined, 44.15
- ,distance from an, 38.4
- free statement, general, 44.23
- further subdivisions using strokes, 44.14-18
- ,intermediate, 44.8-10
- ,miscellaneous - indications, 44.23-25
- ,motion toward stage, 44.3
- not reached, 14.3
- ,off-stage, 44.10, 44.18
- related to space, 44.19
- ,sign/s for, *S*44; 38.4
  - ,application of, 44.3-7
- ,subdivisions of right side, 44.16
- ,toward and away from, 14.3-4
- ,undefined, 44.23

Area (cont.)
- ,unspecified, 44.19-20
  - general sign for, 44.19
- use of narrow, wide signs, 44.9-10

Arena
- front determined for, 43.6
- ,location in circular, 44.25

Arm/s
- approaches body, 25.7
- approximate directions, 48.15
- circles, 18.4
- circular gesture, 48.19
- cross center line, 48.7
- deviates, 48.6, 48.13, 48.16, 48.19, 48.25
- does not arrive at direction, 25.4
- exactly above shoulders, 48.27
- extremity, globe of directions, 16.3
- in area of direction, 48.7
- led by outer side of upper arm, 48.27
- looking under, 48.9
- minor displacements, 16.3-4
- modification of direction, 48.2-3, 48.5, 48.15
- more or less intermediate direction, 48.6
- 'neither flexed nor stretched', 25.11
- pattern related to Standard System of Reference, 36.5
- peripheral path, 3.2
- placement next to center line, 48.1
- rounded position, 48.27
- spatially inward path, 6.5
- 'undercurve' deviation, 48.16
- undeviating path, 48.12

Arrival at designated stage area, 12.9, 44.3, 48.24
- in file, 48.12

Arrow
- at base of polar pin, 23.9
- at base of minor movement pin, 24.7
- double-headed for retracing path, 8.2
- placed in direction symbol, 24.4
- symbol for direction of progression, 24.4

Asymmetrical
- deviations, 10.1-2
- pathway, 10.1

Audience, fixed point in, 46.6
Avoid object, person, 13.2
Awareness of
- contracting, 25.15
- focus of movement, 25.14
- motion away from state, 25.13

Away
- and toward versus destination, S25
- as cancellation, 25.8
- from area, 14.3-4
- from body, 25.7
- from directional point, 25.4-6
- from hot pan, 25.3

Away (cont.)
- from particular stage area, 14.4
- ,hand moves, 25.3
- sign
  - drawn within column, 25.8
  - used as cancellation, 25.8

Axis
- ,double pins indicating, 31.3
- for circles described by pins, 30.1-3
- for tilted circle, 30.3
- outside pelvis, 34.7
- slanted, 31.3

Back to normal sign as cancellation, 24.8
Balanchine, George, n97
Ballet, arm positions, App.B.18-22
Ballroom dancing
- line of dance, 42.1
- Reading Example, 42.4-5

Between
- three cardinal directions, 1.6
- two cardinal directions, 1.2-3

'Bird's eye view
- of elongated circle, 29.7
- of spoke-like movements, 23.4

Black and white circles, 1.7
Body
- as-a-whole, 25.7, 48.23
- Key and minor movements, 16.11
  - for directions, 48.24, n14
  - for vibrating movements, 17.4
- limitations for straight path gestures, 24.12
- 'ripple', 20.2
- section, shifting of, 19.3
- shape, 48.7
- System of Reference, 16.11
- tilt, 48.28
- twist when passing partner, 13.4

Bow
- expressing unity for series of pins, 21.1
- indicates timing of detour, 13.3, 13.5
- indicating duration, 21.1
- indicating temporary departure from normal placement, 21.4
- small linking - for pins, 2.4
- ,tying three directions, 1.6

Bracket
- ,Distal Key placed in, 16.10, 17.3
- placement of step sign in, 12.6
- ,sign for speed placed in, 21.3
- spatial size in, 16.18
- ,spatially small in, 32.8
- ,standard step length in, 37.4
- ,time sign in, 36.8

Breath, intake of, 48.22
Bulge
- at start of gestural path, 10.3
- away from line of travel, 15.8
- out of line, App.B.8

Cancellation
- away sign, 25.8
- general sign, 16.14
- of direction of progression, 24.8
- of Fixed Point Key, 46.3
- of minor displacements, 16.14
- of result of previous motion, 24.8
- of vibrations, 17.6

Cardinal directions
- ,between three, 1.6
- ,between two, 1.2-3

Carets, S47
- foot retains same support, 47.5
- forward reference, 47.24-29
- 'lead into' zed caret, 47.28-29
  - preparatory leg gesture, 47.28
- meaning, 47.1
- motion description, 47.13
- ,same spot, 47.18-20
  - zed, 47.21-23
- ,use of ordinary, 47.1
- ,zed, 47.14-16
  - ,elongated, 47.22

Caribbean dance, actions occuring in, 16.10

Cartwheel paths, 28.5-6
- abbreviated sign, 28.5, 30.2
- ,conical, 28.5
- degree of contraction retained, 32.1
- spiral design, 32.6
- ,surface for, 33.1

Categories of pins, App.B

Ceasé y contraceasé andaluz, 48.25

Center
- line
  - on stage, 45.5-8, 48.18
  - signs placed across, 39.9-10
- of circle as focal point, 41.1
- of gravity, App.A.2
- of weight notation shown in support column, 24.1
- pins used for cancellation, 23.6
- ,return to, 16.14

Central
- displacements, n27
- path/s, S3, 3.3
- to peripheral movement, 6.3

Chair as focal point, 41.1

Change of
- level on third degree pathway 5.2
- front, amount of, 12.11
  - during circle of head, 34.2
  - for torso not included, 34.6

Chart of intermediate directions, App.A.14

Chest-to-waist leans backwards, 48.1

Choreographie, n132

Circle/s (gestures)
- achieved through flexion, extension of the limb, 32.1-2
- ,conical, 27.7
- ,diagonal, 27.5, S30
- drawing a circle on table, 33.2

Circle/s (gestures) (cont.)
- ,freedom in shape, 12.12
- group revolving and traveling, 15.5
- ,horizontal, 27.3, 27.7, 30.3
- ,intermediate range of, 27.5
- ,lateral, 27.4-5, 27.7
- ,modification of shape, 29.2
- of limb, 27.1
- performed with flexed limb, 32.1
- ,planal, 27.2-6
- ,sagittal, 27.4-5, 27.7
- ,size of, S31, 32.2
  - remains constant, 32.8
- ,somersault, 30.2
- specific axis, 30.1-3
- stretched vertically, 29.1
- ,'surface' for, S33
- ,tilted, S30

Circling
- for head and torso, 34.1
- hands, 35.1-4
- head without rotating, 34.3
- movements, minor, S18
- pelvis, 34.7

Circular
- area/arena, established point, 43.9
- displacements, 23.20-21
  - shown with polar pins, 23.20
- movements written with pins, 18.1
- path/s
  - ad lib. sign placed at start, 12.12
  - amount, approximate, 12.11
  - axis used, 30.1-4
  - between cartwheel and somersault, 30.2
  - ,cartwheel, 28.5-6
  - described on surfaces, 33.6
  - deviates, bulges, 15.8
  - ,direction becomes aim of, 15.8
  - ,displacements on, 15.4
  - ,elongated, S29
  - for gestures, S27, S28
  - for hands, knees, S35
  - for head, torso and pelvis, S34,
  - ,horizontal, for gestures, 28.1-3
  - ,lateral, 30.1
  - lying on diagonals, 28.6
  - ,modification to, 12.11-12
  - nature of movement, 3.5
  - sagittal, 30.2
  - shape of, 12.11
  - ,somersault, 28.4
  - traveling into Constant direction, 15.6
- pattern of toe on floor, 18.1

Circus, orientation in, 43.6

Clockwise
- horizontal circular path, 28.1
- movements for polar pins, 22.2-3

Closing laterally, 29.2, 39.9

Cone
- axis, 27.7

Conical
- circles of the limb, 27.1, 27.7
  - angle to axis of circle, 27.1, 27.7
  - definition, 27.7
  - ,size of, 36.2
  - ,spatial placement of, 36.2-3
  - spiral path, 32.5
  - start of, 36.2
- movement horizontal, 28.3
- somersault path, 28.4

Constant
- Cross, 16.13
- Directions Key, 14.2
- Key for
  - group traveling, 14.2, 15.5
  - revolving on straight path, 15.3, 36.6
  - steps and arm movements, 36.6
  - used for circling, 15.10

Contraction
- and extension, destination, 25.11
- motion toward, 25.15
- one increment, n45
- sign with direction of progression, 24.14

Coordinates of vertical circles, n54

Corners
- exaggerate the sharpness, 7.1
- for gestures, sharp or rounded, S7

Counterclockwise movements for polar pins, 22.2-3

Cou de pied position, 48.28

Cross of axes
- for directions for deviations, 9.5
- with distal center, 16.2

Cuboid model, directions based on, App.A.5

Decrease
- in size of step, 37.11
- in speed, 36.9
- of distance, 37.10-13

Defined state
- ,motion toward, away from, 25.12-14

Definition of direction in Labanotation, App.A.2-5

Degree/s
- of circle, 12.11
- of curve (gesture), 6.6
- of deviation, 12.7
- of flexion
  - for circles of limb, 32.1-2
  - is open, 37.12
  - to be achieved, 37.12
- of lateral
  - closing, adduction, 39.9-10
  - spreading, abduction, 39.9
- of sagittal closing, 39.11
- of supporting leg bend, 39.5
- of surface slant, 33.3

Design drawing
- circular patterns on surfaces, 33.6

Design drawing (cont.)
- ,helix written as, 32.8
- laterally elongated circle, 29.1
- retraced, 8.4-5
- spiral paths, 32.6-7
- three-dimensional spiral, 32.9
- to indicate loops, 10.6-8

Destination
- ,action stroke linked with, 21.6
- ,aim of arriving at, 14.5
- ,emphasis on, 21.6
- ,indication of, 26.2
- ,motion versus, S24
- of turn
  - for group, 41.3
  - related to room directions, 41.3, 48.23, 48.31
- ,reaching a, 14.5
- ,toward, away versus, S25

Destinational statement, 25.9-10
- for limb, 24.15, 25.9
- of path of body-as-a-whole, 25.9

Detour to avoid a person or object, S13
- shown on floor plan, 13.6
- path sign, 13.5
- timing, 13.3-6

Deviation/s
- analysis of, S9, 9.5
- asymmetrical deviations, 10.1-2
- at start of movement, 10.1
- bow, curved, 11.2
- 'bulge' from line of path, 15.8
- ,compound symmetrical, 9.10-11
- ,definition of, 9.1-2
- ,degrees of, 12.3, 12.7-8
- ,direction of, 9.6
- duration indicated by bow, 13.5
- for successions, S20
- from horizontal path, 10.12
- from direction of progression path, 24.13
- from path across the floor, Part IV, 12.1-4
- from path of gesture, Part III, 11.4, 16.19
- from standard directions, 10.9-12
- general rule, 11.1
- ,half-way in path, 12.3
- indication, 4.4
- ,jagged, 10.5
- large, 11.3
- leg, 48.28
- local center of directions, 9.11
- loops, 10.6-8
- ,non-centered, 10.3-4
- range in size, 11.1-4, 12.1-5
- ,regressive, 10.5
- ,scales for defining, 11.3-4
- ,single, 9.8-9
- ,size of
  - from path of gesture, S11, 11.2-4
  - unspecified, 12.1-2

Deviation/s (cont.)
- ,sphere of possible, 9.4
- ,three-dimensional, 9.4
- ,two-dimensional, 9.4
- written in path sign, 13.2, 13.5

Diagonal/s
- circles, S30
- ,circular path lying on a, 28.6
- deviation from path, 12.3
- directional pattern, 30.2
- path on stage, 45.9-13
- spatial pattern, 30.2
- spreading, 29.2

Diametral point
- for circular interpretation, 32.3
- ,indication of, 31.2
- ,passing through, 31.1

Direct path, n6

Direction
- based on cuboid model, App.A.5
- from Body Part (DBP), 40.2
- Constant, use of, 14.1
- ,definition of - in Labanotation, App.A.2-5
- in a gesture column, 24.2-3
- in a support column, 24.1
- ,intermediate palm facing, App.A.6-8
- ,modification of a main, 2.2
- of deviation, 9.6
- of path, turn signs related to, 43.4
- of Progression, S24, 24.4-5
  - as cancellation, 24.8
  - ,deviation from, 24.13
  - distance, 24.14
  - level, 24.6-7
  - minor movements, 24.7
  - reference point, 24.4
  - straight, curved, 24.12-13
- of relationship, 16.15-16
- sign
  - arrow placed in, 24.4
  - linked to duration line, 4.2
- symbol/s
  - at end of path sign, 26.2
  - empty, 5.3, 10.11, 8.6
  - ,focal point attached to, 41.8
  - modified by Focal Point Key, 41.7
- system of Labanotation, App.A

Directional point/s
- ,arm movements passing through, 3.2
  - less articulated, 18.4
- ,toward, away from, 25.4-6

Displacement/s
- ,analysis of spoke-like, 23.11-17
- arm, 16.1-4
- ,cancellation of minor, 16.14
- circular, 23.20
- degree from path, 12.7-8
- duration of with vertical bow, 20.2
- for step patterns in place, S14
- from a point, S16; 16.2, 16.19
- from the poles (polar pins), 23.12
- judged from proximal joint, 16.5

Displacement/s (cont.)
- ,momentary, 21.4-5
- paths with turning/circling, S15
- pelvis, 34.7
- pins, 12.1
- ,size of from a point, S22; 16.17-19, 22.1-6
- three-dimensional (from a point), 16.9

Distal
- analysis, 16.3, 16.7, 16.10, 16.17
  - comparison with proximal, 16.8-9
  - disadvantage of, 23.1
- center, 16.2-3
  - at wrist, 16.3
  - description, 18.1
  - for finger, 16.3
  - Key, 16.7, 17.3, n26
  - kinesphere, 16.2
  - located at right elbow, 16.3
  - pins, 16.7
  - pins for rapid arm movements, 48.10
  - System of Reference, 16.2
- displacements, 16.4
  - at right angles to shaft of limb, 16.4
- Key, n26

Distance, Part VIII
- aim of path, S38
- approximate in path sign, 26.6
- between
  - foot and floor, 39.6
  - hands, 40.3
  - heels, steps, 37.3
  - performers, 38.2
- for leg gestures, S39
  - for touching leg gesture, 39.5
  - from center line, 39.9-12
  - in a jump, 39.8
  - off the floor, 39.6-8
- from an area, 38.4
- from an established point, 38.3
- in modification of path (for steps), 12.6-10, 37.8-9
- in step-lengths, 40.4
- for touching leg gestures, 39.1-5
  - level of support, 39.1-2, 39.4
- in terms of
  - foot-lengths, 38.2
  - meters, 38.2
  - units, 38.1-2
- of steps, S37
  - direction and level, 37.1
  - neither long nor short, 37.4
  - rotational state of leg, 37.2
  - standard, 37.3-4
- sign, S40; 40.1
  - combined with box sign, 40.4
  - placed in path sign, 26.6
- traveled left open, 38.1

Dolin, Anton, 48.15, n118

'Door plane', App.A.3

Double
- circle indicating 'each one', 37.8
- ended arrow for retracing a path, 8.2
- pin for intermediate position, App.B.2

Drawing a circle on a horizontal table, 33.2

Duration
- indication of, 21.1-2
- of deviation displacement, 21.4
- of deviation indicated by bow, 13.5
- slow release of weight, 47.4

'Each one', sign for, 37.8
Effort, pressing, 48.21
Elbow facing, 48.1
Elegie, n97
Elongated
- circular paths, S29
- zed caret, 47.22

Emphasis
- on destination, 21.6
- on straight path, 4.6, 24.12

Empty direction sign
- for deviations, 10.11
- for pathways, 5.3
- to show smooth transition, 5.3

Ending state of limb, 24.15
Entrance, (stage), 44.6, 48.3
- ,partial, 44.7
- ,preparations for, 44.12

Enlargement of notation, 21.3
Equal sign for shifts, 19.1
Eshkol, Noa, n127, n130
Exact
- distance of steps, 37.6
- shape of curve not important, 10.11
- size of displacement, 16.17

Exclusion sign, 48.13
Exit (stage), 44.6
Exiting into wings, 45.1, 45.4
Extending, motion toward, 25.15
Extension
- and contraction, destination, 25.11
- and flexion
  - spiral for path, 32.5-7
  - used to create circle, 32.2

Extremity of limb
- displacement of, 19.3
- distal center, 16.2
- follows cartwheel path, 28.5
- ,globe of directions at, 16.3
- head describes circular path, 34.1
- performs horizontal circle, 36.3

Facing each other, 48.30
Feet
- positions, see Positions of feet
- rise without adjusting, 47.11-12
- sliding on floor, 47.7
- slightly apart, 48.19, 48.21

Figure-eight, 29.2

Finger tips
- close to center line, 48.8-10, 48.16
- on center line, 48.10

Fixed
- end of limb
  - ,pins judged from, 2.3
- Point/s
  - cancellation of Key, 46.3
  - direction, 48.31
  - in a defined space, S46
  - in the audience, 46.6
  - judged from center of room, 46.1
  - Key, 46.1, 46.3
  - level, 46.2

Flexion
- action described, 11.2
- and extension
  - for spiral path, 32.5-7
  - used in circular gesture, 32.2
- passing state, 4.3
- degree of - is open, 37.12

Floor
- ,indication of, 44.22
- plan (see also stage area)
  - ,alert reader to, 45.10, n18
  - indication of wings, 45.4
  - ,location of deviation shown, 13.6
  - ,reference to, 12.12
  - use of wedges, 14.5, 15.7

Fluent performance
- use of vertical phrasing bow, 7.1

Focal
- destination for turn, 41.2-4
- point, S41
  - area of room designated, 44.3
  - attached to direction symbol, 41.8
  - center of circle, 41.1
  - ,chair as, 41.1
  - key, 41.6
  - ,moving away from a, 25.2
  - ,moving toward a, 25.2
  - ,orientation in relation to, 41.1
  - placed on turn sign, 41.2
  - ,relationship to, 41.1
  - ,sign for, 41.1
  - System of Reference, 41.5-9

Focus
- for shifting, 24.9
- on a central point, 4.5
- on motion, 25.1

Folding, unfolding, 25.14
Folk dance/s
- passing partner, 13.4

Follow-the-leader dances, 43.1
Foot
- in *cou de pied position*, 48.28
- retains same support, 47.5, 48.30

Forward reference caret, 47.24-29
- affect of leg rotation, 47.24, 47.26

Fourth degree point, performance of, 6.6
Freedom
- in distance traveled, 38.1

Freedom (cont.)
- in duration, 48.23
- in shape of circle, 12.12
- of interpretation
  - for central path, 6.5
  - in motif description, 25.1
- in performance, 48.17

Front
- change of, 12.11
- determined for arena, 43.6
- in relation to path; the periphery, S43
  - Key, 43.2
- orientation, meeting line, 43.6
- oriented to periphery, 43.6-9
- signs, GDP, 42.3

Fügedi, János, App.A.1

Gait, slightly wide, 12.1
Gathering action, 48.8
Geer, Edna, 40.1
General Direction of Progression (GDP), 42.1-5
- front signs, 42.3
- Key, 42.2

Gestural
- circles, timing of, 36.7-9
- path,
  - retracing, 8.1
  - scale of deviations from, 11.3
- statement, 25.6

Gesture/s
- ,indication of circular path for, S28
- saying "no, no", 17.3
- sharpness of corners, 7.1
- smooth the angular transitions, 7.1
- ,steps versus, S24
- toward body, 25.7

Globe of directions around extremity, 16.3
Gorgallata de escuela bolero, 48.28
Gravity and polar pins, 23.2
Group
- becoming smaller, 48.12
- revolving and traveling, 15.5

Half-arrow, 6.3
Halfway point, 1.2
- ,diagram to show, 1.1, 1.3
- ,indication of, S1
- movement to, 22.3
Half-way deviation (path), 12.3
Hand/s
- ,both, 25.3
- circles, 35.1-4
- circling while arm moves, 35.3
- ,circular paths for, S35
- displaced sideward, 19.3
- vibrates, flutters, 17.1-2
Head
- circling without rotating, 34.3
- not included in torso movement, 48.13

Heavy quality, 48.22
Helical paths, 32.8
- written as design drawing, 32.8
Helix, 32.8
- which expands and contracts, 32.9
Horizontal
- axes for - path, 30.3
- circles, 27.3, 27.7
  - starting point, 36.3
  - tilted, 30.3
  - ,understood surface for, 33.1-2
- circular
  - elongated paths, 29.7
  - paths, 28.1-3
  - planal movement, 28.2
- conical movement, 28.3
Hungarian Dance, 48.29-30, *n*28, *n*108

Imaginary lines on stage, 45.5
Inclinations
- of head, very small, 16.6
Increase
- in size sign, 32.9
- in size of steps, 37.11, 37.13
  - for circular path, 37.11
- in speed, 36.8-9
- of distance, 37.10-13
Individual Body Part
- Cross of Axes, 35.1
- Key, 35.2
Infinity sign, 48.24
Intake of breath, 48.22
Intention of performance
- not clear to viewer, 25.5
Intermediate
- areas, 44.8-10
- degrees of slant, 33.3
- directions, 1.1, App.A.9-14
  - arms, 48.25, 48.28
  - chart of directions, App.A.14
  - finer descriptions, *n*3
  - for thighs, 48.21
  - for torso, 48.20
  - for thumb facing, 48.8
  - second deviation pin, App.A.11
- palm facing directions, App.A.6-8
- pins for minor movements, *n*35
- placement of limbs, 18.3
- point
  - ,moving to a, 1.4-5
  - ,shorthand usage, 1.5
- step directions for diagonal path, 45.9
- wings on stage, 45.2
Inward
- path, 4.4
- spoke-like movements, 23.4

Jagdtanz, *n*58
Jazz actions, elbow displacements, 16.10

Key
- ,Body, 16.11

Key (cont.)
- ,Constant Directions, 14.2
- Direction of Path, 43.5
- ,distal center, 16.7, 16.10, 17.3
- ,Fixed Point, 46.1, 46.3
- Focal Point System of Reference, 41.6
- front in relation to direction of path, 43.2
- General Direction of Progression (GDP), 42.2
- Individual Body Part, 35.2
- placed in a bracket, 10.14
- ,Stance, 16.12
- System of Reference Based on the Path, 10.13

Kinesphere
- for distal center, 16.2

Knees
- ,both, 25.3
- ,circular paths for, S35; 35.5
- 'knocking'/trembling, 17.3

Knust, Albrecht, 40.1

Laban, Rudolf von, n127
- SH four-ring 1-7, App.A.4

Lark Ascending, 48.1-10, n110

Lateral
- axis outside pelvis, 34.7
- center line on stage, 45.5-8
- circles, 27.5, 27.7
  - ,where movement starts, 32.4
  - with arm contracted, 32.3
- closing
  - general degree of, 39.9-10
  - with jump, 39.10
- dimension, 27.3-4
- plane, 27.4
- spreading, 29.2-3, 29.6
  - general degree of, 39.9
  - with jump, 39.9
- track, step on backward, 48.30

Laterally elongated circle, 29.1

'Lead into' zed caret, 47.28-29, 48.5, 48.9-10, 48.16, 48.17
- preparatory leg gesture, 47.28

Leeder, Sigurd, n99

Leg gestures
- both rotated to right, 48.30
- degree of kneebend, 39.3
- distance, S39
  - from center line, 39.9-12
  - modifying supporting bend, 39.5
  - off floor, 39.6-8
- lateral closing, 39.10
- lower than normal, 48.26
- touching, 39.1-5

Length of steps, S37 (see also Distance)
- increase or decrease of distance, 37.10-13
- indicated in path sign, 37.8-9

Lester, Keith, n95

Level
- of center of weight cancelled, 25.8
- of fixed point in defined space, 46.2
- of support
  - affecting distance of leg gesture off floor, 39.6
  - with touching leg gestures, 39.1-2, 39.4
- for direction of progression, 24.6
- for minor movements, 16.4

Lilting step, 15.2

Limb/s
- degree of flexion for circle, 32.1
- extremity, ankle, 39.7
- ,performance details for path, S36
- slightly flex or extend, 16.20

Limitations of body when performing a straight path, 24.12

Line/s
- of dance, S42
- of leg to heel, distance from floor, 39.7
- of movement stressed, 26.3
- on stage, S45; 45.5-8
  - diagonal, 45.9-13
  - ,floor plan showing, 45.5
  - lateral, 45.6
  - sign for exact center, 45.7

Location
- and size of circle, S31
- in circular arena, 44.25
- on stage, 44.4

Looking under arm, 48.9

Loops (gestures), 10.6-8

Lower
- arm, planal circles, 27.6
- leg, small circle of, 18.2

'Magnet', area of room acts as, 12.10

Manner of performance
- of spatially central or peripheral paths, 6.4
- of vibration, 17.2

Massine, Léonide, 48.19, n119

Measurement signs
- exact distances, 37.6
- in diamond, 22.1, 22.6

Mediaeval Farandole, 43.1

Meeting line, 41.1, 43.6

Mime gesture
- value of straight path indications, 4.6

Minor
- circling movements, S18
- direction of progression, 24.7
  - cancellation, 24.8
- displacements
  - ,cancellation of, 16.14
  - of whole arm, 16.3
  - successions, 20.2
- modifications of a main direction, S2
- movements, Part V, 16.1, 16.3-4
  - ,Body Key for, 16.11
  - change of level, 24.7

Minor (cont.)
- movements (cont.)
  - described with pins, 16.4
  - described with polar pins, 16.3
  - direction of progression, 24.7
  - ,intermediate pins for, n35
  - without sense of arrival, 25.10
- shifting actions, S19
- tilts, 16.6

Miscellaneous spatial variations, Part X

Modification
- of circular path, 12.11-12
- of directions, Part I
  - with pin, 39.3
- of distance, for gesture, 39.4
- of path, 12.6-10
- of shape of circle, 29.2

Modifying step-length, 37.5
- general scale, 37.5
- specific scale, 37.6-7

Momentary
- displacement, 21.4-5
- regression from main path, 10.5

Monopins, n36

More or less
- center stage, 44.23
- facing audience, 44.23
- facing stage right, 48.23
- second position, 48.11

Motif
- description, 25.1
  - freedom of interpretation, 25.1
  - general location, 44.3
- sign for a step, 12.6, n62, n111

Motion
- away from a defined
  - point, 25.6
  - state of flexion or extension, 25.13-14
- distance not stated, 25.4
- of deviation from path, 12.4
- for gestures, 24.4
- indicated by path sign, 24.10-11
- of approaching, 23.15
- of contracting, 25.15
- toward state of flexion or extension, 25.12
- toward
  - a direction, 48.4-5
  - one degree contraction, 25.12
  - stage area, 44.3
- versus destination, Part VI

Movement/s
- circular by nature, 3.5
- related to Direction of Path, 43.5

Movement Notation, n127, n130

Moving
- away from extended state, 25.14
- to intermediate point, 1.4-5
- to part of the room/stage, 15.9

Narrow sign inside area sign, 44.9
Natural step-length, 37.5

'Neither flexed nor stretched', 25.11
Night Shadow, n97
Nod, 21.4
Non-centered deviations, 10.3-4
Normal
- pace, 37.1
- ,return to, 21.5

'Normal' state, reference point for shifting, 24.9
Numbering walls to indicate specific lines on stage, 45.12
Nutcracker, The, 48.15, n118

Off-stage
- actions, 44.12-13
- area, 44.10, 44.18

'On the spot', 14.1
Orchestra pit, sign for, 44.10, 44.21,
- seating, 46.6

Orientation, Part IX
- in relation to focal point, 41.1

Outward
- movement, emphasis on, 16.10
- spoke-like movements, 23.4

Overlapping successions, 20.3

Palm
- addressing heart, 48.10
- ,displacements of, 23.13-17

'Palms up', App.A.7
Pan, hot, movement away from, 25.3
Pantomimic gestures, 22.1
Parade, 48.19-21, n119
Parallel paths, traveling on, 14.2
Partial entrance on stage, 44.7

Partner
- ,moving away from, 38.3
- ,passing a, 13.4

Passing
- a partner, 13.1, 13.4
- event bow, n31
- flexion, 4.3
- nod of the head, 21.4
- state indicated by vertical bow, 9.7

Passive
- arm accomodation, 23.14
- reaction of hand, 35.4
- reaction of leg, 35.5

Paso de cachucha, 48.27
Paso de tango, 48.26

Path/s (Floor)
- away from focal point, 25.2
- away from an object, 25.2
- combined with circling/turning, S15
- deviating
  - toward another direction, 12.1
  - towards side, 12.4
- diagonal, 45.9-13
- ,front in relation to, S43
- half-way deviation, 12.3
- ,minor deviation in the, 12.2
- modification of, Part IV
  - toward diagonal, 48.2, 48.12

Path/s (cont.)
- ,modifying distance of, 12.6-10
- ,parallel, 14.2
- ,range of deviation from, 12.1-5
- sign/s
  - ,deviation written in, 13.2, 13.5
  - ,step-length placed in, 37.8
- ,third-way deviation on, 12.2
- toward a focal point, 25.2
- toward a stage area, 25.2
- ,veering off normal, S12

Path/s (Gestures), Part VII; 4.6
- ,asymmetrical, 10.1
- bulge at start of path, 10.3
- circle has spatial retention, 36.4
- ,helical, 32.8
- indication of distance, 26.6
- involving unemphasized flexion and extension of the limb, 33.1
- inward, 4.4
- of limb, performance details for, S36
- ,retrace, S8
- sign/s, S24
  - ,distance placed in, 26.6,
  - ,motion indicated by, 24.10-11
- spiral, 32.5-7
- standard analysis, Part III
- to be retraced, 8.3
- to third degree point, 4.2

Pelvis
- circling, 34.7
- shift, 34.7
- to-head tilt backwards, 48.27

Performance
- details for paths of limbs, S36
- larger than pins indicate, 22.2
- left open, 25.13
- of leap, leg gestures, 39.12
- smaller than direction symbols indicate, 22.2

Performers, distance between, 38.2

Peripheral
- arc, 6.6
- circle, 3.2
- curve stressed, 4.7
- displacements, 16.20, n27
- orientation statement, 43.8
- path/s, S3, 3.2, 4.7
  - ,indication of, S4
  - of arm, 24.3
  - stress peripheral curve, 4.7
- to central movement, 6.3

Periphery
- ,around, 44.11
- of area, front sign for, 43.6
- ,outside, 44.11

Phrasing bow for timing, 21.1, n10

Pin/s
- ,active foot indicated with, 47.7
- arm positions, App.B.5, App.B.18-21
- axis of
  - circle, 30.1
  - rotation, App.B.13

Pin/s (cont.)
- ,black, 1.7, App.B.2-5, App.B.12, App.B.18-21
- ,categories of, App.B
- centre - for cancellation, 23.6
- circular movements, 18.1, 18.3
- degree for turn, circling, App.B.12
- deviations, 9.6
  - from path, App.B.9
- direction of
  - relationship, 16.15
  - successions, 20.2
  - vibrations, 17.1
- ,directional definition of, 1.7
- displacement, 12.1
- ,distal center, 16.7, App.B.7-8
- ,double, 31.3
- ,duration line following, 21.1
- fast movement, 21.3
- fixed points in room, App.B.31
- for minor
  - direction of progession, 24.7
  - displacements, App.B.7
  - movements, App.B.8
- General Direction of Progression (GDP), 42.3
- identifying performers, App.B.27-28
- intermediate direction/s, App.A.11, App.B.10
- judged from fixed end of limb, 2.3
- ,level of fixed point in defined space, 46.2
- modifying
  - direction, App.A.10-12
  - parts of room, App.B.30
- not placed in deviation bow, 20.4
- orientation, front signs, App.B.14
- ,polar, S23, App.B33
  - for minor movements, 16.3, 24.7
  - combined forms, 23.8
- proximal analysis, App.B.8
- ,relationship, App.B.2-5
  - indications, App.B.6
  - leg gestures to body, App.B.4
- shifting action, App.B.8
- specific parts of the body, App.B.11
- surfaces for design drawing, App.B.29
- tacks, 1.7
- ,ticks placed on, 16.10
- track pins
  - for arms, App.B.22-26
  - for legs, App.B.15-17
- type of analysis used, 18.2
- used to show loops, 10.6-8
- ,white, 1.7, App.B.12
- with dynamic signs, App.B.32

Placement of
- performers on stage area, 44.11
- sign for distance, 40.3

Planal circles of limb, 28.2, 31.1
- at extremity, 27.7
- cartwheel, 28.5

Planal circles of limb (cont.)
- intermediate, range of, 27.5
- spiral path, 32.5
- three forms, 27.3-5

Point of reference for shifts, 19.2
- establishing in circular area, 43.9

Polar pins, S23
- cancellation, 23.6
- circular displacements, 23.20-21
- clockwise, counterclockwise, 23.6
- ,combined forms, 23.8
- description of sideward shift, 23.14
- displacement from the poles, 23.12
- ,idea of, 23.2-5
- intermediate direction placements, 18.3
- minor movements, 16.3
- motion from where you are, 23.20
- relationship of arrow to base, 23.9
- rising and sinking, 23.6
  - combined with horizontal circular movements, 23.6, 23.8-11
- ,signs for, 23.6-11

Position
- relaxed, 48.22
- signs, App.B.2

Positions of feet
- destination description, 47.13
- motion description, 47.13
- transition from
  - closed to open on two feet, 47.5
  - open to closed on two feet, 47.6-8
  - open to one foot, 47.9-10
  - two feet to one, 47.3
  - weight changes in place, 47.2

Preparations for entrances, 44.12
Preston-Dunlop, Valerie, n67
Proposed intermediate direction system, App.A.10-13

Proximal
- analysis, 2.1-5, 16.6-7
  - comparison with distal analysis, 16.8-9
  - difficulty for moving limb, 23.1
  - disadvantage of, 23.1
  - for movement to side middle, 16.17
- center, 16.5
  - analysis, n25
- joint, focus on, 16.5
- point to judge lower leg circle, 18.2

Quality
- buoyant, uplifted, 48.21
- heavy, 48.22
- relaxed, 48.22
- unemphasized, 48.10

Quarter line on stage, 45.5-6
Quarter stagemarks, 48.3
Quarter-way displacement from path, 12.8
Quick displacement movement, 21.3

Rapid vibrating movements, 17.1

Reaching a destination, 14.5
Reading Examples, S48
- ballroom dance, 42.4-5
- Hungarian Dance, 48.29-30
- *Lark Ascending*, 48.1-10
- *Parade*, 48.19-21
- *Rooms*, 48.22-24
- *Roses*, 48.11
- *Snow Pas*, 48.15-18
- *Sorcerer's Sofa*, 48.12-14
- Spanish Dance, 48.25-28
- *Water Study*, 48.31

Rebound spring, 48.13

Reference
- point for next direction, 24.4
- point for shifting, 24.9
- to Constant Directions for travel, 15.8
- to floor plan, 12.12
- to standard directions, 10.9-12

Regressive, jagged deviations, 10.5

Relationship
- signs used with pins, 16.15
- to focal point, 41.1

Relative
- location for aim of path, 38.3-4
- size of deviation, 11.2

Relaxed, 48.22

Repeat signs
- continuation of movements, 21.3
- circular displacements, 23.21

Repeated small movements, 16.4

Resultant
- bow, 25.9
- turn, 48.11

Resulting location
- distance from area, 38.4

Retained displacement, 20.4

Retention
- of contraction, 32.1
- of spot, 47.17

Retrace path, S8
- arm gesture, 8.4
- hand design, 8.5
- ,indication for, 8.1
- leg gesture, 8.3
- ,shorthand device for, 8.2

Return
- to center, 16.14
- to normal, sudden, 21.5

Reverse spiral pattern, 32.7
Revolving on a straight path (floor), 15.2-3, 48.11
'Rising' movements, 23.2
- ,direction of, 23.3

Rond de jambe, 48.26-28

Room
- area indications, 15.10
- directions (see also Constant directions)
  - destination of turn related to, 41.3

Rooms, 48.22-24, *n*121
Roses, 48.11, *n*114
Rotation sign outside staff, 48.23
Rounded corners for gestures, *S*7
Royal box, sign for, 46.6

Sagittal
- circles (gestures), 27.4-5, 27.7
  - ,surface for, 33.1
- closing
  - degrees of, 39.11
  - during leap, 39.12
  - sign on centered staff, 39.11
- dimension used, 27.3-5
- leg separation, 48.24
- lines on stage, 45.7
- path for head and torso, 34.1
- spreading, 29.2, 29.5-7, 39.11
  - during leap, 39.12

Same spot
- caret, *S*47
  - sign for, 47.18
  - use after springing, 47.20
- zed caret, 47.21-23
  - gesturing leg, 47.21
  - landing on spot, 47.22

'Satellite Center', *n*23
Saying 'no', 17.3
Scale
- for distal analysis displacements, 22.1-4
- for widening steps, 37.7
- of deviations from gestural path, 11.3

Scattering action, 48.8
Schematic drawing for halfway and third-way points, 1.1
Schrifttanz, *n*127
'See floor plan', *n*18
Sense of
- phrasing for minor circular movements, 18.1
- 'unfinished' gesture, 25.5

Sequential movements, 20.2, 25.10
Shape
- angular, 7.2
- of circular path modified, 12.11
- of path, difference in (for gesture), 5.2

Sharp corners for gestures, *S*7
Shawn's Fundamental Exercises, 34.4, *n*57
Shifting action/s, *S*24, 24.9
- anatomical action, 24.9
- body section, 19.3
- minor, *S*19
  - equal sign, 19.1
  - point of reference, 19.2
- of palm, 23.14
- point of reference for, 24.9

Shorthand
- device for retracing a path, 8.2

Shorthand (cont.)
- usage for intermediate point, 1.5
Sign/s for,
- abduction, 39.9
- adduction, 39.9
- any number of people, 43.3
- area, *S*44; 38.4
- away, 25.1
- body-as-a-whole, 25.7
- cartwheel path, 28.5
- degree of flexing left open, 37.12
- distance, *S*40; 40.1
- 'each one', 37.8
- exact center of stage, 45.7
- focal point, 41.1
- 'goes away', 25.8
- 'increase in size', 32.9
- lack of emphasis, 18.4
- looking at audience, 46.6
- modifying distance in paths, 12.6
- much speed, 21.3
- 'neither long nor short', 37.6
- periphery of area, 43.6
- polar pins, 23.6-11
- relating, showing distance, 40.3
- royal box, 46.6
- shifting, 19.1, 23.14
- space measurement, 12.6
  - placed in addition bracket, 22.2
  - placed in diamond, 22.1
- spatial aspects, 7.2
- spatially
  - central, 6.2
  - large, 16.18
  - neither long nor short, 32.8
  - peripheral, 6.2
  - small, 16.18, 32.8
- spectator, audience, 46.6
- spreading, 29.2-3, 29.6-7
- start on either foot, 48.2
- steps, 12.6, 37.13
  - on right foot, 37.9, *n*111
- ,time, 36.8
- toward, 25.1
- turn either right or left, 41.2
- unemphasized performance, 18.4
- unspecified area, 44.19

Single symmetrical deviations, 9.8-9
'Sinking' movements, 23.2
- ,direction of, 23.3
Size
- not precisely measured, 11.4
- of circle (for gestures), *S*31
  - indicated with diametral point, 31.2, 32.4
  - influenced by degree of flexion, 32.1-2
  - remains constant, 32.8
- of conical circle, 36.2
- of deviation, scales of, 11.4
- of deviation from path of gesture, *S*11

Size (cont.)
- of displacement, S22; 11.2
  - clarification, 22.5-6
  - general rule, 22.3
- of distal and proximal displacements, 16.17-19
- of steps, 37.5-11
- of transitional arm deviations, 18.4
  - diminished by using pins, 18.5
- placed in deviation bow, 11.2
- ,spatial, 11.2

Skating, orientation when, 43.6
Slant of surfaces, degrees of, 33.3-4
Slight
- curve, 6.6
- detours from normal path, 9.1
- displacement, 12.7
- sideward deviation, 6.6
- swerve to avoid person or object, 13.2
- 'to and fro' steps, 14.1

Slightly wide gait, 12.1
Small
- circular movements, 16.1
- lateral wrist flexions, 19.3
- linking bow, 2.4
- sideward arm movements, 16.4
- stroke for distal center pins, 16.7

Smooth
- ,arrival at, 12.9
- performance phrasing bow, 21.1

Snow Pas, 48.15-18, *n*118
Sokolow, Anna, 48.22, *n*121
Somersault
- circles, 27.5
- paths, 28.4
  - ,conical backward, 28.4
  - ,elongated, 29.5
  - planal, forward, 28.4

Sorcerer's Sofa, 48.12-14, *n*116
Space
- Harmony
  - directions applied to arm, App.A.4
  - theory, App.A.2
- hold in direction symbol, 36.4
- measurement sign, *n*45, *n*68
  - placed in addition bracket, 22.2
  - placed in diamond, 22.1, 22.6

Spanish Dance, 48.25-28
Spatial
- aspects, sign for, 7.2
- placement of a conical circle, 36.2-3
- points in Space Harmony, App.A.3
- retention, direction of gesture, 36.4
- size, 11.2
  - variation in, 16.18

Spatially
- action - very small, 23.15
- central or peripheral paths, 6.1-5, *n*8
- central, sign for, 6.2
  - abbreviated sign, 6.2
- larger sign, 18.5
- peripheral, sign for, 6.2

Spatially (cont.)
- rounded performance, 7.2
- small sign as pre-sign, 24.14

Specific
- stage diagonals, 45.9
- step length, 37.6

Spectator, audience, sign for, 46.6
Speed
- ,changes in, 36.8-9
- ,indication of, 21.3
- sign in direction symbol, 36.9

Sphere of possible deviations, 9.3
Spherical analysis, App.A.2, App.A.9
Spiral
- design on same plane, 32.6
- paths, 32.5-7
  - reverse pattern, 32.7
  - written with design drawing, 32.6-7
- ,three-dimensional, 32.9

Split (stride), 37.7
Spoke-like
- displacements, 16.20
  - ,analysis of, 23.13-17
  - described using flexion, extension, 23.17
  - of palm, 23.13-17
  - requiring flexion, extension of body part, 23.13
  - using polar pins, 23.16-17
- movements, 23.2, 23.4
  - ,bird's eye view of, 23.4
  - inward, 23.4
  - outward, 23.4

Spot holds, S47
- cancellation, 47.17
- retention of spot, 47.17

Spreading
- diagonally, 29.2
- laterally, 29.2-3, 29.6
- sagittally, 29.2, 29.5-7
- sign with white and black circles, 29.2
- vertically, 29.2-3

Spring, rebound, 48.13
Stage
- area, S44
  - ,above or below, 44.21
  - ,anywhere in, 44.23
  - approximately center stage, 44.23
  - around periphery, 44.11
  - arrival at, 12.9
  - combined to show diagonal, 45.11
  - directions (see also room directions)
  - entrances, exits, 44.6
  - freedom indicated, 44.17, 44.23
  - ,further subdivisions using strokes, 44.14-18
  - ,lines on, 45.5-8
  - offstage, 44.18
  - ,outside, 44.11
  - ,performers distributed over wide, 44.11

Stage (cont.)
- area (cont.)
  - ,placement of performers in relation to, 44.11
  - signs, 44.1-2
  - subdivsions of right side, 44.16
  - terms used, 44.2
  - use of floor plan, 44.6
- diagonals, 45.9-13
  - area signs connected, 45.11
  - ,floor plan showing, 45.10
  - intermediate step directions used, 45.9
  - numbering walls, alphabetizing stage corners, 45.12
  - shallow path (floor), 45.9
  - ,shape of stage affecting, 45.9
- exact center, 45.7
- plan, center line on small, 45.8

Stance Key, 16.12

Standard
- directions
  - ,deviation reference to, 10.9-12
- intermediate direction, App.A.9
- Key for minor circling movements, 18.1
- path (gestures), 3.4-5
  - degrees of distance, 3.4
- points, movement to, 22.3
- step-length, 37.3-4
  - definition, 37.3
  - sign, 37.2
  - ,statement of, 37.4
- System of Reference for Distal Center, 16.2
  - Distal Center Key, 16.7

Start on either foot, sign for, 48.2

Statement
- of arrival, 12.9
- of distance
  - centered in sign, 40.1
  - placed above sign, 40.1
- of spatial size, 24.14

Step/s
- ,crossed, 37.1
- direction judged, 24.1
- length, S37
  - affected by direction and level, 37.1
  - distance indicated in box, 40.4
  - distance to be traveled, 38.1
  - general scale, 37.5
  - ,natural, 37.1-2
  - specific scale, 37.6-7
  - ,standard, 37.1, 37.3-4
- on either foot, sign for, n111
- ,open, 37.1
- patterns in place, displacement, S14
- performed without traveling, 14.1
- scale for widening, 37.7
- sign for, 12.6, n62
  - within bracket, 37.4
- size, 37.4

Step/s (cont.)
- symbols not describing destination, 24.1
- to and fro, 14.1
- versus gestures, S24
- very small, 48.30

Stepping out wider and wider, 37.5, 37.7
Stirring with index finger, 35.4
Straight
- or curved direction of progression, 24.12-13
- path (floor)
  - Constant Key direction, 15.3
  - ,revolving on a, 15.2
- path (gesture), S26; 4.5-6
  - arm gesture, 48.11, 48.13, 48.15, 48.18-19, 48.21
  - body limitations for, 24.12
  - ,emphasis on, 4.6
  - ,indication of, S4
  - ,more than one deviation on, 9.11
  - sign with direction symbol, 26.1
  - ,specific indication of, 6.6
  - to a fourth degree point, 4.5
  - value in mimed gestures, 4.6
  - with direction sign, 24.10

Strong accented movement, 48.24
Successions, 20.2, 25.10
- deviations for, S20
- overlapping, 20.3

'Surface' for a circle, indication of, S33
Sustained transition between pins, 21.1
Swerve (detour), 13.2
Symmetrical
- deviations, 9.5-7, 10.13
- ,single, 9.8-9

System of Reference
- Based on the Path, 10.13-15

Szentpál, Maria, n108

'Table plane', App.A.3
Tacks, 1.7
Taylor, Paul, 48.11-12, n114, n116
Temporary departure from normal placement, 21.4
Third degree point (path), 4.2, n5
Third-way
- deviation, 12.2
- displacement, 16.17, 22.3
- point, 1.8-12
  - advantages of usage, 1.8
  - ,indication of, S1
  - schematic drawing, 1.1
  - two pins in a direction symbol, 1.11

'There and back' pattern, 8.1
Three-dimensional
- displacements, 16.9
- deviations, 9.4
- placement of circle, 31.3
- spiral, 32.9
  - written with design drawing, 32.9

Tick
- added to area signs, 44.14-18
- placed on pin shaft, 16.10

Tilt/s
- of chest disappears, 25.8
- minor movements, 16.6, 19.1

Tilted
- cartwheel, 30.3
- circles, S30
- circular path, 30.4
- somersault path, 30.4

Time sign, 36.8
- for much speed, 48.24

Timing, S21
- ,bow indicating, 21.4
- changes in speed, 36.8-9
- fluent, legato movement, n10
- for destinational state of flexion, 24.15
- for displacement, 18.1
  - of gestural circles, 36.7
- for third degree pathway, S5
- indication of speed, 21.3
- indicating swing, 36.7
- length of bow, 21.4
- of detour, 13.3-6
- of gestural circles, 36.7-9
- sudden return to normal, 21.5
- uneven, 21.5

Tinkel's variations, n4

'To and fro'
- minor movements, 16.1-4
- movement of steps, 14.1
- polar displacements, 23.18-19
- stepping motif, 15.4

Toe sliding in circular pattern, 18.1

Torso
- inclines, degree left open, 48.4
- slumps with heavy quality, 48.22

Touching leg gestures
- distance, 39.1-5
- level of support, 39.1-2, 39.4

Toward
- and away
  - directional point, 25.4-6
  - from an area, 14.3-4
  - from body, 25.7
  - ,hand moves, 25.3
  - versus destination, S25
- sign, n32

Transition to a fourth degree point, 3.6
Transitional arm deviations, 18.4
Trap door location, 44.21

Traveling
- on parallel paths, 14.2
- ,specific, 14.1
- slightly forward, 48.21
- small distance, 48.29
- ,steps performed without, 14.1
- to part of stage, 14.1-2
- to same Constant direction, 15.6

Triangular arm pattern, 7.1
Triple wide sign, 11.3

Turn
- either right or left, 41.2
- focal destination for, 41.2-4
- related to direction of path (floor), 43.4
- to focal point for body part, 41.4

Turning
- combined with displacement paths, S15; 15.2-3
- gradually, 15.2

Two pins in a direction symbol, 1.11

Two-dimensional
- deviations, 9.4
- modification to direction, 2.2

Undeviating path for tilt, 48.28

Unemphasized
- contraction of torso, 48.10
- path, 3.6
- reverse path, 23.19

Uneven timing for a movement, 21.5
Unfolding, 25.14
Uplifted, boyant steps, 48.21
Unqualified 'away' sign, as cancellation 25.13

Use of
- 'center' pin for proximal description, 16.14
- specific directional keys, 16.11-13

Veering
- from forward path, 12.3
- off course gradually, 13.3
- off normal path, S12

Vertical
- ad. lib sign, 25.15, 37.12
- axis
  - for horizontal circular path, 28.1
  - for polar system, 23.5
- bow
  - for deviations, 9.6
  - linking two signs, 12.7
  - to indicate passing state, 9.7
- circles, coordinates for, n54
- deviation bow with small direction symbol, 18.6
- line of gravity, rising and sinking relating to, 23.5
- phrasing bow
  - for fluent performance, 7.1
- planes, 27.5
- spreading, 29.2-3

Very small
- head nods, 16.6
- inclinations/tilts, 16.6

Vibrating actions, S17
- ,cancellation of, 17.6
- of the hand, 17.1-2
- of the knees, 17.3
- pins to indicate direction, 17.1

Wachman, Abraham, n127, n130
Walking a circle performing lateral arm
    circles, 36.5
Waltz-like steps, 15.9
Water
- indication for, 44.22
- surface of, 44.22
Water Study, 48.31
Wavy line to indicate vibrations, 17.1
Wedges
- use in floor plans, 14.5, 15.7, n150
Weight
- shift, 47.10, 47.13
- slightly backward, 48.21
- slow release of, 47.4
Wheeling of the torso, 34.5
White pins, 1.7
Wide sign in area sign, 44.10
Wings on stage, S45, 45.1-3
- ,exiting into, 45.1, 45.4
- ,intermediate, 45.2
- ,number of, 45.3
Writing on a blackboard, 33.2
Wrist
- accommodating articulation, 19.3
- articulation in hand movements, 17.5
- backward fold to indicate start of
    circle, 35.3
- slight lateral flexion, 17.5, 19.3

Zed caret, 47.14-16, n105
- spatial result, 47.15
Zig-zag path, 10.5

Useful Contact Information

Language of Dance Centre
17 Holland Park
London W11 3TD
United Kingdom
Tel: +44 (0) 20 7229 3780
Fax: +44 (0) 20 7792 1794
web: http://www.lodc.org
email: info@lodc.org

Language of Dance Center
1972 Swan Pointe Drive
Traverse City
MI 49686
USA
Tel: +1 231 995 0998
Fax: +1 231 995 0998
email: Tinalodc@aol.com

Dance Notation Bureau
151 West 30th Street, Suite 202
New York NY 10001
USA
Tel: +1 212 564 0985
Fax: +1 212 904 1426
web: http://www.dancenotation.org
email: notation@mindspring.com

Dance Notation Bureau Extension
The Ohio State University
Department of Dance
1813 N. High Street
Columbus OH 43210-1307
USA
Tel: +1 614 292 7977
Fax: +1 614 292 0939
web: http://www.dance.ohio-state.edu
email: marion.8@osu.edu

The Labanotation Institute
The University of Surrey
Guildford
Surrey GU2 5XH
United Kingdom
Tel: +44 (0) 1483 259 351
Fax: +44 (0) 1483 300 803
email: J.Johnson-Jones@Surrey.ac.uk

Andy Adamson
Department of Drama and Theatre Arts
University of Birmingham
P.O. Box 363
Birmingham B15 2TT
United Kingdom
email: a.j.adamson@bham.ac.uk